Handbook of Economic Evaluation of HIV Prevention Programs

AIDS Prevention and Mental Health

Series Editors:

David G. Ostrow, M.D., Ph.D.
Howard Brown Health Center and Illinois Masonic Medical Center, Chicago, Illinois

Jeffrey A. Kelly, Ph.D.
Medical College of Wisconsin, Milwaukee, Wisconsin

Evaluating HIV Prevention Interventions
Joanne E. Mantell, Ph.D., M.S.P.H., Anthony T. DiVittis, M.A.,
and Marilyn I. Auerbach, A.M.L.S., Dr. P.H.

Handbook of Economic Evaluation of HIV Prevention Programs
Edited by David R. Holtgrave, Ph.D.

Methodological Issues in AIDS Behavioral Research
Edited by David G. Ostrow, M.D., Ph.D., and Ronald C. Kessler, Ph.D.

Preventing AIDS: Theories and Methods of Behavioral Interventions
Edited by Ralph J. DiClemente, Ph.D., and John L. Peterson, Ph.D.

Women and AIDS: Coping and Care
Edited by Ann O'Leary, Ph.D., and
Lorretta Sweet Jemmot, R.N., Ph.D., F.A.A.N.

Women at Risk: Issues in the Primary Prevention of AIDS
Edited by Ann O'Leary, Ph.D., and Loretta Sweet Jemmott, R.N., Ph.D.

A Continuation Order Plan is available for this series. A continuation order will bring delivery of each new volume immediately upon publication. Volumes are billed only upon actual shipment. For further information please contact the publisher.

Handbook of Economic Evaluation of HIV Prevention Programs

Edited by

David R. Holtgrave, Ph.D.

Center for AIDS Intervention Research
Medical College of Wisconsin
Milwaukee, Wisconsin

Plenum Press • New York and London

Library of Congress Cataloging-in-Publication Data

Handbook of economic evaluation of HIV prevention programs / edited by
David R. Holtgrave.
        p.   cm. -- (AIDS prevention and mental health)
    Includes bibliographical references and index.
    ISBN 0-306-45749-0
    1. AIDS (Disease)--Prevention--Cost effectiveness. 2. AIDS
(Disease)--Government policy--United States--Cost effectiveness.
I. Holtgrave, David R. II. Series.
RA644.A25H3665 1998
362.1'9697'92--dc21   98-39090
                                                                  CIP

ISBN 0-306-45749-0

© 1998 Plenum Press, New York
A Division of Plenum Publishing Corporation
233 Spring Street, New York, N.Y. 10013

http://www.plenum.com

10 9 8 7 6 5 4 3 2 1

Printed in the United States of America

To Lorie Holtgrave, for her encouragement during the hardest moments—she truly made completion of this effort possible; Dr. John Graham, for teaching me policy analysis; Dr. Jim Curran, for showing me policy making; and Buddy and Katie Lynn, for their endless supply of infectious happiness

Contributors

Paul R. Abramson ● Department of Psychology, University of California, Los Angeles, Los Angeles, California 90024

Charles Begley ● Center for Health Policy Studies, School of Public Health, The University of Texas at Houston, Houston, Texas 77030

Heather Cecil ● Department of Psychiatry and Behavioral Medicine, Center for AIDS Intervention Research (CAIR), Medical College of Wisconsin, Milwaukee, Wisconsin 53202

Julie Denison ● School of Hygiene and Public Health, Johns Hopkins University, Baltimore, Maryland 21205

Wayne J. DiFranceisco ● Department of Psychiatry and Behavioral Medicine, Center for AIDS Intervention Research (CAIR), Medical College of Wisconsin, Milwaukee, Wisconsin 53202

Paul G. Farnham ● Department of Economics, Georgia State University, Atlanta, Georgia 30303; and Division of Prevention Research and Analytic Methods, Epidemiology Program Office, Centers for Disease Control and Prevention (CDC), Atlanta, Georgia 30333

Andrew Fourney ● Center for Health Policy Studies, School of Public Health, The University of Texas at Houston, Houston, Texas 77030

Robin D. Gorsky ● Late of Division of HIV-AIDS Prevention, National Center for HIV, STD, and TB Prevention, Centers for Disease Control and Prevention, Atlanta, Georgia 30333; and Department of Health Management and Policy, University of New Hampshire, Durham, New Hampshire 03824

Anne Haddix ● Prevention Effectiveness Activity, Centers for Disease Control and Prevention (CDC), Atlanta, Georgia 30333

David R. Holtgrave ● Department of Psychiatry and Behavioral Medicine, Center for AIDS Intervention Research (CAIR), Medical College of Wisconsin, Milwaukee, Wisconsin 53202

James G. Kahn ● Center for AIDS Prevention Studies, Institute for Health Policy Studies, and Department of Epidemiology and Biostatistics, School of Medicine, University of California, San Francisco, San Francisco, California 94109

Edward H. Kaplan ● School of Management, Yale University, New Haven, Connecticut 06520-8200

Jeffrey A. Kelley ● Department of Psychiatry and Behavioral Medicine, Center for AIDS Intervention Research (CAIR), Medical College of Wisconsin, Milwaukee, Wisconsin 53202

Robert F. Martin ● Department of Economics, University of Chicago, Chicago, Illinois 60637

Anna Johnson Masotti ● Center for AIDS Intervention Research (CAIR), Medical College of Wisconsin, Milwaukee, Wisconsin 53202

Paul Masotti ● Center for Health Policy Studies, School of Public Health, The University of Texas at Houston, Houston, Texas 77030

Richard L. Melchreit ● Connecticut Department of Public Health, Hartford, Connecticut 06134-0308

Edward C. Norton ● Department of Health Policy and Administration, University of North Carolina at Chapel Hill, Chapel Hill, North Carolina 27599-7400

Douglas K. Owens ● VA Palo Alto Health Care System, Palo Alto, California 94304; and Section on Medical Informatics, Department of Medicine, and Department of Health Research and Policy, Stanford University, Stanford, California 94305

A. David Paltiel ● School of Medicine, Yale University, New Haven, Connecticut 06520

Kathryn A. Phillips ● Center for AIDS Prevention Studies (CAPS), University of California, San Francisco, San Francisco, California 94105

Steven D. Pinkerton ● Department of Psychiatry and Behavioral Medicine, Center for AIDS Intervention Research (CAIR), Medical College of Wisconsin, Milwaukee, Wisconsin 53202

L. Yvonne Stevenson ● Department of Psychiatry and Behavioral Medicine, Center for AIDS Intervention Research (CAIR), Medical College of Wisconsin, Milwaukee, Wisconsin 53202

Aaron A. Stinnett ● Department of Health Care Organization and Policy, University of Alabama, Birmingham, Alabama 35294

Michael D. Sweat ● School of Public Hygiene and Public Health, Johns Hopkins University, Baltimore, Maryland 21205

Mary E. Turk ● Department of Psychiatry and Behavioral Medicine, Center for AIDS Intervention Research (CAIR), Medical College of Wisconsin, Milwaukee, Wisconsin 53202

Wendee M. Wechsberg ● Research Triangle Institute, Research Triangle Park, North Carolina 27709

Beth Weinstein ● Connecticut Department of Public Health, Hartford, Connecticut 06134-0308

Anna Fay Williams ● Consultant, Houston, Texas 77005

Preface

If resources for HIV prevention efforts were truly unlimited, then this book would be entirely unnecessary. In a world with limitless support for HIV prevention activities, one would simply implement all effective (or potentially effective) programs without regard to expense. We would do everything useful to prevent the further spread of the virus that has already claimed hundreds of thousands of lives in the United States and millions of lives worldwide.

Unfortunately, funding for HIV prevention programs is limited. Even though the amount of available funding may seem quite large (especially in the United States), it is still fixed and not sufficient to meet all needs for such programs. This was very well illustrated in the summer of 1997 when over 500 community-based organizations applied for a combined total of $18 million of HIV prevention funding from the U.S. Centers for Disease Control and Prevention (CDC). Less than one-fifth of these organizations received support via this funding mechanism. Hence, although $18 million may seem like a large amount of money at first blush, it is not enough to meet all of the prevention needs that could be addressed by these community-based organizations.

This point is true even more generally. In total, U.S. federal support for HIV prevention efforts is measured in the hundreds of millions of dollars per year. These funds are used to support the efforts of state, local, and territorial health departments; national and regional minority organizations; the community-based organizations noted previously; and a wide variety of other governmental and nongovernmental organizations. The programs funded with these monies include HIV counseling and testing services, health education and risk reduction, public information, and other HIV prevention interventions.

Of course, even this seemingly large sum is also limited and not sufficient to meet all HIV prevention needs in the United States. Therefore, any use of this money entails an opportunity cost—a dollar spent on one program is a dollar unavailable for others. A decision to spend $100,000 on HIV counseling and testing services in a state might mean that a street outreach program for injection drug users might go unfunded. These resource allocation choices are very real and highly consequential.

HIV prevention resource allocation decisions are made in a highly volatile context of politics, activism, science, personal values, and community norms. Some resource allocation decisions are made subject to constraints, such as congressional earmarks. Others are made after comprehensively considering the costs and consequences of funding decisions across a variety of communities. To capture the wide diversity of ways in which HIV prevention allocation decisions are made would require the development of a variety of descriptive models of decision making.

This book is focused on one general type of resource allocation decision making. We take as a starting point that HIV prevention resources are limited, that funding one program instead of another can have real effects on the course of the epidemic and on individual morbidity and mortality, and that it is desirable to avert the maximum number of HIV infections possible given a limited set of resources. Indeed, we assume in this book that the major goal of HIV prevention programs is the prevention of HIV infection (a seemingly obvious yet controversial and consequential assumption). We assume that to achieve this goal, it is necessary to balance carefully the relative costs and consequences of HIV prevention efforts.

This "balancing act" must be done explicitly (so that the resource allocation process may be transparent to observers and more easily justified), and it must be done carefully and comprehensively. Because of these desiderata, the techniques of cost and cost-effectiveness analysis are useful. Cost analysis allows us to answer the question: What resources does it take to deliver a particular type of HIV prevention intervention to a specific group of clients? Cost-effectiveness analysis allows us to answer the related question: What does it cost to deliver a particular type of HIV prevention intervention to achieve one unit of some outcome measure (e.g., cost per HIV infection averted)? When applied across a variety of HIV prevention intervention types, cost-effectiveness analysis helps us to begin to answer the question: Which HIV prevention interventions are most cost-effective? When applied across a variety of HIV prevention interventions and programs in other disease areas (such as cancer prevention and the treatment of heart disease) and when using a common outcome measure (such as cost per quality-adjusted life-year saved), cost-effectiveness analysis helps us to begin to answer the question: Is HIV prevention a cost-effective expenditure of funds relative to investments in programs in other disease areas?

When used with care and skill, the techniques of cost and cost-effectiveness analysis constitute important decision aiding devices to those persons charged with HIV prevention resource allocation. *This book is an in-depth discussion of the methods, applications, and utilization of cost and cost-effectiveness analysis in HIV prevention resource allocation decision making.*

The book is divided into three major sections. The first section, consisting of three chapters, is devoted to the methods of cost and cost-effectiveness analysis. Kathryn Phillips and colleagues provide a detailed definition of some important economic evaluation terms. Further, they provide a brief description of some standards for doing cost and cost-effectiveness analysis that have recently been established by a blue-ribbon panel convened by the U.S. Public Health Service.

Next, in a pair of chapters Steve Pinkerton and colleagues provide an overview of a methodological framework for doing cost-effectiveness analysis in the context of HIV prevention. They note that calculation of the "cost-utility ratio" depends on four key parameters: program cost, the number of HIV infections prevented, medical costs saved when an HIV infection is prevented, and the number of quality-adjusted life-years saved when an HIV infection is prevented. (When cost-effectiveness analysis is focused on the cost per quality-adjusted life-year saved, it is called "cost-utility analysis.") They describe progress made in identifying methods to estimate each of these four key parameters. An entire chapter is devoted to the special topic of estimating the number of HIV infections prevented by a program that is empirically assessed by behavioral but not biological outcomes.

The methodological section of the book provides a relatively brief overview of the methods required to perform HIV prevention cost and cost-effectiveness analyses. It is not a complete tutorial on these topics, although it is a potential guide to further learning on these topics.

The second section of the book (six chapters) is devoted to reviews of cost-effectiveness analyses of particular types of HIV prevention interventions. In a 1996 *Annual Review of Public Health* paper, Holtgrave and colleagues reviewed the literature for all economic evaluations of HIV-related programs (both prevention and treatment). They found that most of the studies located were focused on interventions for persons who inject drugs and on HIV counseling and testing interventions (for a wide variety of populations).

This emphasis in the literature is reflected in the second portion of the book. Jim Kahn comprehensively reviews the cost-effectiveness analysis of interventions for persons who inject drugs. In a complementary pair of chapters, Paul Farnham and Doug Owens review the literature on HIV counseling and testing. Dr. Farnham describes his review of over forty studies of the cost-effectiveness of HIV counseling and testing, and he provides an interesting taxonomy of the literature based on the observation that counseling and testing may have a variety of purposes (e.g., case finding, behavioral change, and so on). He notes that the perceived purpose of the counseling and testing services can have important implications for the analytic methods used to assess cost-effectiveness. Dr. Owens focuses on studies in which testing has been used for screening purposes, especially for screening health care workers, their patients, and pregnant women.

The previous review by Holtgrave and colleagues identified several gaps in the economic evaluation literature. In fact, a number of extremely important types of HIV prevention interventions then had not been assessed via cost-effectiveness (and some still have not). In this book, Mike Sweat and Julie Denison describe a centrally important level of intervention, namely, interventions delivered at the societal level (e.g., policy and law changes). At a recent NIH Consensus Development Conference, societal level interventions were cited as having been especially effective at changing HIV-related risk behavior in international settings and were heralded as holding great promise for the United States. In his chapter, Dr. Sweat describes these international experiences and domestic possibilities, emphasizing economic and economic evaluation issues.

Next, Holtgrave and Pinkerton review some very recent studies of the cost-effectiveness of other especially effective types of interventions, small group and community-level interventions. In the final chapter in this section, Holtgrave proposes a comprehensive list of the myriad types of possible HIV prevention interventions and provides a brief sense of what is known or still needs to be known about the cost-effectiveness of each type of intervention.

The third section of the book, composed of six chapters, addresses issues of how the results of cost-effectiveness analyses are used or might be used. In the first, David Paltiel discusses the potential and pitfalls of comparing HIV prevention programs to interventions in other disease areas. Although many policy makers are interested in this central question because they need to decide whether to allocate money to HIV prevention or elsewhere, answering the question can be done correctly only if many methodological cautions are heeded. Dr. Paltiel provides guidance for proceeding in this area.

Beth Weinstein and Richard Melchreit provide a challenging state health department perspective on using cost-effectiveness analysis for real-world decision making. They feel that the use of such information is important, yet in practice is met with many barriers. This chapter is extremely important because only by understanding these barriers can we begin to address them.

Anna Fay Williams and colleagues describe in detail their experiences in assessing the cost of local HIV prevention interventions delivered by community-based organizations. Dr. Williams describes the ideal methods for collecting cost information, identifies practical challenges in conducting such evaluative activities in the field, and proposes a realistic, compromise methodology.

Ed Kaplan addresses the issue of using cost-effectiveness analysis in HIV prevention community planning processes. He notes that some of the data are lacking for completely utilizing cost-effectiveness analysis for community planning purposes, yet he describes a methodology that draws on the expert judgment of community planning group members to supply missing pieces of information. This chapter is the first complete description of a comprehensive, practical methodology for using cost-effectiveness analysis in community planning.

It is sometimes difficult in practice to determine the number of HIV infections averted by a prevention program. In their chapter, however, Ed Norton and colleagues show that a technique called threshold analysis can often be used to answer the question: How many HIV infections would a particular program have to prevent for it to be considered cost-effective? Answering this question may be a satisfactory (even if temporary) proxy to answering the more detailed question: How cost-effective is this particular HIV prevention program?

In the final chapter of the book, Holtgrave provides a number of personal observations about the use (or lack thereof) of cost-effectiveness information in federal, state, and community resource allocation decision making. He proposes some practical approaches for using economic evaluation in real-time decision making. He also attempts to assess candidly where the field stands in terms of its accomplishments and its ability to truly inform HIV prevention resource allocation decisions.

There are four appendices to the book. The first is a reprint of a seminal article on performing cost analysis in HIV prevention programs. This article was written by Robin Gorsky, who died tragically in an airplane crash in 1995. No book on HIV prevention and economic evaluation would be complete without a contribution from our dear friend and inspirational colleague, Dr. Gorsky. Indeed, she provided much leadership in this field before her untimely death. She is much missed by the other authors who contributed to this book.

The second appendix by Holtgrave and Pinkerton is a reprint of a journal article that provides the latest updates on estimates of the cost of treating a case of HIV disease and on estimates of the number of quality-adjusted life-years saved when an HIV infection is averted. The third appendix by Pinkerton and colleagues is a full length, detailed example of how to conduct a cost-utility analysis of an HIV primary prevention intervention (a summary of this full-length report will be published shortly in the *American Journal of Public Health*). It is provided here so that persons interested in performing this economic evaluation technique for the first time can follow one entire worked example. The final appendix by Mary Turk and colleagues lists and describes World Wide Web sites of particular utility to persons doing economic evaluation work in public health.

In summary, assessment of the cost and cost-effectiveness of HIV prevention is an emerging field. It is a clearly definable, yet still relatively small and specialized, body of knowledge. The field has many challenges to meet (in terms of methodology and acceptance). However, the analytic findings to date have real policy and program management implications. Because the stakes are so high in both human and fiscal terms, we must take a careful look at the cost-effectiveness information currently available and the uses to which it has been put and must challenge the field to produce even more relevant studies in the future. The purpose of this book is to take that hard look at the rigor and relevance of HIV prevention cost-effectiveness analysis.

Acknowledgments

The editor wishes to thank the National Institutes of Mental Health for supporting the preparation of this book via grants P30-MH52776, R01-MH55440, and R01-MH56830. The editor also thanks the Center for AIDS Intervention Research (CAIR), Medical College of Wisconsin, for providing the opportunity to pursue the completion of this volume, and he thanks Dr. Steve Pinkerton for unending intellectual stimulation during the completion of this volume. The editor thanks Lori Holtgrave for her support in the preparation of this work. Finally, the editor thanks the series editors Drs. Jeff Kelly and David Ostrow and the acquisitions editor Ms. Mariclaire Cloutier for their strong support of this book.

Contents

Chapter 4. Economic Evaluation of Primary HIV Prevention in Injection Drug Users
James G. Kahn

Chapter 5. Economic Evaluation of HIV Counseling and Testing Programs: The Influence of Program Goals on Evaluation
Paul G. Farnham

Chapter 6. Economic Evaluation of HIV Screening Interventions
Douglas K. Owens

Chapter 7. Changing Public Policy to Prevent HIV Transmission: The Role of Structural and Environmental Interventions

Michael D. Sweat and Julie Denison

Chapter 8. The Cost-Effectiveness of Small Group and Community-Level Interventions

David R. Holtgrave and Steven D. Pinkerton

Chapter 9. The Cost-Effectiveness of the Components of a Comprehensive HIV Prevention Program: A Road Map of the Literature

David R. Holtgrave

Chapter 10. Resource Allocation and the Funding of HIV Prevention

A. David Paltiel and Aaron A. Stinnett

Chapter 11. Economic Evaluation and HIV Prevention Decision Making: The State Perspective

Beth Weinstein and Richard L. Melchreit

Chapter 12. Adapting Cost Analytic Techniques to Local HIV Prevention Programs

Anna Fay Williams, Charles Begley, Andrew Fourney, Paul Masotti, and Anna Johnson Masotti

Chapter 13. Economic Evaluation and HIV Prevention Community Planning: A Policy Analyst's Perspective

Edward H. Kaplan

Chapter 14. Threshold Analysis of AIDS Outreach and Intervention

Edward C. Norton, Robert F. Martin, and Wendee M. Wechsberg

Chapter 15. A Few Reflections on the Practicality of Economic Evaluation Methods and Conclusions
David R. Holtgrave

Appendix A. A Method to Measure the Costs of Counseling for HIV Prevention
Robin D. Gorsky

Appendix B. Updates of Cost of Illness and Quality of Life Estimates for Use in Economic Evaluations of HIV Prevention Programs
David R. Holtgrave and Steven D. Pinkerton

Appendix C. Cost-Effectiveness of a Community-Level HIV Risk Reduction Intervention

Steven D. Pinkerton, David R. Holtgrave, Wayne J. DiFranceisco,
* L. Yvonne Stevenson, and Jeffrey A. Kelly*

Appendix D. HIV Prevention and Cost-Effectiveness Resources on the World Wide Web

Mary E. Turk, Steven D. Pinkerton, David R. Holtgrave, and Heather Cecil

An Overview of Economic Evaluation Methodologies and Selected Issues in Methods Standardization

KATHRYN A. PHILLIPS, ANNE HADDIX, and DAVID R. HOLTGRAVE

INTRODUCTION

Economic evaluations are becoming increasingly important tools for assisting in health services decision making. Program managers and other decision makers often need to compare different programs and set priorities for resource allocation. Economic evaluations can be helpful by providing information about the costs and benefits of various alternatives. For evaluations to be comparable, however, they must be conducted by similar methods. Economic evaluation for AIDS prevention and prevention generally is a relatively new concept, and therefore methods for conducting such studies are still being developed.

Recently, two major efforts have addressed the methodological issues in conducting economic evaluations. First, the Centers for Disease Control and Prevention (CDC) published a practical guide to prevention effectiveness in 1994,[1] which was also published as a book in 1996.[2] These publications were developed to provide information about currently available methods for addressing complex public health policy questions and to provide an introduction to methods in prevention effectiveness for practitioners who conduct studies and for persons who make decisions on the basis of study results.

Second, the U.S. Public Health Service convened the "Panel on Cost-Effectiveness in Health and Medicine" in 1993, resulting in a 1996 book.[3] The Panel was charged with assessing the current state-of-the science of the field and with providing recommendations for conducting studies to improve their quality and encourage their comparability. The Panel's creation was motivated by (1) the keen interest of the Public Health Service in using cost-effectiveness analyses to enhance perspectives for health-related decisions and

KATHRYN A. PHILLIPS • Center for AIDS Prevention Studies (CAPS), University of California, San Francisco, San Francisco, California 94105.   *ANNE HADDIX* • Prevention Effectiveness Activity, Centers for Disease Control and Prevention (CDC), Atlanta, Georgia 30333.   *DAVID R. HOLTGRAVE* • Department of Psychiatry and Behavioral Medicine, Center for AIDS Intervention Research (CAIR), Medical College of Wisconsin, Milwaukee, Wisconsin 53202.

Handbook of Economic Evaluation of HIV Prevention Programs, edited by Holtgrave. Plenum Press, New York, 1998.

by (2) its accompanying discomfort with the variability of the range of techniques used in these analyses. The Panel focused on cost-effectiveness and cost-utility analysis rather than cost-benefit analysis, and we reflect that emphasis in this chapter.

The purpose of this chapter is to examine the implications of the Panel and CDC recommendations for cost-effectiveness and cost-utility analyses of AIDS prevention. We begin by briefly reviewing basic economic evaluation concepts. Then we examine three major recommendations that are particularly relevant to AIDS prevention and provide examples of how the recommendations are applied to AIDS prevention.

A REVIEW OF ECONOMIC EVALUATION CONCEPTS

The purpose of economic evaluation is to identify, measure, value, and compare the costs and consequences of alternate interventions, strategies, or policies. Cost analysis (CA) is the measurement or estimation of the resources consumed, here, by a particular HIV prevention program. CA is essential for policy makers to decide whether they have sufficient resources to afford a particular type of intervention. When several interventions are equally effective, cost-minimization analysis (CMA) is used to determine the least costly of the interventions. Some might refer to CMA as "comparison shopping" among otherwise equally attractive alternatives.

When HIV prevention interventions vary both in terms of costs and consequences, three methods of economic evaluation are especially relevant: cost-benefit analysis, cost-effectiveness analysis, and cost-utility analysis. Cost-benefit analysis (CBA) expresses both the costs of interventions and their consequences in monetary terms, and a determination is made whether the cost of a given intervention is outweighed by the monetary benefits. Because assigning a monetary value to a consequence, such as a human life saved, is especially difficult, CBA is controversial. As noted, we follow the lead of the Panel on Cost-effectiveness in Health and Medicine and emphasize cost-effectiveness and cost-utility analysis in this chapter.

Cost-effectiveness analysis (CEA) compares the costs of interventions per health outcome achieved. In comparison to cost-benefit analysis, a monetary value is not assigned to outcomes. Rather, results are presented in the form of cost per health outcome, such as "cost per HIV infection averted" or "cost per life year saved." CEA is most useful when the goal of the analysis is to identify the most cost-effective intervention from a set of alternatives that produce a common type of outcome (for instance, comparing various HIV prevention programs to each other in terms of "cost per HIV infection averted").

Cost-utility analysis (CUA) is a specific kind of CEA. In CUA, the results are usually reported as "cost per quality-adjusted, life-years (QALYs) gained." Therefore, CUA takes into account the impact of interventions on the quality and the quantity of life. (For instance, one year in perfect health is seen as equally desirable as two years with a 50% diminished quality of life, or three years with quality of life diminished by two-thirds.) CUA is most appropriate when quality of life is an important outcome and when the intervention affects both morbidity and mortality. [The Panel on Cost-effectiveness in Health and Medicine recommends using the QALY measure even though the disability-adjusted life year (DALY) is widely used in economic evaluation of HIV prevention interventions conducted outside of the U.S.[4]]

The majority of economic evaluations of AIDS prevention strategies have been CEAs.

In a recent review of HIV prevention programs, Holtgrave et al. found 93 studies that could be considered HIV/AIDS economic evaluations.[5] Of these, 40% were on behavioral change interventions, 39% were on HIV testing, and 21% were on care and treatment. Examining only studies on behavioral change or testing, 71% were CEAs, 22% were CBAs, and 5% were CUAs.

Steps in conducting an economic evaluation can be summarized as follows:[1]

1. Define the audience for the evaluation
2. Define the problem or question to be analyzed
3. Indicate the strategies being evaluated
4. Specify the perspective of the analysis
5. Define the relevant time frame and analytic horizon
6. Determine the analytic methods
7. Determine whether the analysis is to be a marginal or incremental analysis
8. Identify the relevant costs
9. Identify the relevant outcomes
10. Specify the discount rate
11. Identify the sources of uncertainty and conduct sensitivity analyses
12. Determine the summary measures to be reported
13. Analyze the distributional and ethical effects

The Panel and CDC recommendations include checklists for evaluating studies, as do several other books and articles.[1–3,6]

The Panel's recommendations focus on a concept called the "Reference Case". The Reference Case is a standard set of methodological practices that an analyst follows to improve the comparability of economic evaluations. Although a particular study may use other assumptions and methods that best serve the purpose of the analysis, the inclusion of a Reference Case analysis allows each study to contribute to a broader pool of information. The recommendations that follow outline some of the requirements for a Reference Case analysis.

(Editor's Note: The reader not interested in technical issues about methodological standardization but who desires an overview of a practical way to perform economic evaluations of HIV prevention interventions may proceed at this point to the chapter by Pinkerton and Holtgrave in this volume,[7] without loss of continuity.)

MAJOR RECOMMENDATIONS PARTICULARLY RELEVANT TO AIDS PREVENTION

We discuss three major topics addressed by the Panel and CDC recommendations. First, we discuss the expanded use of CUA. The Panel recommended that CUA, using quality-adjusted life years, be used whenever an analysis is intended to contribute to decisions on the broad allocation of health resources. However, CUA has traditionally been little used in assessing HIV prevention interventions (although, as will be seen throughout this book, that trend is changing rapidly). Furthermore, several of the recommendations made for CUA are controversial or contrary to current practice, and therefore it is important to examine their application to AIDS prevention (e.g., the use of community preferences to develop QALYs). Here, we discuss some of the theoretical and methodological issues with the Panel's recommendations on CUA. Later in this book, Pinkerton and Holtgrave describe a practical approach to the use of CUA in the evaluating HIV prevention programs.[7]

Second, we discuss the measurement of costs. The issues in determining which costs to measure and how to measure them is critical to economic evaluation and are covered in detail in the Panel's recommendations. Many issues in measuring costs, however, have been highly controversial, particularly the treatment of productivity losses. We examine the relevance of these issues for AIDS prevention.

Third, we discuss discounting. The discounting of future costs and benefits to their present value may appear relatively straightforward, and it is a topic with relatively fewer recommendations from the Panel and CDC than in other areas. However, the conceptual basis of discounting and how it is applied continues to be controversial. Furthermore, discounting particularly affects prevention, so it is important to understand its implications for AIDS prevention.

Cost-Utility Analysis and Quality of Life Measurement

As noted above, the Panel recommended the use of cost-utility analysis in the Reference Case analysis. Further, they suggested that the analyses employed quality-adjusted life years (QALYs). Quality of life, according to the Panel, should be measured empirically. It should be measured by surveying a representative cross section of the community at large. This is a particularly consequential recommendation. As an illustration, suppose that an analyst needs to obtain a quality of life for end-stage renal disease. The analyst would not go directly to a sample of patients experiencing this disease stage and inquire about their quality of life. Rather, the analyst would develop a description of the disease stage and (using accepted measurement methods), present the description to a cross section of the community, and ask their perceptions of the quality of life in this disease stage.

The community in general, many members of which are not currently experiencing the disease stage of immediate interest, may have perceptions of the quality of life much higher or lower than persons living in the disease stage, that is, community members might not perceive that a particular disease state is so bad (e.g., vertigo may seem inconsequential until one experiences it). Alternatively, community members may believe that a disease stage (such as late-stage AIDS) is particularly undesirable, yet persons experiencing the disease stage may find that they can cope with the disease and, over time, perceive that their quality of life is quite high. Empirical research on this topic is needed.

Conforming strictly to the Panel's recommendation of community-representative quality of life assessment would be expensive and logistically difficult to implement routinely in analyses. Proxy measures may need to be used (although empirical work assessing the correlation between various proxy measures and community wide perceptions of quality of life would be informative). Holtgrave and Pinkerton recently reviewed all available, empirical studies that attempted to measure the quality of life across the various stages of HIV disease.[8] They found that no available studies meet the Panel's recommendations because one study used physician proxies and the remaining studies focused on the quality of life perceptions of patients living with HIV disease.

Holtgrave and Pinkerton used the available quality of life information to estimate the number of quality-adjusted, life years saved each time an HIV infection is prevented (for a person at a given age).[7,8] Although the available studies do not meet the Panel's recommendations, it is reassuring to note that estimates of the number of QALYs saved each time an HIV infection is averted are not particularly sensitive to the quality of life measurements. This finding results from the fact that the major contributor to estimates of the number of QALYs lost when a person becomes HIV infected is the years of life lost prematurely (the mortality effect) rather than the exact quality of life in the particular disease stages.

In summary, there is much work to be done in HIV prevention economic evaluation research to be in full compliance with the Panel's recommendation for communitywide quality of life measurement, and it is conceptually important to do this work. However, because HIV disease causes a person (on average) to lose such a large number of years of life prematurely, this mortality effect overwhelms any measurement error in assessing the quality of life during the HIV disease stages between infection and death.[8] Hence, although this topic is conceptually important, it does not have a major, practical impact on CUAs of HIV prevention interventions. Certainly, CUAs of HIV prevention programs can proceed while such empirical research goes on. Indeed, any CUA of an HIV prevention intervention can include a sensitivity analysis to gauge the robustness of study results to the variance in quality of life estimates.

Measuring Costs

An important component in any economic evaluation is estimating costs. Costs comprise the numerator of all cost-effectiveness and cost-utility ratios. Misspecification, exclusion, or faulty measurement of costs may lead to flawed conclusions about the cost-effectiveness of HIV/AIDS interventions. Thus, both the Panel and the CDC have paid special attention to the issues associated with specifying and measuring costs. This section on measuring costs describes the two sets of recommendations, discusses their relevance for AIDS studies by examining cost estimation in the current body of CEA literature, and concludes with recommendations for proceeding with comprehensive, rigorous, and comparable studies. First we examine the Panel's recommendations.

The Panel recommends valuing all changes in resource use associated with a health intervention in monetary terms, and these should appear in the numerator of the cost-effectiveness ratio. These costs include and are limited to the direct medical and nonmedical costs of the intervention and participant costs, including the participant time to seek and obtain treatment associated with the intervention, the medical and nonmedical costs of treating the health condition, the costs associated with caregiving, and the costs associated with the nonhealth impacts of the intervention. Further, the estimates of resource use included in a CEA are restricted to the population that is actually affected by the intervention. This set of recommendations provides the most comprehensive guidance for specifying, measuring, and reporting costs in CEAs that appears in the literature to date.

In addition to specifying which costs should be included in CEAs, the Panel's recommendations provide guidance for their measurement. Specifically, resources should be valued on the basis of their opportunity cost. Opportunity cost is the value of a resource in its highest use or the value of foregone alternative uses. Prices may be used to value resources to the extent that they reflect opportunity costs. When prices do not reflect opportunity costs because of market imperfections, as is frequently the case with health care resources, they should be adjusted accordingly. For example, one frequently used method for adjusting hospital prices is to use published cost-to-charge ratios to convert hospital charges to costs. When it is not possible to adjust prices and substantial bias is suspected, more suitable proxies for opportunity costs should be used. The Panel also recommends reporting all costs in constant dollars but does not recommend the use of a specific inflation adjuster. However, it is recommended that if the prices in question change at a rate different than that of general inflation, a more appropriate adjuster should be used. For example, the Consumer Price Index (CPI) for all items is frequently used for adjusting for general inflation, but because the prices of many health care services have risen at faster rates, many analysts adjust health care costs using the CPI medical care component.

The Panel also makes specific recommendations for valuing participant, volunteer, and caregiver time costs. For people in the labor force, they recommend that wages are a generally acceptable measure. When the use of wage rates for a specific target population may influence the conclusions of the analysis, the Panel recommends conducting sensitivity analyses to describe the influence. The Panel provides the least guidance for valuing the time for individuals not in the compensated labor force and for leisure time. They recommend using wages as proxies but adjusting them to reflect the full opportunity cost, but they do not recommend methods for making such an adjustment. Because this recommendation applies to vulnerable populations, children, the elderly, and the unemployed, ethical concerns arise about this method for time valuation.

The Panel's recommendations for estimating costs in CEAs are similar to but narrower than the CDC recommendations which also include productivity losses associated with morbidity and premature mortality from the intervention, i.e., side effects and the health condition. The Panel specifically excludes productivity losses (often referred to as indirect costs) because they maintain that these effects are captured in the outcome measure, QALYs, which appear in the denominator. Including them in the numerator would result in double counting. There is still some debate, however, whether QALYs fully capture the value to society of the productivity lost from the health condition.

The discordance in the two sets of recommendations appears in the formulation of the CE ratios. The Panel recommends reporting the results only with the direct medical and nonmedical costs whereas the CDC recommends reporting two ratios: the first in which the numerator includes the direct medical and nonmedical costs and a second ratio in which the productivity losses or indirect costs are included. Because the Panel classifies participant time costs as a direct cost and CDC classifies them as productivity costs, however, the numerators for direct cost ratios will be different. If participant costs are a large component of the intervention costs, substantially different conclusions may be drawn.

Relevance for AIDS Research

In a recent review of cost-effectiveness analyses of HIV prevention strategies, the quality of cost estimation was evaluated.[9] The review of twenty-five studies examined the extent to which the costs used in the analysis were specified and measured. The author reported that the quality of the cost assessment in the studies varies considerably. Only two studies specified and only one study measured the cost of participant time. Many studies excluded relevant costs, such as the cost to achieve behavioral changes. Costs were often aggregated so that individual costs could not be identified or valued. In eight studies only the intervention costs were included. HIV and AIDS treatment costs which were avoided because of the effectiveness of the intervention were excluded. The author recommends that for useful and comparable studies from which policy and program decisions can be made studies must attempt to measure and value resource use accurately. Using the amount paid or charges for a service may distort the resource value. In addition, the author points out that researchers are often faced with the challenges of sorting out shared costs. For example, HIV counseling and testing are frequently offered as one component of a visit for treatment of another sexually transmitted disease. All of the problems identified in this review were addressed in the recommendations for cost estimation made by the Panel.

The HIV prevention studies for which it will be the most difficult to fully comply with the Panel's recommendations are those in which the cost-effectiveness of proposed, but not yet implemented, interventions is examined. These studies generally construct models of hypothetical situations. Parametric estimates are rarely drawn from primary cost data but either are based either on estimates in the existing literature or use estimates of equivalent services from existing programs. Of course, available costs in the literature may not comply with the Panel's recommendations, but because of the need to make decisions prior to implementing programs, such CEAs frequently must be undertaken. Such a study recently appeared in the literature examining the economic impact of treating HIV-positive pregnant women and their newborns with zidovudine.[10]

The costs included in the CEA by Mauskopf et al. were comprehensively specified and measured. The authors included the costs of the intervention, counseling and testing costs, zidovudine costs, and associated medical costs, and the costs of infant HIV infections prevented. The cost of an infant HIV infection included the costs of hospital days; emergency room, outpatient, and home care visits; and dental and drug costs. Because of lack of information, the authors specified but did not measure caregiver costs. Rationales were provided for all costs which were excluded from the analysis, and the nature of any exclusion bias was described. For example, no infant HIV test costs were included because the authors considered that this cost would have occurred regardless of whether the intervention was delivered. To obtain the value of the resource use, the authors converted billing record data to costs using cost-to-charge ratios. The authors converted the costs to 1994 dollars using an inflation factor but did not specify whether they used the Consumer Price index for all items or only the medical care component. This study is a good example of one which met most of the criteria set by the Panel for cost estimation.

To comply with the new standards for cost measurement in CEA and CUA, we make five recommendations. First, the Panel's recommendations must extend to other forms of economic evaluation, particularly to cost analyses published in the literature. Because the majority of CEAs and CUAs rely to some extent on cost data from the literature, unless these data are in line with the Panel's recommendations, new CEAs will not meet the new Reference Case standards.

Secondly, researchers must begin to collect participant costs routinely, both individuals' time to participate in interventions and out-of-pocket expenses. Thirdly, time costs, whether for participants or for caregivers, must be reclassified as direct costs. These costs have previously been lumped with productivity losses associated with morbidity and premature mortality which are not included in the Panel's recommendation for the numerator of CEAs. Fourthly, research must be initiated to develop better methods for valuing time. The Panel recommends valuing time using the person's wage rate. This recommendation presents both conceptual and ethical problems, particularly related to valuing time for vulnerable populations. More work developing alternative methodologies needs to be undertaken.

Finally, researchers must begin to specify in detail the costs used in their analyses and their valuation methods so that consumers of cost and cost-effectiveness analyses can evaluate the comprehensiveness and accuracy of the costs. This will facilitate the adoption of cost-effectiveness studies to similar interventions in other settings. Increasing the utility and the comparability of CE studies will aid both programmatic and policy decision making.

Discounting

Discounting, the process by which future costs and health consequences are converted to their present values, is a commonly accepted practice in economic evaluations.[6,11-13] Discounting reflects the decision maker's time preference for present over future outcomes. For example, because most people prefer being given $100 today rather than $100 one year from now, discounting is used to adjust $100 in the future to its current value ($95 at a 5% discount rate). The formulae for performing discounting are readily available in the literature and are available as preinstalled functions in most computer spreadsheet programs.[1-3]

Despite the almost "cookbook" approach to discounting, there is actually a great deal of controversy about its empirical and conceptual underpinnings.[3,14-20] In particular, this controversy focuses on: (1) the appropriate discount rate and (2) discounting of nonmonetary benefits.

Both the Panel and CDC recommended discounting costs and health outcomes at the same rate. The Panel recommended a rate of 3%, with sensitivity analyses using 5%, 0%, and 7%.[3] The 1995 CDC guide recommended a rate of 5%, with sensitivity analyses using 0% and 8%, although the 1996 book recommended either 3% or 5%.[1,2] Rates are in real or constant dollars, that is, not adjusted for future inflation.

The Panel report includes an extensive review of the conceptual basis for selecting a discount rate. To summarize, two broadly different strategies for selecting a discount rate have been debated: one based on the political process and one based on preferences revealed in the marketplace. Within the latter approach, the Panel adopted the "shadow-price-of-capital" alterative, based on the social rate of time preference. based on this conceptual approach and relevant empirical studies, the Panel recommends a rate of 3%. They recommend that the standard discount rate be reexamined over time but that the base rate of 3% be retained for at least 10 years.

The Panel report also includes an extensive review of the conceptual basis for setting the discount rate for health effects equal to those for costs. They begin by reviewing two major rationales in support of setting the discount rate for health effects equal to that of costs (technically, the consistency argument[13] and the Keeler–Cretin paradox[21]). Then the Panel reviews the numerous challenges that have been raised. We discuss two challenges that are particularly relevant to AIDS prevention: that prevention is "different" and that individual time preferences are not consistent with a discount rate for effectiveness equal to the market rate.

Because the benefits of prevention occur primarily in the future whereas costs occur primarily in the present, the process of discounting particularly affects the cost-effectiveness of prevention.[16] This is particularly true if the discount rate is high (e.g., 10%), and benefits and costs are discounted. There are also philosophical arguments which challenge how discounting is used in economic evaluations of prevention. Discounting may not reflect the way people want government to act in their behalf.[17,18] It has been asserted that programs which reduce future risks, such as prevention, should have a low discount rate because they provide a social good.[22]

Both the Panel and CDC examined this issue and concluded that if the benefits of prevention are undervalued, the solution may be to quantify the benefits of prevention more comprehensively, not to manipulate the discount rate.

Many studies have found that individual time preferences are not consistent with a discount rate based on social time preference. Individual's discount rates are variable both between and among individuals, individuals do not discount future events using a constant-rate model, and preferences are subject to change. The Panel concludes that despite the descriptive evidence that individuals' discount rates are not consistent with a social discount rate, there are compelling reasons for continuing to use a social discount rate. These reasons include the following: (1) that the purpose of CEA is to serve as a prescriptive or normative tool, not to describe individuals' behavior; and (2) to base a normative theory on a foundation of dynamically shifting preferences is to abandon a fundamental tenet of welfare economics, the stability of preferences. Therefore, it is reasonable to assume that individuals' discount rates on average are comparable to a social discount rate. The Panel does provide, however, a preliminary method for incorporating individual time preferences and notes the need for further theoretical and empirical work in this area.

Relevance to AIDS Prevention

An example of the importance of discounting to AIDS prevention is provided by Guinan et al.[23] This analysis estimates the medical cost savings for a case of HIV prevented, which is necessary for assigning a systematic economic value to an HIV infection averted in economic evaluations. The estimate of medical cost savings has been subsequently updated by Holtgrave and Pinkerton.[7,8] Guinan and colleagues note that the time interval over which these costs are incurred and the discount rate used can have a substantial impact on the resulting cost-savings estimates. By using cost data previously published but undiscounted,[24,25] epidemiological assumptions about the course of HIV infection, and a 5% discount rate, they estimated the present value of future cost savings for a case of HIV prevented at from $56,000 (in 1992 dollars) to $80,000 (in 1991 dollars). Undiscounted, these costs are $94,000 and $135,000, respectively.

An example of an HIV prevention study that used a range of discount rates is provided by Villari et al.[26] This economic evaluation of HIV testing among intravenous drug users in Italy used 5% as the base rate, with sensitivity analyses using 0% and 8%. They found that at an initial HIV prevalence of 0.05, any discount rate showed that a testing program is cost saving. However, at an initial HIV prevalence of 0.60, the cost per year of life gained ranged from $15,000 (0% rate) to $50,000 (8% rate) (Italian lire converted to U.S. dollars).

Two reviews of economic evaluations of AIDS prevention examined the use of discounting. Holtgrave et al.[5] examined 93 studies published between 1990 and early 1995. Of the 22 CEAs of domestic, behavioral-change prevention interventions, only one study reported the discount rate used (8%), 55% did not report a discount rate, and for the remaining studies discounting was not applicable (i.e., all costs and benefits occurred in the present). Sisk et al.[9] examined 25 domestic studies published between 1984 and 1995 (note that there was some overlap with [Holtgrave, 1996][5] in the studies reviewed). Fifty-six percent of the studies reviewed did not report a discount rate, 28% discounted both costs and benefits, 8% discounted costs but not benefits, and for the remainder of the studies, discounting was not applicable or there was missing information. Of the nine studies which used discounting, five used a rate of 5%, two used a rate of 6%, one used a rate of 3%, and one a rate of 4%.

Therefore, our first conclusion is that discounting may be very relevant in economic evaluations of AIDS prevention, but that the majority of prior studies have neglected to consider discounting. It is very important that authors explicitly state the rate used for discounting costs and benefits or why discounting is not applicable.

Our second conclusion is that the majority of the prior studies of AIDS prevention that discounted used a rate of 5%. It is likely to prove difficult to change the use of 5% as the standard discount rate.

Our third conclusion is that some economic evaluations of AIDS prevention do not discount health effects and costs. For some of these studies, the discounting of health effects would have a minimal impact on the results (e.g., Phillips, 1994;[27] Lurie, 1994[28]). Analysts should, however, either discount health effects or discuss why they did not.

More complex are the issues surrounding whether AIDS prevention is "different." AIDS is often perceived to be "different" because it is an infectious disease which usually results in death and because of its tremendous toll on younger individuals. Therefore, society and individuals may place a higher value on the benefits of AIDS prevention than is indicated by the discounted benefits. For example, society may value the benefits to future generations of a "cure" for AIDS much more than would be indicated by the discounted benefits.

Another complex issue for AIDS prevention is the variability of individuals' time preferences. To our knowledge there have not been any studies of individuals' time preferences specifically for AIDS prevention. For example, individuals may place a very high value on avoiding AIDS, whether it is one year in the future or five years in the future. Future research in this area would be useful.

As noted in the recommendations, however, the issues of whether prevention is "different" and the variability of individuals' time preferences do not invalidate the need for discounting. Economic evaluations of AIDS prevention should use discounting when appropriate or should explicitly state why discounting was not used. Analysts need to be aware, however, of the controversies surrounding discounting and not assume that discounting is a simple methodological trick that can be done mechanically. Because AIDS prevention programs often incur costs in the present but the benefits are in the future, they are often particularly affected by discounting.

CONCLUSIONS

In this chapter, we defined some of the basic terminology of economic evaluation and discussed some current issues in methodological standardization. In particular, we focused on issues of employing quality of life measurements, cost assessment, and discounting. For each of the three areas, we provided some thoughts as to needed, further research.

We also note that the Panel and CDC made their recommendations about methodological standardization general so as to be relevant to many areas of health and medicine, not just HIV prevention. We observe that methodological standardization must also occur within a disease area, that is, analysts working on HIV prevention issues should come to some agreement on key parametric values used in all of their studies (e.g., the estimate of lifetime treatment costs for HIV disease). Holtgrave and Pinkerton[7,8] have begun to work on such standardization within HIV prevention, but more work remains to be done.

It is important to take our methodological discussion in the proper spirit. Economic evaluation methods in HIV prevention can be further refined but can already be put into practice in rigorous and programmatically relevant ways. This will be demonstrated throughout this volume. A number of analysts have successfully employed economic evaluation techniques *rigorously* in assessing HIV prevention interventions. Some have even developed streamlined methods for rapidly answering breaking policy questions in real time. Methodological standardization will make their future studies even more comparable to each other, and this comparability is a key issue in making the research even more usable to decision makers.

REFERENCES

1. Teutsch S, Haddix A, eds. *A Practical Guide to Prevention Effectiveness: Decision and Economic Analysis.* Atlanta, Georgia: Centers for Disease Control and Prevention; 1994.
2. Haddix AC, Teutsch SM, Shaffer PA, Duñet DO, eds. *Prevention Effectiveness: A Guide to Decision Analysis and Economic Evaluation.* New York: Oxford University Press; 1996.
3. Gold MR, Siegel JE, Russell LB, Weinstein MC, eds. *Cost-effectiveness in Health and Medicine.* New York: Oxford University Press; 1996.
4. World Bank. *World Development Report 1993: Investing in Health.* New York: Oxford University Press; 1993.
5. Holtgrave DR, Qualls NL, Graham JD. Economic evaluation of HIV prevention programs. *Annu Rev Public Health* 1996; 17:467–488.
6. Drummond M, Stoddard G, Torrance G. *Methods for the Economic Evaluation of Health Care Programmes.* New York: Oxford University Press, 1987.
7. Pinkerton SD, Holtgrave DR. Assessing the cost-effectiveness of HIV prevention interventions: A primer. In Holtgrave DR, ed. *Handbook of Economic Evaluation of HIV Prevention,* New York: Plenum.
8. Holtgrave DR, Pinkerton SD. Updates of cost of illness and quality of life estimates for use in economic evaluations of HIV prevention programs. *J Acquired Immune Defic Syndr Hum Retrovirol,* in press.
9. Sisk J. *The effectiveness of AIDS prevention efforts.* The Office of Technology Assessment, 1995.
10. Mauskopf J, Paul J, Wichman D, White A, Tilson H. Economic impact of treatment of HIV-positive pregnant women and their newborns with zidovudine. *JAMA* 1996; 276(2):132–138.
11. Drummond M, Brandt A, Luce B, Rovira J. Standardizing methodologies for economic evaluation in health care. *Int J Technol Assessment Health Care* 1993; 9(1):26–36.
12. Warner K, Luce B. *Cost-Benefit and Cost-Effectiveness Analysis in Health Care.* Ann Arbor, Michigan: Health Administration Press, 1982.
13. Weinstein M, Stason W. Foundations of cost-effectiveness analysis for health and medical practices. *N Engl J Med* 1977; 296(13):716–721.
14. Phillips KA, Holtgrave D. Using cost-effectiveness/cost-benefit analysis to allocate health resources: A level playing field for prevention? *Am J Preventive Med,* 1997; 13(11):18–25.
15. Ganiats T. Discounting in cost-effectiveness research. *Medical Decision Making* 1994; 14(3):298–303.
16. Krahn M, Gafni A. Discounting in the economic evaluation of health care interventions. *Medical Care* 1993; 31(5):403–418.
17. Sheldon T. Discounting in health care decision-making: Time for a change? *J Public Health Med* 1992; 14(3):250–256.
18. Robinson J. Philosophical origins of the social rate of discount in cost-benefit analysis. *The Milbank Q* 1990; 68(2):245–265.
19. Ganiats T. On sale: Future health care. *West J Med* 1992; 156:550–553.
20. Anonymous. Discounting health care: Only a matter of timing? *Lancet* 1992; 340:148–149.
21. Keeler E, Cretin S. Discounting of life-saving and other nonmonetary effects. *Manage Sci* 1983; 23: 300–306.
22. Horowitz J, Carson R. Discounting statistical lives. *J Risk Uncertainty* 1990; 3:403–413.

23. Guinan ME, Farnham PG, Holtgrave DR. Estimating the value of preventing an HIV infection. *Am J Preventive Med* 1994; 10:1–4.
24. Hellinger F. Forecasts of the costs of medical care for persons with HIV: 1991–1995. *Inquiry* 1992; 29: 356–365.
25. Hellinger F. The lifetime cost of treating a person with HIV. *JAMA* 1993; 270:474–478.
26. Villari P, Fattore G, Siegle J, Paltiel A, Weinstein M. Economic evaluation of HIV testing among intravenous drug users. *Int J Technol Assessment Health Care* 1996; 12(2):336–357.
27. Phillips KA, Lowe R, Kahn J, Lurie P, Avins A, Ciccarone D. The cost-effectiveness of HIV testing of physicians and dentists in the United States. *JAMA* 1994; 271(11):851–858.
28. Lurie P, Avins A, Phillips KA, Kahn J, Lowe R, Ciccarone D. The cost-effectiveness of voluntary counseling and testing of hospital inpatients for HIV infection. *JAMA* 1994; 272(23):1832–1838.

The Bernoulli-Process Model of HIV Transmission

Applications and Implications

STEVEN D. PINKERTON and PAUL R. ABRAMSON

INTRODUCTION

Evaluation of HIV prevention programs is complicated by challenges at the biomedical, societal, and individual levels. Although the transmission of HIV is a discrete event, rarely can the outcome of a particular opportunity for transmission be ascertained with certainty. When seroconversion occurs, it is delayed by several weeks or even months from the time of infection. Moreover, most cases of HIV infection are detected only much later in the course of disease progression, after the manifestation of symptoms associated with deterioration of the immune system. Because of this uncertainty, from an analytic perspective HIV transmission is best viewed as a stochastic process. Thus, we might assume that there is a certain probability of HIV transmission each time a susceptible person has unprotected sex or engages in other HIV-risk behaviors. Or instead, we might consider each new sexual relationship as posing some definite HIV risk. In either case, risk is quantified as a probability of HIV transmission. Although the focus herein is on the sexual transmission of HIV, analogous models for drug injection-related risks also exist.[1,2]

Within this probabilistic framework, the effectiveness of an HIV prevention strategy, such as condom promotion, can be assessed by estimating the expected reduction in the probability of transmission, and therefore the expected reduction in the number of infections, attributable to the prevention program.[3] This exercise can be carried out either at a theoretical level, comparing hypothetical prevention interventions to determine which would have the greatest expected impact if implemented, or as an adjunct to retrospective evaluations of existing programs. These estimates of the expected or actual effectiveness of one or more HIV prevention programs can then be combined with information on the cost of implementing the program(s), permitting evaluation of the relative cost-effectiveness of alternative HIV prevention interventions.[4] Cost-effectiveness analyses provide important information that aids public health decision makers in deciding how to allocate limited health-related resources to maximize the overall well-being of the public.[5]

STEVEN D. PINKERTON • Department of Psychiatry and Behavioral Medicine, Center for AIDS Intervention Research (CAIR), Medical College of Wisconsin, Milwaukee, Wisconsin 53202. PAUL R. ABRAMSON • Department of Psychology, University of California, Los Angeles, Los Angeles, California 90024.

Handbook of Economic Evaluation of HIV Prevention Programs, edited by Holtgrave. Plenum Press, New York, 1998.

In the Bernoulli-process model of sexual HIV transmission examined here, each act of sexual intercourse is treated as an independent stochastic trial (rather like the flip of a coin) that is associated with a very small probability of HIV transmission. The model provides a bridge between self-reported sexual behavior and the associated risk of transmission, and therefore permits effectiveness evaluation of HIV prevention programs targeting sexual risk behaviors.[3] Advantages of the modeling approach include the ability to examine consequences of alternative scenarios and to assess the dependence of results on specific programmatic assumptions or characteristics of the target population. Moreover, difficulties associated with biological monitoring of HIV transmission have thus far precluded the implementation of large-scale intervention studies using HIV seroconversion as an endpoint. These factors suggest that modeling will remain an important tool for evaluating HIV prevention programs.[6]

Although this area of HIV modeling is relatively new, several analyses have already appeared in the literature. In this chapter, we describe the Bernoulli model in considerable detail, highlight some of the main theoretical findings that have been obtained with regard to HIV prevention effectiveness, examine selected assumptions and variants of the model, and apply the model to a simple illustrative cost-effectiveness analysis of a hypothetical intervention.

THE BERNOULLI-PROCESS MODEL

In the basic Bernoulli-process model, each act of (vaginal or anal) intercourse is treated as an independent event with a small, fixed probability of HIV transmission from an already infected person to an uninfected partner. (In this model HIV transmission and infection are assumed equivalent, i.e., transmission always leads to infection.) The small, per-act probability of transmission is known as the *infectivity* of HIV and is usually denoted by the Greek letter alpha (α). As discussed later, a number of factors are believed to influence the infectivity of HIV, including the particular sex act engaged in (e.g., penile-vaginal or penile-anal intercourse), the sex role (insertive or receptive), and the stage of disease progression of the infected partner. For now, however, we shall assume a constant infectivity of 0.001 for male-to-female transmission during unprotected penile-vaginal intercourse and an infectivity of 0.01 for unprotected receptive penile-anal intercourse.[7] Although these per-act probabilities are fairly small, they compound rapidly when the number of contacts is increased. For multiple contacts with an infected partner, the cumulative probability of transmission is given by

$$P = 1 - (1 - \alpha)^n \tag{1}$$

where α is the infectivity (i.e., the per-contact probability of transmission) and n is the number of contacts.

One way to reduce this risk, of course, is to use condoms consistently. A recent meta-analysis conducted by the present authors found that, in practice, condoms reduce the infectivity of HIV by a minimum of between 90 and 95%.[8] Assuming the more conservative estimate of 90% condom effectiveness, the reduced infectivity for condom-protected intercourse is

$$\alpha_k = (1 - 0.9)\alpha_n = 0.1\alpha_n \tag{2}$$

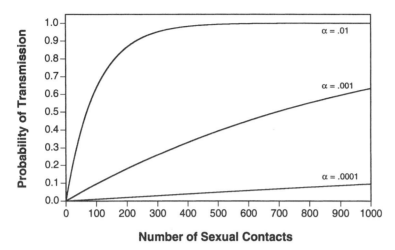

Figure 1. Probability of HIV transmission from an infected individual to an uninfected partner as a function of the number of sexual contacts, for several infectivity values α.

where α_k and α_n are the infectivities of protected and unprotected intercourse, respectively. If, as assumed above, the infectivity of unprotected intercourse is $\alpha_n = 0.01$ or 0.001, then the infectivity when condoms are used is reduced to $\alpha_k = 0.001$ or 0.0001.

Figure 1 illustrates how the cumulative probability of HIV transmission grows with increasing numbers of sexual contacts, for three infectivity conditions: $\alpha = 0.01$ (unprotected anal intercourse), $\alpha = 0.001$ (protected anal intercourse or unprotected vaginal intercourse), and $\alpha = 0.0001$ (protected vaginal intercourse). As shown, the cumulative probability rises quickly as the number of contacts increases. For example, the probability of transmission exceeds one-half after only 100 contacts in the high infectivity, anal intercourse condition ($\alpha = 0.01$). For vaginal intercourse ($\alpha = 0.001$) the impact of consistent (i.e., 100%) condom use is substantial and reduces the risk of transmission by about 90%. For anal intercourse the reduction in risk is limited by ceiling effects caused by the rapid accumulation of risk.

The large risks evident in Fig. 1 arise from sexual contacts with a partner who is known to be infected with HIV. Under most circumstances, whether or not a particular partner is infected is unknown. To take this uncertainty into account, an additional factor must be introduced that reflects the probability that a randomly selected partner is infected. For simplicity, this probability is usually approximated by the prevalence of infection (denoted π) in the population from which partners are selected. (Because greater than average sexual activity is a risk factor for HIV infection, π may underestimate the actual probability of selecting an infected partner. Conversely, HIV disease, and especially AIDS, may adversely affect sexual activity levels, decreasing this probability.) For n contacts with a partner of unknown infective status, the cumulative probability of HIV transmission is given by

$$P = \pi[1 - (1 - \alpha)^n] \qquad (3)$$

which is simply the joint probability that (1) the partner is infected and (2) transmission would occur given that the partner is infected (this form of the equation has been examined by Hearst and Hulley,[9] Pinkerton and Abramson,[10] and others).

Because Eq. 3 differs from Eq. 1 by only a multiplier, the shape of the corresponding probability curves is identical to those shown in Fig. 1, and only the magnitude differs. Thus, for example, in the high infectivity case ($\alpha = 0.01$), the probability of transmission rapidly rises toward its maximum value (π) as the number of contacts grows into the hundreds (notice that Eq. 1 reflects the special case of Eq. 3 in which π equals 1.0). As before, consistent condom use reduces the risk of transmission by about 90% in the low infectivity case ($\alpha = 0.001$) and also in the high infectivity condition, provided that the number of contacts is not too great.

The more general situation of multiple (simultaneous or sequential) partners is slightly more complex. For someone with m different sexual partners who has n_i unprotected and k_i protected contacts with partner i ($i = 1 \ldots m$), the cumulative probability of infection is given by[3-11]

$$P = 1 - \prod_{i=1}^{m} \{1 - \pi[1 - (1 - \alpha_n)^{n_i}(1 - \alpha_k)^{k_i}]\} \tag{4}$$

This equation can be simplified greatly by introducing additional assumptions about the distribution of sexual contacts among sexual partners (*for now assume that all contacts are unprotected*). For example, if the contacts are evenly distributed among the m partners (i.e., each $n_i = n$), then Eq. 4 simplifies to[10,12-14]

$$\begin{aligned} P &= 1 - \{1 - \pi[1-(1 - \alpha)^n]\}^m \\ &= 1 - [(1 - \pi) + \pi(1 - \alpha)^n]^m \end{aligned} \tag{5}$$

Whereas, the risk arising from n sex contacts with a main partner and m "one-night stands" with other partners is given by

$$P = 1 - [(1 - \pi) + \pi(1 - \alpha)^n](1 - \pi\alpha)^m \tag{6}$$

Obviously, many other combinations are possible. (Equation 4 can also be generalized to incorporate multiple risk behavior, such as anal *and* vaginal intercourse, and condom use for some but not all partners or contacts—see later.)

RESULTS FROM THE BASIC MODEL

The Bernoulli-process model can be used to address a number of fundamental questions about HIV risk and effective risk reduction strategies. Examples of such questions include the following: What is the best way to limit the probability of transmission, using condoms consistently or decreasing the number of sexual partners? What if condoms are not used consistently, but only occasionally? Is it better to use condoms consistently with some partners and not at all with other partners, or to use them occasionally with all partners? Under what circumstances is "serial monogamy" a risky behavior?

We begin with the simple assertion that the probability of infection arising from $(k + j)$ contacts with a single partner is less than that from k contacts with one partner and j contacts with another.[10] Thus, having only one partner is always safer than having two. From this it follows naturally that the safest way to allocate a "sex budget" of n total acts is to have n contacts with a single partner, and the riskiest is to have n "one-night stands" with n different partners.

Not surprisingly, the risk of infection increases with both the number of contacts and the number of partners. But if both are fixed, what then is the optimal strategy for "allocating" sexual contacts among sexual partners? To make the problem a bit more concrete, consider a person with a fixed sex budget of n contacts, divided among m partners.[15] As it turns out, the risk is maximal when the contacts are evenly distributed among the partners i.e., there are n/m contacts per partner and minimal when there are $(n - m + 1)$ contacts with one partner and one contact each with the remaining $(m - 1)$ partners (mathematical proofs are provided in Ref. 10). Thus, having one steady partner together with some number of "one-night stands" is safer than having several sexual relationships of similar intensity.

Both the number of partners and the distribution pattern of sexual contacts matter. But just how much do they matter? Figure 2 illustrates the two extreme cases, "serial monogamy" in which sexual contacts are evenly distributed among partners (see Eq. 5), and "almost monogamy" in which there is a main partner who accounts for most of the contacts, plus some number of "one-night stands" (see Eq. 6). (This figure assumes an HIV prevalence of $\pi = 0.1$. However, similar figures are obtained for prevalence levels from $\pi = 0.001$ to $\pi = 0.5$.) As shown in the figure, the risk associated with "serial monogamy" is substantially larger than that of "almost monogamy." According to the results cited previously, all other strategies for allocating sexual contacts among m partners necessarily produce levels of risk intermediate to these extremes. Notice, however, that the bulk of the risk for "serial monogamy" is incurred for the first ten or twenty partners in the high infectivity condition ($\alpha = 0.01$) and for the first few in the low infectivity condition ($\alpha = 0.001$). For "almost monogamy" each additional partner contributes a very small increment to the overall probability of infection. Thus, the number of partners beyond the first few, though important, is not necessarily a primary determinant of risk.[12] Instead, as argued further later, the infectivity of the particular act (moderated, perhaps, by the use of condoms) plays a stronger role in determining the level of risk.

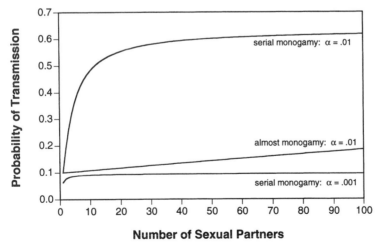

Figure 2. Probability of HIV transmission from 1,000 sexual contacts with one or more partners, m, drawn from a population with HIV prevalence $\pi = 0.1$ for two infectivity values α. For "serial monogamy" the sexual contacts are evenly distributed among the m partners, whereas in "almost monogamy" there are $(1,000 - m + 1)$ contacts with a single main partner and $(m - 1)$ "one night stands."

Of course, most people do not consciously allocate sexual contacts among different partners according to a preplanned sex budget. Nevertheless, this result highlights a possible shortcoming of HIV prevention messages that advocate reducing the number of partners as a primary means of diminishing HIV risk. Such messages were especially common early in the epidemic, when many public health officials, educators, and other commentators called on sexually active Americans (and gay men in particular) to decrease the number of partners with whom they had sex, in the hope that such reductions would markedly diminish their susceptibility to HIV.[14] Messages promoting sexual partner reductions (and especially monogamy and abstinence), however, were viewed by some gay activists as both antisexual and homophobic (i.e., as an attempt to remake gay sexuality in the image of heterosexuality). In contrast, *How to Have Sex in an Epidemic*[16] and other early, gay-authored HIV educational materials stressed substituting safer sexual practices, including condom use and nonpenetrative activities, for riskier ones. Once "safer sex" has been embraced the need for limiting partners becomes less clear. In general, it is often difficult to convince people who have already made one modification to their sexual lifestyles that additional sacrifices are needed.[17] Thus, although from an ivory tower it is clear that the best advice is to decrease the number of partners *and* use condoms, for many people the relevant decision is instead whether to decrease the number of partners *or* use condoms.[10,14] Which is the better strategy?

Figure 3 provides a partial answer to this question. This figure illustrates two distinct ways by which a person in the high infectivity ($\alpha = 0.01$), all "one-night stands" condition could reduce the risk of becoming infected. The person could either reduce the infectivity to $\alpha = 0.001$ by using condoms consistently, or instead could switch to monogamy. From Fig. 2, it is clear that the former scenario is always preferable to the latter (the low-infectivity curve for all "one-night stands" is always lower than the high-infectivity curve for monogamy). Thus, under the conditions examined here, even the most drastic change in the

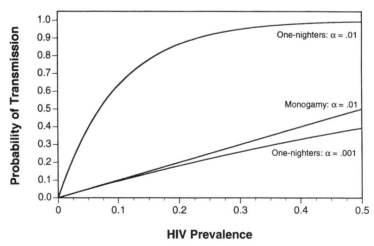

Figure 3. Probability of HIV transmission assuming 1,000 sexual contacts with either a single partner ("monogamy") or 1,000 different partners ("one-nighters"), drawn from a population with HIV prevalence π, for two infectivity values α.

number of partners (from one thousand partners to a single partner) does not reduce the risk of infection as much as the consistent use of 90% effective condoms.[9,10,14]

Clearly, for condoms to provide *maximum* protection requires that they be used consistently, that is, for every sexual contact. Unfortunately, many people use condoms only occasionally, rather than consistently, if they use them at all.[18,19] Does this lack of consistency negate or substantially lessen the benefits of condom use as implied by educational messages stressing 100% consistent condom use and not just increased condom use? According to the perspective implicit in such messages, anything less than consistent usage is unacceptable, presumably because any act of unprotected sexual intercourse puts one at some risk of infection. Indeed, the HIV/AIDS literature contains numerous case reports of individuals who became infected with HIV as the result of a single or very few acts of unprotected intercourse with an infected partner.[20–22]

Compared to other common STDs (e.g., syphilis and gonorrhea), however, HIV is not easily transmitted under most circumstances. Therefore, the significance of a single act of unprotected sex is relatively minor. For example, Fig. 4 illustrates how the probability of transmission varies as a function of the percentage of condom use for 100 contacts with partners drawn from a population in which the prevalence of HIV is $\pi = 0.1$ (the general shape of the curves, however, does not depend strongly on the prevalence). In all three of the behavioral patterns considered in this figure ("monogamy," "serial monogamy," and all "one-night stands"), the risk of infection decreases approximately linearly as the proportion of condom-protected contacts increases. For example, using condoms 50% of the time reduces the risk about half as much as does using condoms 100% of the time. Thus, even occasional condom use can provide a substantial reduction in the risk of infection.[13] Because some people are either unwilling or unable to use condoms for every act of intercourse, HIV/AIDS prevention messages are needed that focus on the importance of situation-specific

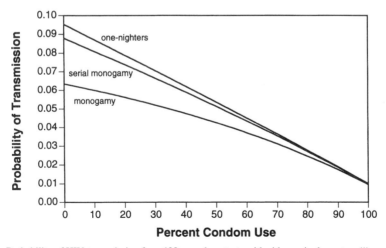

Figure 4. Probability of HIV transmission from 100 sexual contacts with either a single partner ("monogamy"), 100 different partners ("one-nighters"), or 5 different partners ("serial monogamy"), drawn from a population with HIV prevalence $\pi = 0.1$, as a function of the percentage of contacts that are condom-protected, assuming an infectivity of $\alpha = 0.01$.

condom use (e.g., with a new partner) or that simply encourage people to use condoms more frequently.

If condoms are used only occasionally, rather than consistently, the question arises as to how condom use should optimally be distributed. Is it better to use condoms consistently with some partners and not at all with others or to use them some of the time with all partners? The answer, by analogy to the problem of distributing contacts over a fixed number of partners, is that the greatest reduction in risk occurs when condom use is targeted, rather than applied evenly. The general rule is that overall risk is maximal when the component risks arising from different partnerships are equal. Thus, for example, "serial monogamy" (in which contacts are evenly distributed among partners) is much riskier than having a single main partner and several "one- night stands." Unfortunately, the long-term sexual behavior pattern of many sexually active adults closely resembles "serial monogamy." The prevailing ideal in America and other Western nations is, of course, lifelong monogamy. But, for many people this ideal, however appealing, is simply unattainable. For such people, life is a series of committed but ultimately transitory monogamous relationships. The Bernoulli model suggests that this pattern could be dangerous because frequent partnership changes increase the likelihood of becoming involved with an infected person, whereas the extended duration of the (more or less monogamous) relationships provides ample opportunity for HIV to be transmitted in the absence of consistent condom use.

We are aware that readers may find this discussion far too rational. After all, people fall in love or are ensnared by lust, according to emotional, physical, and myriad other factors, rather than according to an esoteric calculus of HIV risk. Nevertheless, there are important implications here for HIV prevention efforts. For one, increasing condom use—even occasional condom use—should be a top priority. Accordingly, additional research is needed on the situational determinants of occasional condom use. Moreover, because HIV-infected individuals may be much more infectious in the first few weeks or months following infection than during the long asymptomatic period that follows, delaying sexual activity or consistently using condoms during the first few months of new relationships could have disproportionately large protective effects.[23] Messages that encourage people to reduce the number of partners with whom they have sex or that emphasize only the benefits of *consistent* condom use should be carefully targeted to ensure that they do not interfere with the important goal of increasing condom use by setting what may seem an unattainable standard.

A similar shortcoming is evident in admonishments to "know your partner" (i.e., choose only partners who are likely to be uninfected). Although we have focused previously on the infectivity of HIV and the number of different partners, it is evident from Eq. 3 that, in fact, the most significant determinant of risk is π, the probability that a given partner is HIV-infected.[9] In the previous exposition, the prevalence of HIV in the population (or community) from which partners are drawn has been taken as an estimate of π, and it has been assumed that partners are selected *at random* from this population. Clearly, any nonrandom selection technique that reduces the probability of selecting an infected partner should be employed whenever possible. This observation led Hearst and Hulley, on the basis of risk estimates obtained from a Bernoulli-process model of monogamy, to recommend that people "not have sex with anyone known to be seropositive or with anyone in a high-risk group who has not stopped all high-risk activities for at least six months and subsequently tested negative for HIV antibody."[9,p.2431]

Although this is generally sound advice, it is unclear how practical it is when applied to real-life sexual relationships.[24] Having unprotected intercourse with an infected person is obviously risky, yet many committed life partners of infected people do exactly that. Provided that the number of contacts is not too large and, especially, that condoms are used regularly, the ensuing risk may be viewed as acceptable within a personal calculus of utilities that places great value on continued physical and emotional intimacy.[17,25] For casual or nascent relationships there is the additional difficulty of identifying potentially infected partners or members of "high-risk" groups. If gay men, in toto, comprise a high-risk group, then for gay men this advice constitutes a de facto proscription of *all* sexual intercourse. The defining features of high-risk groups, including "promiscuity," same-gender sex, and IV drug use, are all socially deprecated activities, and therefore not likely to be readily admitted to a potential sex partner. Finally, the very concept of a "high-risk" group invites people to deny their own risk and creates an environment of stigmatization. For these and numerous other reasons,[26,27] advising potentially at-risk individuals to avoid having sex with members of high-risk groups is likely to be counterproductive.

Moreover, the importance of prevalence as a determinant of HIV risk diminishes rapidly as the number of partners is increased. This is illustrated in Fig. 5, which shows the effect on transmission probabilities of decreasing either the HIV prevalence or the infectivity by 90% for 1,000 contacts divided equally among one or more partners (notice that a 90% reduction in infectivity can be achieved through consistent condom use). As shown, diminishing by 90% the probability that a partner is infected leads to a greater reduction in risk than does consistent condom use, but the difference is substantial only when the number of partners is relatively small. Because Hearst and Hulley emphasized the monogamous case, for which there is a substantial difference, their findings are not necessarily applicable to more realistic scenarios. From this example and those presented before, it

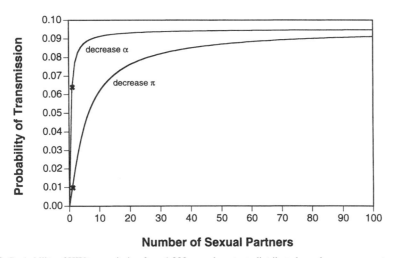

Figure 5. Probability of HIV transmission from 1,000 sexual contacts distributed evenly among m partners drawn from a population with HIV prevalence $\pi = 0.1$ or 0.01, assuming an infectivity of $\alpha = 0.01$ without condoms or $\alpha = 0.001$ if condoms are used consistently. The two conditions are (1) "decrease α"—consistent condom use in higher prevalence population ($\alpha = 0.001$, $\pi = 0.1$); and (2) "decrease π"—no condom use in lower prevalence population ($\alpha = 0.01$, π 0.01). The corresponding probabilities for the monogamous condition ($m = 1$) are marked with the symbol ×.

should be clear that although the Bernoulli model provides an excellent analytic tool for conceptualizing and examining alternative HIV risk reduction strategies, the public policy implications of the ensuing results are not always unambiguous.

BERNOULLI MODEL OF SECONDARY TRANSMISSION

The Bernoulli-process model described previously can be used to estimate the probability that an uninfected person would become infected with HIV based on his or her sexual activity pattern, and to evaluate the impact of various behavioral risk reduction strategies. Considering instead the viewpoint of an *infected* individual, analogous models can be developed that focus on preventing "secondary" transmission from HIV-infected persons to their partners. (The difference between "primary" and "secondary" transmission, as used here, is wholly one of assumed perspective.) In this section we develop the secondary transmission equations corresponding to those presented before for primary transmission.

Obviously, the main difference between the primary and secondary transmission models is that the latter concerns itself with the susceptibility of the index person's partners, rather with the susceptibility of the index person. Thus, for example, the probability of transmission from an infected person to a monogamous partner, assuming n unprotected contacts, is given by

$$P = (1 - \pi)[1 - (1 - \alpha)^n] \tag{7}$$

This equation differs from Eq. 3 only in the substitution of $(1 - \pi)$ for π, where $(1 - \pi)$ is the probability that the partner is susceptible (in this model we ignore the possibility of an already infected person becoming infected with additional strains of HIV). By extension, the expected number of secondary infections among the partners of an infected person who has n sexual contacts with each of m partners is given by[28]

$$R = m(1 - \pi)[1 - (1 - \alpha)^n] \tag{8}$$

For example, Fig. 6 shows the expected number of secondary infections for an infected person who had 1,000 sexual contacts divided evenly among one or more partners ("serial monogamy") drawn from a population in which the prevalence of HIV is 0.1. As shown, the number of secondary infections rises quickly as a function of the number of partners in the high infectivity condition ($\alpha = 0.01$) but is relatively flat in the low infectivity condition ($\alpha = 0.001$). This figure also reemphasizes the utility of consistent condom use, in that 10 condom-protected contacts with each of 100 partners results in fewer secondary infections than does 1,000 unprotected contacts with a single partner. In fact, provided that condoms are used consistently, 1,000 "one-night stands" produce about the same number of secondary infections as does monogamy in which condoms are not used at all (similar results obtain when infectivity estimates of 0.001 and 0.0001 are assumed for unprotected and condom-protected sex, respectively).

The number of secondary infections is also extremely important from an epidemiological standpoint. Clearly, for the HIV epidemic to sustain itself requires that each infected person pass the virus to at least one other person, on average. That is, the expected number of secondary infections R must be greater than one. Because R is inversely related to the prevalence of infection (see Eq. 8), as more people become infected it is increasingly more difficult to sustain an epidemic. Thus, R is greatest early in the epidemic, when essentially

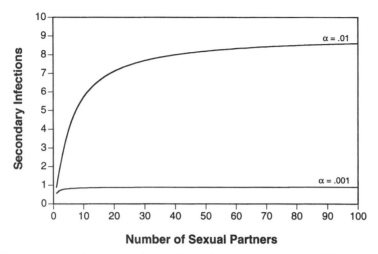

Figure 6. Expected number of secondary infections for an infected individual having 1,000 total sexual contacts divided evenly among one or more partners drawn from a population with HIV prevalence $\pi = 0.1$, for two infectivity values α.

everyone can be assumed susceptible (i.e., $\pi = 0$). (When $\pi = 0$, the expected number of secondary infections, treated as a population parameter, is known as the "reproductive rate of HIV infection."[28]) According to Eq. 8, the expected number of secondary infections for 1,000 "one-night stands" with 1,000 susceptible partners is $R = 1,000\alpha$, which, for $\alpha = 0.001$ equals 1.0 when condoms are used consistently. In contrast, just 100 contacts with each of 10 partners results in more than six secondary infections when condoms are not used ($\alpha = 0.01$).

NOTES ON MODEL PARAMETERS, APPROXIMATIONS, AND VARIANTS

Before proceeding further, a few brief comments are in order about the parametric values utilized herein. Recent estimates of HIV prevalence among high-risk heterosexuals, men who have sex with men, and injection drug users (IDUs) in the 96 U.S. metropolitan areas with populations over 500,000 suggest that about 10% of such persons are currently infected with HIV.[29] Thus, the prevalence value assumed in most of the previous examples, $\pi = 0.1$, represents a fairly high-risk population. However, the results given before and illustrated in the figures do not, in general, depend strongly on the prevalence. Similar results are obtained for very low prevalences (e.g., $\pi = 0.001$) and, to a lesser extent, very high prevalence populations (e.g., $\pi = 0.5$), although as the prevalence increases, the number of sexual partners becomes a more important determinant of HIV risk.

In contrast, many of the results do depend on the infectivity of HIV and may not necessarily hold if the infectivity is much greater than assumed here. Two infectivity estimates are used in the figures and examples considered previously, $\alpha = 0.01$ and $\alpha = 0.001$, which very roughly correspond to the per-contact probability of transmission for unprotected receptive anal and vaginal intercourse, respectively. These estimates are subject to substantial uncertainty. Several factors are believed to influence the infectivity of HIV beyond the particular sex act and role, including the stage of disease progression of the infected partner, the particular strain of HIV, and the presence of additional biological cofactors, including sexually transmitted diseases and genital lesions.[30–33] In particular, infectivity may be much higher during (1) the brief phase of primary infection before seroconversion and (2) following the development of AIDS-defining symptoms (see Ref. 23 for a review and discussion). During these periods of high infectivity, the per-contact probability of transmission could be as great as 0.3 for receptive anal intercourse,[34] which would make HIV roughly as contagious as gonorrhea.[35] Fortunately, the (putative) high infectivity phase of primary infection is believed to be relatively short-lived, lasting a few weeks to a few months.

Although this hypothesis of phase-dependent increased infectivity has not yet been empirically verified, we can nevertheless assess the more obvious implications, such as the heightened importance of consistent (as opposed to occasional) condom use and the advisability of limiting the number of sexual partners, as illustrated in Fig. 7. *If*, as now seems possible, HIV is highly infectious under certain circumstances, then it may be necessary to reconsider existing HIV prevention strategies and to develop novel strategies that specifically address those circumstances under which HIV is highly infectious.[23]

For many applications of the Bernoulli-process model, it is helpful to simplify the mathematics via approximations to the formulas provided earlier. For instance, as is evident in many of the figures (e.g., Fig. 1), the probability of HIV transmission is essentially a linear function of the infectivity and the number of contacts, provided that these values are sufficiently small. In particular, if $\alpha n < 1$, then the probability that an uninfected person becomes infected as the result of n contacts with an infected person can be approximated by the product αn.[10] Thus,

$$1 - (1 - \alpha)^n \approx \alpha n \tag{9}$$

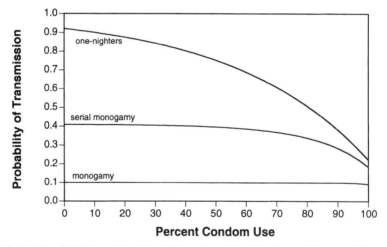

Figure 7. Probability of HIV transmission from 100 sexual contacts with either a single partner ("monogamy"), 100 different partners ("one-nighters"), or 5 different partners ("serial monogamy"), drawn from a population with HIV prevalence $\pi = 0.1$, as a function of the percentage of contacts that are condom-protected, assuming a very high infectivity ($\alpha = 0.25$).

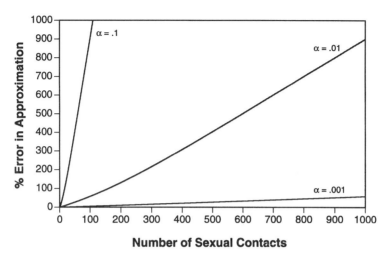

Figure 8. "Error" in approximating via Eq. 9 the probability of HIV transmission from an infected individual to an uninfected partner as a function of the number of sexual contacts, for several infectivity values α.

(This approximation is derived from the familiar binomial expansion,

$$(1 - \alpha)^n \approx 1 - n\alpha + \frac{n(n-1)\alpha^2}{2!} - \frac{n(n-1)(n-2)\alpha^3}{3!} + \ldots \qquad (10)$$

which is valid for α < 1.) Figure 8 illustrates the accuracy of this approximation as a function of the number of sexual contacts n and the infectivity α (the "error in approximation" is defined as $1 - A/E$, where E is the standard estimate and A is the approximation). As shown, the error in approximating the probability of transmission from Eq. 9 grows rapidly with the number of contacts, especially with higher infectivity. Indeed, the error exceeds 10% except when n is less than about 0.2α (e.g., $n = 2$, 20, and 200 in Fig. 8). Therefore care must be exercised applying this and other linear approximations.

Similar caution is warranted when approximating the effect of condom use on transmission probabilities. For example, in the standard model, the probability of transmission resulting from n total contacts, x percent of which are protected, with an infected partner is given by

$$P = 1 - (1 - \alpha)^{n(1-x)} (1 - f\alpha)^{nx} \qquad (11)$$

where f is the failure rate of condoms to prevent HIV transmission (as discussed before, the examples presented here assume $f = 0.1$). This quantity can be approximated by

$$P = 1 - \{1 - [1 - (1 - f)x]\alpha\}^n \qquad (12)$$

(similar approximations appear in Refs. 24 and 36). As Fig. 9 demonstrates, this approximation is close only when the proportion of condom use is either very low or extremely high, or when the infectivity is minimal (α < 0.001). In all other instances, Eq. 12 greatly underestimates the risk of transmission relative to the standard model.

The previous models assume that condom use effectively reduces the per-contact probability of transmission, α (see Eq. 2). Thus, 90% effective condoms diminish the

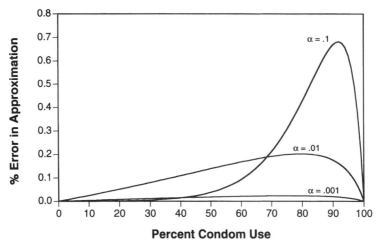

Figure 9. "Error" in approximating via Eq. 12 the probability of HIV transmission from 100 sexual contacts with an infected partner, as a function of the percentage of contacts that are condom-protected, for several infectivity values α.

infectivity by a factor of ten (e.g., from 0.1 to 0.01). Alternately, we could assume that condoms provide perfect protection 90% of the time, and offer no protection the remaining 10% of the time. (In other words, condom protection and failure are all-or-none.) Under this assumption, condoms effectively reduce the number of risky contacts, but the contacts that remain are at full risk. Then, the probability of transmission for n unprotected and k condom-protected contacts with an infected partner is given by

$$P = 1 - (1 - \alpha)^{n+fk} \tag{13}$$

rather than

$$P = 1 - (1 - \alpha)^n (1 - f\alpha)^k \tag{14}$$

as in the standard model (where f is the condom failure rate). Figure 10 compares the probabilities estimated from the standard model (Eq. 14) with those obtained via Eq. 13. The two methods yield essentially the same results when the percentage of condom use is not too great or the infectivity is low but diverge somewhat in the high infectivity condition ($\alpha = 0.1$) when the condom use percentage exceeds 90% or so (in any case, Eq. 13 always produces larger estimates of transmission risk). To our knowledge, this model of discrete, all-or-none condom success and failure has not been previously examined in the literature.

There is yet another variant of the Bernoulli model, in which the basic unit of behavior is the sexual partnership, rather than the sexual contact. In this variant, each sexual partnership is associated with a fixed probability of HIV transmission β from an infected person to an uninfected partner. As the number of partnerships m increases, the cumulative probability of transmission grows according to the following formula:[37,38]

$$P = 1 - (1 - \beta)^m \tag{15}$$

Notice that this equation is identical to the corresponding equation for the per-contact model (Eq. 1), except that per-contact infectivity (α) has been replaced by per-partnership infec-

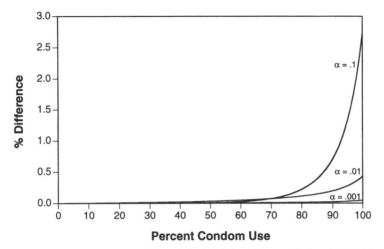

Figure 10. Percentage difference in transmission probabilities derived from standard model (Eq. 14) and alternative model (Eq. 13) of condom action, as a function of the percentage of contacts that are condom-protected. Estimates assume 100 sexual contacts with an infected partner.

tivity (β), and number of partners (m) has been substituted for number of contacts (n). If partners are drawn at random from a population with prevalence π, then the appropriate per-partnership formula is given by

$$P = 1 - [(1 - \pi) + \pi\beta]^m \tag{16}$$

(see Eq. 5). As discussed later, empirical evidence from studies of sexual transmission in HIV-serodiscordant couples favors the per-partnership model over its per-contact counterpart.[37] The per-contact model is somewhat more appealing logically, however, because it makes relationship intensity (duration or number of contacts) explicit, rather than confounding it with infectivity.[28] As Anderson and May note, "the rough equivalence between estimates of β from male homosexual partnerships and for monogamous heterosexual partnerships may be because the transmission probability per act is higher for the former, but the average duration (and number of acts) per partnership is compensatingly higher for the latter."[39, p.516] In practice, the effectiveness estimates (see below) obtained from the per-contact and per-partner models for a particular data set are often quite similar.[40–42]

ESTIMATING INTERVENTION EFFECTIVENESS

In the previous sections the Bernoulli-process model has been utilized to analyze the theoretical efficacy of various HIV risk reduction strategies, such as the consistent (or occasional) use of condoms or decreasing the number of sex partners. This same model, together with specialized variants and extensions, can also be applied to analyzing data from actual HIV prevention interventions to estimate programmatic effectiveness.[3,43] In particular, the model can be used to estimate the number of infections averted by a specific behavioral intervention to reduce HIV transmission (such as a program to increase condom use). This information can be combined with economic data on the cost of the intervention to determine its cost-effectiveness relative to other HIV prevention programs or other health care services.[4,38,40–42,44]

Consider, for example, a behavioral intervention that seeks to decrease risky sexual behavior among a cohort of people, some of whom may be infected with HIV. More precisely, suppose that there are N uninfected and M infected people enrolled in the intervention and that the participants are surveyed twice, once just before the intervention commences and again six months later, about their sexual behavior during the preceding six-month period. Focusing on the uninfected participants first, the Bernoulli model (e.g., Eqs. 3–6) can be used to translate the sexual behavior reported in the surveys into pre- and postintervention risk estimates, the difference between which provides an estimate of the decrease in individual risk that can theoretically be attributed to the intervention.[3] For example, suppose that the average intervention participant's cumulative probability of infection decreases from 0.25 for the six-month period preceding the intervention to 0.2 for the six-month follow-up period. The probability that any one participant becomes infected is therefore reduced by 0.05, and correspondingly, the number of infections that could be expected to arise among uninfected participants in any six-month period drops from $0.25N$ to $0.2N$. Thus, it can reasonably be claimed that the intervention averted $0.05N$ infections during the six-month period assessed by the survey, assuming that preintervention behavioral patterns would have persisted in the absence of intervention (ideally, a comparison group would be available to help control for nonintervention-related factors, such as secular trends, that might have contributed to the observed reduction in risk). Notice that this procedure produces a very conservative estimate of the number of infections averted, in that it is assumed that the effect of the intervention disappears completely once behavior has been assessed at the end of the intervention. In practice, one would expect a much more gradual deterioration of intervention effects.

Similarly, the number of infections averted among the sexual partners of infected participants can be estimated using the Bernoulli-process model of secondary HIV transmission (Eqs. 7 and 8).[3] For example, for an intervention with M infected participants, each of whom modifies his or her behavior sufficiently to reduce the number of partners to whom he or she would be expected to pass the virus from 0.5 to 0.3, the number of secondary infections averted by the intervention is $0.2M$. If this were the same intervention as described in the preceding paragraph, then the estimated total number of infections averted, both primary and secondary, would be $0.05N + 0.2M$, or an average of $(0.05N + 0.2M)/(N + M)$ infections averted per intervention participant, regardless of HIV status. Because averting infections is the main goal of most HIV prevention interventions, this measure, the average number of infections averted per intervention participant, constitutes a meaningful index of programmatic effectiveness.[43,45] Moreover, if the average per-participant cost of the intervention is known, then a cost-effectiveness or cost-utility ratio can easily be computed, permitting assessment of the relative cost-effectiveness of the program using established methodologies[4] (see also the chapter by Pinkerton and Holtgrave in the present volume).

To illustrate this estimation technique, imagine a hypothetical HIV prevention intervention that stresses condom use and sexual negotiation skills. Suppose that 200 people participate in the intervention, that the prevalence of HIV infection among this group and their partners is 10%, and that the average participant changes condom use frequency from 60% at baseline to 80% at six-month follow-up, with an average of two partners and 20 contacts per partner over each six-month assessment period. Assume that increased condom use is the only effect of the intervention, that this effect lasts only for the six-month period assessed at follow-up, and that HIV risk would have remained constant at baseline levels in the absence of intervention.

If there were no intervention, then for each of the $10\% \cdot 200 = 20$ already infected "participants," the expected number of secondary infections would be given by

$$R = m(1 - \pi)[1 - (1 - \alpha_n)^n(1 - \alpha_k)^k]$$
$$= 2 (1 - 0.1)[1 - (1 - \alpha_n)^8(1 - \alpha_k)^{12}]$$

where n and k are the number of unprotected and protected acts of intercourse, respectively, and α_n and α_k are the corresponding infectivities (see Eq. 8). With $\alpha_n = 0.01$ and 90% effective condoms ($\alpha_k = 0.001$), the expected number of secondary infections per person is $R = 0.16$, and the total number of secondary infections is 3.2.

Similarly, the expected number of primary infections among each of the 180 previously uninfected "participants" is given by

$$P = 1 - \{1 - \pi [1 - (1 - \alpha_n)^n(1 - \alpha_k)^k]\}^m$$
$$= 1 - \{1 - 0.1 [1 - (1 - \alpha_n)^8(1 - \alpha_k)^{12}]\}^2$$

(see Eq. 5), which equals 0.02 when α_n and α_k are as given previously. Thus, the total number of expected primary infections is 3.6, and the overall number of infections, both primary and secondary, expected during the six-month period in the absence of intervention is 6.8. The intervention decreases these estimates to $R = 0.13$ and $P = 0.01$ (replace 8 by 6 and 12 by 14 in the preceding equations), and therefore averts a total of $6.8 - 4.4 = 2.4$ infections.

According to one analysis, society should be willing to spend up to about \$400,000 to avert a single HIV infection, based on considerations of the lifetime medical care costs of treating a case of HIV disease and society's willingness to pay for other health-related programs and procedures.[46] The hypothetical intervention described would therefore be cost-effective for society to implement, provided that it cost less than about \$1 million.

SUMMARY, LIMITATIONS, AND FUTURE DIRECTIONS

Effectiveness evaluation of HIV prevention programs is needed to ensure that limited economic and other resources are used wisely, in ways that help maximize the prevention potential of these resources. The mathematical modeling techniques described constitute an important tool that can be used by program planners, analysts, and decision makers to evaluate the actual or expected effectiveness of different intervention strategies and to investigate how different programmatic characteristics affect the effectiveness of these strategies. Thus, these methods can aid decision makers in answering the following meaningful questions: (1) Is intervention A or intervention B more effective at reducing HIV transmission in a particular population? (2) Which is more cost-effective? (3) How would the answers to (1) and (2) be changed if the prevalence of infection in the target population were halved or doubled? And so on.

In the present chapter, the Bernoulli-process model of HIV transmission has been used to illustrate one approach to effectiveness modeling. Elsewhere, other mathematical models of HIV transmission and epidemiology (notably differential equation and compartmental models) have been applied to effectiveness and cost-effectiveness evaluation of HIV prevention programs.[47–49] Among the principal advantages of the Bernoulli model are its relative simplicity, generalizability, and intuitive appeal. That the risk of transmission should increase with repeated contacts with an infected partner is intuitively rather obvious. Therefore, it is somewhat surprising that several empirical studies of transmission in serodiscordant couples have failed to find a significant association between the number of contacts and the probability of transmission.[21,50,51] Some commentators have cited this as evidence of a fundamental flaw in the constant-infectivity, per-contact Bernoulli-process model.[37,50–52] Data bearing on this issue, however, remain limited and inconclusive.[37] Blower and Boe suggest that the nature of the relationship between the number of sex acts and the number of partners may obscure the true relationship between the number of contacts and the acquisition of HIV.[15; see also 28] Alternatively, the apparent independence of the number of sexual contacts and the probability of transmission could be due to variability in infectiousness, either between or within individuals, that is, perhaps some people are especially infectious or especially susceptible, or perhaps infectiousness varies over the course of illness (both of these possibilities are likely). Although a preliminary investigation of the impact of temporal variability in infectiousness on modeling results has recently appeared in the literature,[23] additional research is clearly needed, especially to characterize possible interpersonal variability.

Carefully controlled empirical studies are also needed to validate (or invalidate) the Bernoulli-process model directly and to evaluate the sensitivity of the basic model to changes in fundamental assumptions. If infectiousness is positively correlated with plasma viral titers, as many believe,[23] then it might be possible to use newly developed methods of viral load monitoring to investigate the complex relationship, postulated by the Bernoulli model linking the number of contacts, infectiousness, and probability of transmission, and to characterize interpersonal variability in infectiousness. Even in the absence of empirical studies, however, it may be possible to examine these issues through computer simulation.[53]

Additional assumptions of the Bernoulli model are also amenable to empirical examination. For example, in the simplified model described before, the number of infections averted by an HIV prevention intervention is estimated under the assumption that sexual behavior is uniform across participants. Thus, the average number of sexual partners, the average number of contacts, and average levels of condom use are first calculated for intervention participants, and then these data are used to estimate the probability that a hypothetical "average" participant would become infected. Alternatively, if individual level behavioral data are available, we can calculate a separate infection probability for each participant and from these probabilities infer the expected number of infections averted by the intervention.[3]

To-date, the Bernoulli model has been successfully applied to a variety of questions concerning the effectiveness of sexual and drug-injecting risk reduction intervention strategies,[1,2,9,10,12–14,24,28,36,38,40–42,44] to issues of condom effectiveness,[8] and to vaccine effectiveness and coverage.[54,55] Future refinements and extensions to the basic model promise to increase the applicability of the model to other areas of research, such as non-HIV STD prevention and the interaction between sexual and drug-injection related risks for HIV infection. Although the Swiss mathematician Jakob Bernoulli's pioneering investigations into the theory of probability were motivated by an interest in the lifeless topics of gaming and gambling, one cannot help but believe that he would approve of these newfound uses for his discoveries.

REFERENCES

1. Kahn JG, Washington AE, Showstack JA, Berlin M, Phillips K. *Updated Estimates of the Impact and Cost of HIV Prevention in Injection Drug Users.* Final report prepared for the Centers for Disease Control and Prevention. San Francisco: Institute for Health Policy Studies, University of California at San Francisco; 1992.
2. Holtgrave DR, Pinkerton SD, Jones TS, Lurie P, Vlahov D. Cost and cost-effectiveness of increasing access to sterile syringes and needles as an HIV prevention intervention in the United States. *J Acquired Immune Defic Synd Hum Retrovirol* 1998; 18(Suppl. 1):S133–S138.
3. Pinkerton SD, Holtgrave DR, Leviton L, Wagstaff D, Abramson PR. Model-based evaluation of HIV prevention interventions. *Evaluation Rev* 1998; 22:155–174.
4. Pinkerton SD, Holtgrave DR. A method for evaluating the economic efficiency of HIV behavior risk reduction interventions. *AIDS and Behavior*, in press.
5. Gold MR, Siegel JE, Russell LB, Weinstein MC, eds. *Cost-effectiveness in Health and Medicine.* New York: Oxford University Press; 1996.
6. NIH Consensus Development Conference Consensus Statement. *Interventions to Prevent HIV Risk Behaviors.* Washington DC: Government Printing Office; 1997.
7. Mastro TD, de Vincenzi I. Probabilities of sexual HIV-1 transmission. *AIDS* 1996; 10(Suppl. A):S75–S82.
8. Pinkerton SD, Abramson PR. Effectiveness of condoms in preventing HIV transmission. *Soc Sci Med* 1996; 44:1303–1312.
9. Hearst N, Hulley SB. Preventing the heterosexual spread of AIDS. *JAMA* 1988; 259:2428–2432.
10. Pinkerton SD, Abramson PR. Evaluating the risks: A Bernoulli process model of HIV infection and risk reduction. *Evaluation Rev* 1993; 17:504–528.
11. Eisenberg B. The number of partners and the probability of HIV infection. *Stat Med* 1989; 8:83–92.
12. Fineberg HV. Education to prevent AIDS: Prospects and obstacles. *Science* 1988; 239:592–596.
13. Pinkerton SD, Abramson PR. Occasional condom use and HIV risk reduction. *J Acquired Immune Defic Syndr Hum Retrovirol* 1996; 13:456–460.
14. Reiss IL, Leik RK. Evaluating strategies to avoid AIDS: Number of partners vs. use of condoms. *J Sex Res* 1989; 26:411–433.
15. Blower SM, Boe C. Sex acts, sex partners, and sex budgets: Implications for risk factor analysis and estimation of HIV transmission probabilities. *J Acquired Immune Defic Syndr* 1993; 6:1347–1352.
16. Berkowitz R, Callen M. *How to Have Sex in an Epidemic.* New York: News from the Front Publications; 1983.
17. Abramson PR, Pinkerton SD. *With Pleasure: Thoughts on the Nature of Human Sexuality.* New York: Oxford University Press; 1995.
18. Catania JA, Coates TJ, Stall R, Turner H, Peterson J, Hearst N, Dolcini MM, Hudes E, Gagnon J, Groves R. Prevalence of AIDS-related risk factors and condom use in the United States. *Science* 1992; 258:1101–1106.
19. Pleck JH, Sonenstein FL, Ku LC. Adolescent males' condom use: Relationships between perceived cost-benefits and consistency. *J Marriage Family* 1991; 53:733–745.
20. Johnson AM, Petherick A, Davidson SJ, Brettle R, Hooker M, Howard L, McLean KA, Osborne LEM, Robertson R, Connex C, Tchamouroff S, Shergold C, Adler MW. Transmission of human immunodeficiency virus to sexual partners of hemophiliacs. *AIDS* 1989; 3:367–372.
21. Peterman TA, Stoneburner RL, Allen JR, Jaffe HW, Curran JW. Risk of human immunodeficiency virus transmission from heterosexual adults with transfusion-associated infections. *JAMA* 1988; 259:55–58.
22. Staszewski S, Schieck E, Rehmet S, Helm EB, Stille W. HIV transmission from male after only two sexual contacts. *Lancet* 1987; 2:628.
23. Pinkerton SD, Abramson PR. Implications of increased infectivity in early-stage HIV infection: Application of a Bernoulli-process model of HIV transmission. *Evaluation Rev* 1996; 20:516–540.
24. Wittkowski KM. Preventing the heterosexual spread of AIDS: What is the best advice if compliance is taken into account? *AIDS* 1988; 3:143–145.
25. Pinkerton SD, Abramson PR. Is risky sex rational? *J Sex Res* 1992; 29:561–568.
26. Cochran SD, Mays VM. Sex, lies, and HIV. *N Engl J Med* 1990; 322:774–775.
27. Crimp D. How to have promiscuity in an epidemic. In Crimp D, ed. *AIDS: Cultural Analysis, Cultural Activism.* Cambridge, MA: MIT Press; 1988.
28. Pinkerton SD, Abramson PR. An alternative model of the reproductive rate of HIV infection: Formulation, evaluation, and implications for risk reduction interventions. *Evaluation Rev* 1994; 18:371–388.
29. Holmberg SD. The estimated prevalence and incidence of HIV in 96 large US metropolitan areas. *Am J Public Health* 1996; 86:642–654.

30. Holmberg SD, Horsburgh CR Jr., Ward JW, Jaffe HW. Biologic factors in the sexual transmission of human immunodeficiency virus. *J Infect Dis* 1989; 160:116–125.
31. Nicolosi A. Human immunodeficiency virus (HIV-1): Infectivity transmission, risk behaviours and host susceptibility. *Functional Neurology* 1992; 7:13–29.
32. O'Brien TR, Busch MP, Donegan E, Ward JW, Wong I, Samson SM, Perkins HA, Altman R, Stoneburner RL, Holmberg SD. Heterosexual transmission of human immunodeficiency virus type 1 from transfusion recipients to their sex partners. *J Acquired Immune Defic Syndr* 1994; 7:705–710.
33. Royce RA, Seña A, Cates W Jr., Cohen MS. Sexual transmission of HIV. *N Engl J Med* 1997;336:1072–1078.
34. Jacquez JA, Koopman JS, Simon CP, Longini IM Jr. Role of primary infection in epidemics of HIV infection in gay cohorts. *J Acquired Immune Defic Syndr* 1994; 7:1169–1184.
35. Hooper RR, Reynolds GH, Jones OG, Zaidi A, Wiesner PJ, Latimer KP, Lester A, Campbell AF, Harrison WO, Karney WW, Holmes KK. Cohort study of venereal disease I: The risk of gonorrhea transmission from infected women to men. *Am J Epidemiol* 1978; 108:136–144.
36. Weinstein MC, Graham JD, Siegel JE, Fineberg HV. Cost-effectiveness analysis of AIDS prevention programs: Concepts, complications, and illustrations. In Turner CF, Miller HG, Moses LE, eds. *AIDS: Sexual Behavior and Intravenous Drug Use*. Washington DC: National Academy Press; 1989.
37. Kaplan EH. Modeling HIV infectivity: Must sex acts be counted? *J Acquired Immune Defic Syndr* 1990; 3: 55–61.
38. Moses S, Plummer FA, Ngugi EN, Nagelkerke NJD, Anzala AO, Ndinya-Achola JO. Controlling HIV in Africa: Effectiveness and cost of an intervention in a high-frequency STD transmitter core group. *AIDS* 1991; 5:407–411.
39. Anderson RM, May RM. Epidemiological parameters of HIV transmission. *Nature* 1988; 333:514–519.
40. Holtgrave DR, Kelly JA. Preventing HIV/AIDS among high-risk urban women: The cost-effectiveness of a behavioral group intervention. *Am J Public Health* 1996; 86:1442–1445.
41. Holtgrave DR, Kelly JA. The cost-effectiveness of an HIV/AIDS prevention intervention for gay men. *AIDS and Behavior* 1997; 1:173–180.
42. Pinkerton SD, Holtgrave DR, Valdiserri RO. Cost-effectiveness of HIV prevention skills training for men who have sex with men. *AIDS* 1997; 11:347–357.
43. Holtgrave DR, Leviton LC, Wagstaff D, Pinkerton SD. The cumulative probability of HIV infection: A summary risk measure for HIV prevention intervention studies. *AIDS and Behavior* 1997; 1:169–172.
44. Pinkerton SD, Holtgrave DR, DiFranceisco WJ, Stevenson LY, Kelly JA. Cost-effectiveness of a community-level HIV risk reduction intervention. *Am J Public Health*, in press.
45. Pinkerton SD, Abramson PR. Not all behavior change is equivalent. *Am J Public Health* 1998; 88:864.
46. Holtgrave DR, Qualls NL. Threshold analysis and HIV prevention programs. *Medical Decision Making* 1995; 15:311–317.
47. Brandeau ML, Owens DK, Sox CH, Wachter RM. Screening women of childbearing age for human immunodeficiency virus: A model-based policy analysis. *Manage Sci* 1993; 39:72–92.
48. Kaplan EH. Economic analysis of needle exchange. *AIDS* 1995; 9:1113–1119.
49. Kaplan EH, Abramson PR. So what if the program ain't perfect? A mathematical model of AIDS education. *Evaluation Rev* 1989; 13:107–122.
50. Downs AM, de Vincenzi I. Probability of heterosexual transmission of HIV: Relationship to the number of unprotected sexual contacts. *J Acquired Immune Defic Syndr* 1996; 11:388–395.
51. Wiley JA, Herschkorn SJ, Padian NS. Heterogeneity in the probability of HIV transmission per sexual contact: The case of male-to-female transmission in penile-vaginal intercourse. *Stat Med* 1989; 8:93–102.
52. Jewell NP, Shiboski SC. Statistical analysis of HIV infectivity based on partner studies. *Biometrics* 1990; 46:1133–1150.
53. Pinkerton SD, Holtgrave DR. Combination antiretroviral therapies for HIV: Some economic considerations. In Ostrow DG, Kalichman SC, eds. *Psychosocial and Public Health Impacts of New HIV Therapies*. New York: Plenum Press, 1998.
54. Pinkerton SD, Abramson PR. HIV vaccines: A magic bullet in the fight against AIDS? *Evaluation Rev* 1993; 17:579–602.
55. Pinkerton SD, Abramson PR. A magic bullet against AIDS? *Science* 1993; 262:162–163.

Assessing the Cost-Effectiveness of HIV Prevention Interventions
A Primer

STEVEN D. PINKERTON and DAVID R. HOLTGRAVE

As demonstrated in a number of chapters in this book,[1] HIV prevention interventions can be highly cost-effective for society. In many instances, HIV prevention is actually cost-saving, meaning that the cost of the prevention intervention is more than offset by the savings in medical care costs. The *net cost*, therefore, is negative. (As discussed further later on, this is actually a very conservative interpretation of "cost saving" since it omits other important benefits of prevention, such as averting productivity losses.) Cost-saving programs represent unquestionably sound societal investments, because economic resources are conserved in the long run by implementing such programs. As a consequence, society should be willing to fund all cost-saving programs.

Two pieces of information are needed to determine the overall savings in averted future HIV/AIDS-associated medical care costs resulting from a prevention intervention: first, an estimate of the lifetime cost of medical care per case of HIV disease and AIDS, and second, an estimate of the total number of infections averted by the intervention. Then, the net intervention cost is obtained by subtracting the product of the number of infections averted (A) and the per-case cost of treatment (T), from gross program costs (C). In symbols, Net cost = $C - AT$. If the net cost is negative, then the intervention is cost-saving.

Of course, most health care procedures (e.g., open-heart surgery, antibiotic therapy for the common cold) have a net economic cost to society. Loosely, a health-related intervention, procedure, or program is considered "cost-effective" if it achieves an acceptable overall balance of costs to consequences (this vague definition reflects the vagaries and multidimensionality of human decision making, in which economic considerations may or may not be paramount). Competition for limited economic resources is implicit in the notion of cost-effectiveness, which thus involves a comparison between or among programs. Therefore cost-effectiveness is defined within the context of a particular resource allocation problem, from which it is inseparable. Nevertheless, it is convenient to speak of a program, procedure, or intervention as "cost-effective" in isolation, without explicit reference to competing uses for the same economic resources.

STEVEN D. PINKERTON and DAVID R. HOLTGRAVE • Department of Psychiatry and Behavioral Medicine, Center for AIDS Intervention Research (CAIR), Medical College of Wisconsin, Milwaukee, Wisconsin 53202.

Handbook of Economic Evaluation of HIV Prevention Programs, edited by Holtgrave. Plenum Press, New York, 1998.

For example, in cost-utility analysis (a special form of cost-effectiveness analysis in which health outcomes are measured in quality-adjusted life year [QALYs]—see the Phillips and Holtgrave chapter, this volume), a convention can be adopted based on Kaplan and Bush's observation that programs costing less than about $40,000 per QALY saved are generally considered "cost-effective by current standards," whereas the cost-effectiveness of a program with a cost-utility ratio in excess of $180,000/QALY is "questionable in comparison with other health care expenditures" (programs with intermediate cost-utility ratios are "possibly controversial, but justifiable by many current examples").[2,p.74] (The cost per QALY estimates provided here were updated from Kaplan and Bush's original ratios to 1996 dollars using the medical care component of the Consumer Price Index.[3])

Thus, to evaluate the cost-effectiveness of an HIV prevention intervention within a cost-utility framework requires, in addition to an indication of the net program cost, an estimate of the total number of QALYs saved by preventing cases of HIV infection. This estimate can be obtained by multiplying an estimate of the number of QALYs saved for each prevented HIV infection (Q) by the number of infections averted by the intervention (A, as before). Then the overall cost per QALY saved, or cost-utility ratio, can be expressed as

$$\text{Cost-utility ratio} = \frac{\text{Net cost}}{AQ} = \frac{C - AT}{AQ}$$

Although (as noted before) it is difficult to judge an intervention in isolation, on the basis of conventional standards, programs with cost-utility ratios less than about $110,000 per QALY saved (the midpoint of the $40,000 to $180,000 range) represent potentially cost-effective interventions (see also Paltiel and Stinnett, this volume).

To summarize, the main steps in conducting a cost-utility analysis of an HIV prevention intervention are (1) determining the overall cost of implementing the program; (2) estimating the number of infections averted by the intervention; (3) estimating the lifetime medical care cost of treating a case of HIV/AIDS; (4) calculating the number of QALYs saved when someone is prevented from becoming infected; (5) combining these components into a cost-utility ratio and conducting supplementary sensitivity analyses, in which key analytic parameters are varied over a range of plausible values, to assess how uncertainty in these parameters affects the results.[4–6] These steps are described further later on, followed by a brief discussion of how this methodology is extended to cost-benefit analysis.

ASSESSING THE COST OF THE INTERVENTION

The cost of the intervention can be determined either prospectively (while the intervention is ongoing) or retrospectively (after the intervention has concluded). In a retrospective analysis, information about intervention costs is obtained from available records and interviews with program administrators, key staff, and participants. Because pertinent records may have been lost or destroyed in the interim (assuming they existed in the first place) and because important details may be imperfectly recalled or overlooked completely, retrospective cost analyses can sometimes under- or overestimate true intervention costs. For this reason, uncertainty in intervention cost estimates should be acknowledged and appropriate sensitive analyses undertaken to ensure that any inaccuracies in the cost estimates do not lead to erroneous conclusions regarding the overall cost-effectiveness of the intervention.

Most of the HIV prevention economic analyses conducted to date have employed the retrospective strategy.

In a prospective cost analysis, relevant data are collected while the intervention is being conducted. This permits greater accuracy in assessing resource quantities consumed but increases the cost of performing the analysis. In a prospective analysis, personnel costs might be assessed, for example, by having intervention staff maintain time diaries or by observing staff and recording the amount of time they spend on the intervention. Although prospective data collection is potentially more accurate, sensitivity analyses are still necessary to assess the impact of possible measurement error in determining intervention costs.

When performing a cost analysis from the societal perspective (in which all costs are included, regardless of who pays or incurs the cost), costs borne by the intervention participants (e.g., transportation, day care, lost wages) and any additional costs associated with adverse or beneficial side effects of the intervention (e.g., syringe/needle disposal costs) must be included in addition to the direct cost of implementing the program (e.g., staff salary, materials, laboratory tests, etc.).[3] The main categories of intervention costs include, but are not limited to, staff compensation (salary or hourly rate, plus fringe benefits); facility-related costs (rent, utilities); materials (videos, syringe sterilization kits, condoms, printed matter, such as pamphlets); participant incentives (money, bus passes, etc.); and overhead (often assessed as a fixed percentage of overall operating expenses).[3] Standard techniques of cost analysis can be used to estimate these program costs.[7-9]

To reflect general societal preferences for receiving benefits in the present while deferring costs to the future, any program costs or benefits that arise beyond the first year of implementation should be discounted.[10] Although previous analyses have utilized various annual discount rates (usually not exceeding 5%), the Panel on Cost-Effectiveness recommends using a 3% discount rate in the "Reference Case" analysis and conducting sensitivity analyses at 0% and 5%.[4]

ESTIMATING THE NUMBER OF INFECTIONS AVERTED

One of the most important and perhaps the most difficult to obtain of the several parameters needed to perform a cost-utility analysis of an HIV prevention intervention is an estimate of the number of HIV infections actually prevented by the intervention. Obviously, the preferred method for determining the number of infections averted would be to compare the number of seroconversions among intervention participants with the number expected in the absence of the intervention. Unfortunately, in most instances this strategy is precluded by the small size and time frame of the intervention relative to the expected seroconversion rate.[11] Indeed, in many cases fewer than a single seroconversion could be expected during the intervention time frame even in the absence of the intervention program.

However, as described in the chapter by Pinkerton and Abramson,[12] mathematical modeling techniques can be used to translate behavioral risk reduction data (e.g., changes in condom use frequency or needle sharing behavior) into estimates of the number of infections averted by the intervention.[3,12-15] For example, suppose that P_B and P_F are the probabilities derived from an "average" intervention participant's self-reported behavior prior to and immediately following the intervention, respectively, and assume that there would have been no behavioral change in the absence of intervention. The difference, $P_B - P_F$, is a measure of intervention effectiveness that is easily converted to an estimate of the number of infections averted by the intervention.[15,16] In particular, the intervention reduces the expected number of seroconversions among N uninfected intervention participants from NP_B to NP_F, a reduction if $N(P_B - P_F)$ "primary" infections during the brief intervention period. Similarly, the number of "secondary" infections that would arise among the sexual or injection-equipment sharing partners of already infected intervention participants can be estimated. The total number of infections averted by the intervention is the sum of the primary infections prevented among intervention participants and the secondary infections prevented among their partners.[12] (Ideally, information about the behavior of intervention participants and a control group would be available for both baseline and follow-up assessments. In this case, P_B and P_F would be replaced by differences in the probabilities of infection arising from behaviors reported at the two behavioral assessment points.)

The probabilities themselves can be obtained from mathematical models of HIV transmission. For example, in one popular model, the probability of transmission in any one act of sexual intercourse (often denoted by the Greek letter α) is assumed constant, and the individual acts of intercourse are assumed probabilistically independent. The cumulative probability of transmission arising as a result of n unprotected and k protected acts of receptive anal intercourse (for example) with each of m partners can be modeled via the equation,

$$P = 1 - [(1 - \pi) + \pi(1 - \alpha_n)^n(1 - \alpha_k)^k]^m,$$

where π is the probability that any one of the partners is infected and α_n and α_k denote the per-contact probability of transmission of unprotected and protected intercourse, respectively.[12,15,17–19] More and less complex models can also be constructed, of course, as can models of injection-associated HIV transmission risk.[20,21] Alternatively, HIV transmission risk can be estimated using a "per-partner" model, in which the probability of transmission is assessed on a per-partnership rather than per-act basis.[12,22,23]

HIV/AIDS-ASSOCIATED MEDICAL TREATMENT COSTS AND QALYs SAVED

The analytic parameters discussed previously (intervention cost and number of infections averted) clearly depend on the specifics of the intervention being evaluated. In contrast, the cost of treating HIV/AIDS and the number of QALYs saved when a case of HIV disease is prevented are essentially independent of the particular intervention.

The overall cost of treating a case of HIV disease and AIDS includes drug-related costs for antiretroviral therapy (e.g., reverse transcriptase and protease inhibitors) and opportunistic infection prophylaxis and treatment (e.g., pentamidine, ganciclovir); regular viral load and CD4 cell count monitoring; hospital and/or hospice charges; and general medical care charges for office visits, nursing assistance, and so on. The overall impact of protease inhibitor combination therapies on the lifetime cost of treating HIV disease is not yet known. Such therapies are relatively expensive (around $10,000 per year in drug costs alone), but may decrease in-patient hospital utilization over the long term. Unfortunately (from an analytic standpoint only), continuing advances in the medical management of

HIV disease make estimating the lifetime cost of treating HIV a difficult task, akin to hitting a moving target.

A similar difficulty arises when attempting to determine the number of QALYs saved by HIV prevention (or equivalently, the number lost when a person becomes infected). HIV reduces the number of QALYs remaining in an infected person's life both by foreshortening life expectancy and by decreasing the quality of life during years spent living with HIV (in the QALY framework each year of life is associated with a utility weight that represents the quality of life during that period, where 1.0 denotes perfect health and 0.0 represents death). Therefore the number of QALYs lost to HIV depends on the age of the person at the time of infection.[3]

To increase comparability across economic evaluation studies of HIV prevention interventions, standardized values of the treatment cost and QALY parameters should be used whenever possible.[24] Moreover, because different medical care regimens are associated with different costs and also with different health and quality of life outcomes, it is important that analysts consider ⟨treatment cost, QALY⟩ *pairs*, rather than separately incorporating treatment cost and QALY considerations into their analyses.

Recently, Holtgrave and Pinkerton conducted a thorough review of the available literature on HIV/AIDS treatment costs and the impact of medical care on AIDS-related mortality and quality of life.[24] This analysis produced three different <treatment cost, QALY> pairs corresponding to different medical care regimens, as shown in Table 1 for a patient who was infected at 26 years of age (the corresponding QALY values for other ages are presented elsewhere[3]). In the low cost, poor access to care scenario, they assumed that the infected individual is unaware of the infection for the first six years, at which time zidovudine monotherapy is initiated (this scenario was included for compatibility with previous analyses;[25] it no longer represents an acceptable level of care in the United States). The intermediate level of care scenario was based on the 1996 guidelines of the International AIDS Society—USA Panel on antiretroviral therapy,[26] which, for many patients, recommended the initiation of combination therapy with a pair of nucleoside analog reverse transcriptase inhibitors, as soon as infection is detected, and the addition of a protease inhibitor when the patient's CD4 count falls below 500/mm³. In the high level of care scenario, triple-drug combination therapy with two reverse transcriptase inhibitors and a protease inhibitor is initiated just after seroconversion. In addition, both the intermediate and high level of care scenarios assume that viral load is monitored every six months following detection of infection.

Table 1. HIV/AIDS-Related Medical Care Costs and QALYs Saved[a]

Level of Care Scenario	Medical Care Costs (QALYs Saved)[b]		
	0% Discount Rate	3% Discount Rate	5% Discount Rate
Low	$118,892 (26.85)	$87,045 (13.18)	$71,143 (8.57)
Intermediate	$274,766 (23.87)	$195,188 (11.23)[c]	$157,348 (7.10)
High	$424,763 (20.37)	$296,844 (9.34)	$239,945 (5.87)

[a]From Holtgrave and Pinkerton (1997).[24]
[b]1996 dollars; number of QALYs saved for individual infected at 26 years of age.
[c]Recommended base-case values.

Holtgrave and Pinkerton recommend that the intermediate scenario ⟨$195,188, 11.23 QALYs saved⟩ be used in all base-case analyses.[24] However, recent treatment guidelines developed by the IAS Panel suggest that many patients (especially those with viral load levels in excess of 5,000 to 10,000 copies/mL) would benefit from initiating triple combination therapy as soon as infection is detected.[27] Therefore it is important to conduct sensitivity analyses that incorporate all three level of care scenarios.

COMBINING PARAMETERS AND PERFORMING SENSITIVITY ANALYSES

Once the cost of the intervention (C) has been assessed, the number of infections averted (A) has been estimated, and the number of QALYs (Q) saved and medical care costs averted (T) per prevented case of HIV infection have been determined, this information can be combined to form a single measure of economic efficiency, the *cost-utility ratio*:

$$\text{Cost-utility ratio} = \frac{C - AT}{AQ} = \frac{C/A - T}{Q}$$

As discussed previously, three rather ill-defined regions of "intervention space" can be discerned. According to Kaplan and Bush, interventions with cost-utility ratios less than about $40,000/QALY saved are probably cost-effective by current standards, those with cost-utility ratios between $40,000/QALY and $180,000/QALY are possibly cost-effective, and those with ratios in excess of about $180,000/QALY are probably not cost-effective in comparison with other health care expenditures.[2]

Sensitivity analyses should be performed around all key parameters (C, A, T, Q, and their constituents) to determine the impact of uncertainty in the exact values of these parameters and to increase the generalizability of the results to similar interventions or to other populations (which might differ in HIV prevalence, for example, and therefore in the expected number of infections averted by the intervention). Holtgrave and Pinkerton provide three distinct scenarios for T and Q (see Table 1) that can be used in sensitivity analyses.[24] The range of plausible values for C and A that should be included in sensitivity analyses depends on the particular intervention being evaluated and the data collection and estimation procedures used.

In addition to performing sensitivity analyses in which the values of key parameters are varied over a range of plausible values, it is also helpful to conduct *threshold analyses* to determine critical parametric values at which the intervention switches, for example, from cost-saving to not cost-saving or from being cost-effective to not cost-effective. For instance, from the previous equation it is clear that the intervention is cost-saving if and only if $C/A < T$. This inequality provides threshold conditions on C, A, and T that can be evaluated by fixing any two of the three parameters and solving for the third.

AN EXTENSION TO COST-BENEFIT ANALYSIS

In cost-benefit analysis the common metric of dollars is used to value both the cost and consequences of an intervention. Although the outcome of a cost-benefit analysis can be expressed as a ratio of intervention costs to monetized benefits (cost-benefit ratio), it is not always clear whether a particular economic component (e.g., averted medical care costs) should be counted as a benefit or as a negative cost. Differential placement of components in the numerator or the denominator can critically affect the value of the resulting ratio.[4,28,29] To avoid the possibility of ambiguity, many analysts prefer the net present value approach in which monetary benefits are subtracted from program costs:

$$\text{Net present value} = C - AS,$$

where S denotes society's willingness to pay to avert an HIV infection. A negative net present value indicates that the intervention is cost-saving to society.

Willingness to pay is a comprehensive measure of the perceived benefits of preventing illness that represents the amount of money that society, as a whole, would be willing to pay (or forgo) to eliminate a single case of HIV disease and AIDS. Ideally, S should reflect society's recognition of and desire to avoid the myriad deleterious consequences of HIV infection, including substantial medical care costs, lost productivity, decreased longevity, diminished quality of life, increased disability, and pain and suffering. Notice in particular that net present value subsumes the elements appearing in the numerator of the cost-utility ratio (program costs and averted medical care costs) and incorporates additional important benefits of preventing HIV infection. An intervention that is cost-saving in the cost-utility sense (i.e., that has a negative cost-utility ratio) therefore is also cost-saving in the net present value sense, but not conversely.

The two primary techniques for determining willingness to pay are inference and direct measurement. In the second (usually favored) technique, a samples of individuals—possibly patients, doctors, or informed members of the public—are asked how much money they would be willing to pay or forgo to decrease their risk of incurring a particular adverse health condition. Then an estimate of society's overall willingness to pay can be inferred from these individual responses.

Unfortunately, no direct survey data exist at present regarding people's willingness to pay to avoid HIV infection. However, inferential evidence of society's willingness to pay to save a QALY is available and can be used to estimate overall willingness to pay to prevent HIV. As discussed before, society appears generally willing to support health-related programs that cost less than \$40,000 per QALY saved and unwilling to finance those that cost more than \$180,000 per QALY.[2,3] These approximate threshold values can be combined with the estimated number of QALYs saved by preventing HIV infection (see Table 1) to derive willingness-to-pay estimates for HIV prevention.[30,31] The results of this exercise for an individual infected at age 26 and receiving an intermediate level of care are displayed in Table 2. Thus, for example, if society is willing to spend \$110,000 (the mean of \$40,000 and \$180,000) to save a single QALY, then it should also be willing to spend \$1,235,300 (discounted at 3%) to prevent a 26-year-old from becoming infected with HIV. Both smaller and larger willingness-to-pay estimates have appeared in the literature,[32] and, as is evident from Table 2, a substantial range of values could plausibly be justified. Therefore cost-benefit analyses employing this approach should include sensitivity analyses in which willingness to pay is varied over a wide range of values.

SUMMARY

A methodology for conducting cost-utility and cost-benefit analyses of HIV prevention interventions is outlined (a thorough description has appeared elsewhere[3]). This methodology has previously been used to assess the cost-effectiveness of small group and community-level sexual risk reduction interventions for gay men,[33–35] and multisession

Table 2. Inferred Willingness to Pay to Prevent HIV Infection

Value of QALY	Low Level of Care			Intermediate Level of Care			High Level of Care		
	0%[a]	3%	5%	0%	3%	5%	0%	3%	5%
$40,000	$1,074,000	$527,200	$342,800	$954,800	$499,200	$284,000	$814,800	$373,600	$234,800
$110,000	$2,953,500	$1,449,800	$942,700	$2,625,700	$1,235,300	$781,000	$2,240,700	$1,027,400	$645,700
$180,000	$4,833,000	$2,372,400	$1,542,600	$4,296,600	$2,021,400	$1,278,000	$3,666,600	$1,681,200	$1,056,600
QALYs Lost[b]	26.85	13.18	8.57	23.87	11.23	7.10	20.37	9.34	5.87

[a]Discount rate.
[b]Age at infection = 26 years.

cognitive-behavioral HIV risk reduction interventions for at-risk, inner-city women[36] (see also the Holtgrave and Pinkerton chapter, this volume). A variant of this methodology has also been used to evaluate the economic efficiency of postexposure prophylaxis following either occupational or sexual exposure to HIV.[37–39]

To apply this methodology requires four items of information: the cost of, and number of infections averted by, the intervention; the number of QALYs saved each time an infection is prevented; and an estimate of the lifetime medical care costs associated with HIV disease and AIDS. The first two of these parameters are intervention-specific, whereas the latter two are independent of the particular intervention (provided that the average age of intervention participants is known). The existence of standardized values of HIV and AIDS-related medical care costs and QALYs saved[24] increases comparability across economic evaluation studies and reduces data requirements for performing such studies.

As the cost and effectiveness of HIV/AIDS treatments change, so too does the cost-effectiveness of prevention interventions, in accordance with the relationship expressed in the equation for the cost-utility ratio. Future developments in the medical management of HIV disease might cause prevention interventions to appear either more or less cost-effective. Thus, the cost-effectiveness of a particular intervention is not static but changes with advances in HIV therapeutics. This suggests that it might be desirable to update previously completed economic analyses to reflect current treatment options and their impact on the longevity and quality of life of persons with HIV. To facilitate such a program requires only that analysts report separately the overall intervention costs and numbers of infections averted and that the standardized values of HIV-related medical care costs and QALYs saved be updated as necessary.

Furthermore, it is easily shown that the cost-utility ratio of Intervention #1 exceeds that of Intervention #2 if and only if the *gross* cost per infection averted (*C/A*) of Intervention #1 also exceeds that of Intervention #2.[3] Thus, it is only necessary to consider this simpler ratio when comparing the relative cost-effectiveness of different HIV prevention interventions for the same population. This observation provides the basis for an obvious extension of the methodology to the conduct of cost-effectiveness analyses.

As argued throughout the present volume, subjecting HIV prevention interventions to rigorous economic evaluation is critical to ensure appropriate targeting of limited HIV prevention resources (and health-related resources more generally). The methodology reviewed herein provides one means for assembling the data needed by HIV prevention decision makers. By facilitating appropriate resource allocation decisions, hence maximizing the impact of spending on HIV prevention, it is hoped that this methodology helps, however indirectly, to inhibit the further spread of HIV.

ACKNOWLEDGMENTS. Preparation of this chapter was supported by grants U62/CCU513481-01 from the Centers for Disese Control and Prevention; grants R01-MH55440 and R01-MH42908 from the National Institute of Mental Health (NIMH); and by NIMH Center grant P30-MH52776.

REFERENCES

1. Holtgrave DR, ed. *Handbook of Economic Evaluation of HIV Prevention Programs*. New York: Plenum Press; 1998.

2. Kaplan RM, Bush JW. Health-related quality of life measurement for evaluation research and policy analysis. *Health Psychol* 1982; 1:61–80.

3. Pinkerton SD, Holtgrave DR. A method for evaluating the economic efficiency of HIV behavioral risk reduction interventions. *AIDS and Behavior*, in press.

4. Gold MR, Siegel JE, Russell LB, Weinstein MC, eds. *Cost-effectiveness in Health and Medicine*. New York: Oxford University Press; 1996.

5. Haddix AC, Teutsch SM, Shaffer PA, Duñet DO, eds. *Prevention Effectiveness: A Guide to Decision Analysis and Economic Evaluation*. New York: Oxford University Press; 1996.

6. Weinstein MC, Stason WB. Foundations of cost-effectiveness analysis for health and medical practices. *N Engl J Med* 1977; 296:716–721.

7. Gorsky RD, Haddix AC, Shaffer PA. Cost of an intervention. In Haddix AC, Teutsch SM, Shaffer PA, Duñet DO, eds. *Prevention Effectiveness: A Guide to Decision Analysis and Economic Evaluation*. New York: Oxford University Press; 1996.

8. Moreau W, Hager CJ. Determining the Unit Cost of Services: A Guide for Estimating the Cost of Services Funded by the Ryan White Care Act of 1990. Washington, DC: U.S. Department of Health and Human Services; 1993.

9. Schmid GP. Understanding the essentials of economic evaluation. *J Acquired Immune Defic Syndr Hum Retrovirol* 1995; 10(Suppl. 4):S6–S13.

10. Shaffer PA, Haddix AC. Time preference. In Haddix AC, Teutsch SM, Shaffer PA, Duñet DO, eds. *Prevention Effectiveness: A Guide to Decision Analysis and Economic Evaluation*. New York: Oxford University Press; 1996.

11. Pinkerton SD, Holtgrave DR, Leviton LC, Wagstaff DA, Cecil H, Abramson PR. Toward a standard sexual behavior data set for HIV prevention evaluation. *Am J Health Behavior*, in press.

12. Pinkerton SD, Abramson PR. The Bernoulli-process model of HIV transmission: Applications and implications. In Holtgrave DR, ed. *Handbook of Economic Evaluation of HIV Prevention Programs*. New York: Plenum Press; 1998.

13. Kahn JG, Washington AE, Showstack JA, Berlin M, Phillips K. *Updated Estimates of the Impact and Cost of HIV Prevention in Injection Drug Users*. Final report prepared for the Centers for Disease Control and Prevention. San Francisco: Institute for Health Policy Studies, University of California at San Francisco; 1992.

14. Weinstein MC, Graham JD, Siegel JE, Fineberg HV. Cost-effectiveness analysis of AIDS prevention programs: Concepts, complications, and illustrations. In Turner CF, Miller HG, Moses LE, eds. *AIDS: Sexual Behavior and Intravenous Drug Use*. Washington DC: National Academy Press; 1989.

15. Pinkerton SD, Holtgrave DR, Leviton L, Wagstaff D, Abramson PR. Model-based evaluation of HIV prevention interventions. *Evaluation Rev* 1998; 22:155–174.

16. Holtgrave DR, Leviton LC, Wagstaff D, Pinkerton SD. The cumulative probability of HIV infection: A summary risk measure for HIV prevention intervention studies. *AIDS and Behavior* 1997; 1:169–172.

17. Hearst N, Hulley SB. Preventing the heterosexual spread of AIDS. *JAMA* 1988; 259:2428–2432.

18. Pinkerton SD, Abramson PR. Evaluating the risks: A Bernoulli process model of HIV infection and risk reduction. *Evaluation Rev* 1993; 17:504–528.

19. Reiss IL, Leik RK. Evaluating strategies to avoid AIDS: Number of partners vs. use of condoms. *J Sex Res* 1989; 26:411–433.

20. Kahn JG. Are NEPs cost-effective in preventing HIV infection? In Lurie P, Reingold AL, eds. *Public Health Impact of Needle Exchange Programs in the United States and Abroad*. Berkeley: School of Public Health, University of California, 1993.

21. Holtgrave DR, Pinkerton SD, Jones TS, Lurie P, Vlahov D. Cost and cost-effectiveness of increasing access to sterile syringes and needles as an HIV prevention intervention in the United States. *J Acquired Immune Defic Synd Hum Retrovirol* 1998; 18(Suppl. 1):S133–S138.

22. Holtgrave DR, Kelly JA. Preventing HIV/AIDS among high-risk urban women: The cost-effectiveness of a behavioral group intervention. *Am J Public Health* 1996; 86:1442–1445.

23. Kaplan EH. Modeling HIV infectivity: Must sex acts be counted? *J Acquired Immune Defic Syndr* 1990; 3: 55–61.

24. Holtgrave DR, Pinkerton SD. Updates of cost of illness and quality of life estimates for use in economic evaluations of HIV prevention programs. *J Acquired Immune Defic Syndr Hum Retrovirol* 1997; 16:54–62.

25. Guinan ME, Farnham PG, Holtgrave DR. Estimating the value of preventing a human immunodeficiency virus infection. *Am J Preventive Med* 1994; 10:1–4.

26. Carpenter CCJ, Fischl MA, Hammer SM, Hirsch MS, Jacobsen DM, Katzenstein DA, Montaner JSG,

Richman DD, Saag MS, Schooley RT, Thompson MA, Vella S, Yeni PG, Volberding PA. Antiretroviral therapy for HIV infection in 1996: Recommendations of an international panel. *JAMA* 1996; 276:146–154.

27. Carpenter CCJ, Fischl MA, Hammer SM, Hirsch MS, Jacobsen DM, Katzenstein DA, Montaner JSG, Richman DD, Saag MS, Schooley RT, Thompson MA, Vella S, Yeni PG, Volberding PA. Antiretroviral therapy for HIV infection in 1996: Updated recommendations of the International AIDS Society—USA Panel. *JAMA* 1997; 277:1962–1969.

28. Drummond MF, Stoddart GL, Torrance GW. *Methods for the Economic Evaluation of Health Care Programmes*. New York: Oxford University Press; 1987.

29. Clemmer B, Haddix AC. Cost-benefit analysis. In Haddix AC, Teutsch SM, Shaffer PA, Duñet DO, eds. *Prevention Effectiveness: A Guide to Decision Analysis and Economic Evaluation*. New York: Oxford University Press; 1996.

30. French MT, Mauskopf JA, Teague JL, Roland EJ. Estimating the dollar value of health outcomes from drug-abuse interventions. *Medical Care* 1996; 9:890–910.

31. Holtgrave DR, Qualls NL. Threshold analysis and HIV prevention programs. *Medical Decision Making* 1995; 15:311–317.

32. McKay NL, Phillips KM. An economic evaluation of mandatory premarital testing for HIV. *Inquiry* 1991; 28:236–248.

33. Holtgrave DR, Kelly JA. Preventing HIV/AIDS among high-risk urban women: The cost-effectiveness of a behavioral group intervention. *Am J Public Health* 1996; 86:1442–1445.

34. Pinkerton SD, Holtgrave DR, DiFranceisco WJ, Stevenson LY, Kelly JA. Cost-effectiveness of a community-level HIV risk reduction intervention. *Am J Public Health*, in press.

35. Pinkerton SD, Holtgrave DR, Valdiserri RO. Cost-effectiveness of HIV prevention skills training for men who have sex with men. *AIDS* 1997; 11:347–357.

36. Holtgrave DR, Kelly JA. The cost-effectiveness of an HIV/AIDS prevention intervention for gay men. *AIDS and Behavior* 1997; 1:173–180.

37. Pinkerton SD, Holtgrave DR, Pinkerton HJ. Cost-effectiveness of chemoprophylaxis after occupational exposure to HIV. *Arch Intern Med* 1997; 157:1972–1980.

38. Pinkerton SD, Holtgrave DR, Bloom FR. Cost-effectiveness of post-exposure prophylaxis following sexual exposure to HIV. *AIDS* 1998; 12:1067–1078.

39. Pinkerton SD, Holtgrave DR, Bloom FR. Is postexposure prophylaxis for sexual or injection-associated exposure to HIV cost-effective? *N Engl J Med* 1997; 337:500–501.

Economic Evaluation of Primary HIV Prevention in Injection Drug Users

JAMES G. KAHN

INTRODUCTION

IDUs and the AIDS Epidemic

In 1998, injecting drug users are the most important risk group in the AIDS epidemic. Injecting drug users (IDUs) themselves account for 26% of all newly reported AIDS cases[1] and are estimated to represent 50% of new HIV infections.[2] In addition, HIV infections in IDUs spread in quantitatively important ways to other population groups. For example, women whose risk factor is being the sex partner of IDUs constitute 4% of all new AIDS cases.[1] These women may in turn transmit the virus to other sex partners and to their off-spring.

A varied mix of HIV prevention strategies has been implemented in IDUs. Some strategies are similar to those applied in other population groups because they are designed to identify and reduce HIV risk of any type. These include HIV counseling and testing, extended counseling (e.g., detailed risk assessment and skills building), peer education, outreach, and partner notification.[3–5] Some HIV prevention strategies specific to IDUs focus on drug use or the mechanics of injecting.[6] These are drug treatment, bleach distribution, and needle exchange. HIV prevention in IDUs has succeeded in large measure, decreasing the prevalence of risk behavior (e.g., needle sharing) and thereby reducing annual HIV incidence from rates as high as 15–20% in the early 1980s to 7% or less in the 1990s.[7,8] Nonetheless, substantial risk remains, and there is little understanding of how to select among prevention strategies.

Feasibility of Economic Evaluation in IDUs

Economic evaluation of HIV prevention in IDUs is an area replete with opportunity but also poses substantial technical challenges. The opportunity derives from the broad range of prevention strategies used in IDUs and the relatively extensive behavioral evaluation literature. The large number of behavioral evaluations reflects the fact that illicit drug use was considered a problem warranting intervention long before the arrival of HIV, so that

JAMES G. KAHN • Center for AIDS Prevention Studies, Institute for Health Policy Studies, and Department of Epidemiology and Biostatistics, School of Medicine, University of California, San Francisco, San Francisco, California 94109.

Handbook of Economic Evaluation of HIV Prevention Programs, edited by Holtgrave. Plenum Press, New York, 1998.

there was an established drug research community and even some studies conducted before HIV that remain relevant today. In addition, more so than for other groups, some interventions for IDUs (e.g., needle exchange) are suitable for economic evaluation on the basis of process measures (e.g., numbers of needles exchanged) rather than behavioral outcome studies.

The technical issues are both epidemiological and economic. The epidemiology of HIV is always difficult to model and is critically important to the accuracy of economic evaluation. In IDUs the epidemiology of HIV is particularly challenging for two reasons. First, IDUs transmit HIV both sexually and via needle sharing. In the early part of the epidemic, needle sharing risk probably predominated. More recently, however, with decreases in needle sharing, sex may account for a third or more of HIV transmission among IDUs.[9] Secondly, IDUs are responsible for the spread of HIV to other populations, in particular, sex partners and offspring. Thus, each infection in an IDU may lead to one or more infections in others. The economic challenges are also twofold. First, the economic role of IDUs in society is more mixed than that of other groups. Although many IDUs work, a significant proportion rely on illegal income. Thus, preventing an HIV infection may actually increase the economic burden to society (unless the technique is to end the use of illegal drugs). This negative effect of prevention raises ethical issues regarding the prevailing criterion for prevention: minimizing disease burden vs. maximizing economic well-being. Secondly, for interventions that do lead to cessation of drug use, there is a joint product problem: costs must be apportioned to the benefits of reduced HIV infection and reduced drug use.

Preview of Chapter

The remainder of this chapter is primarily a structured review of the existing literature on the economic evaluation of HIV prevention in IDUs, first a description of the pattern of findings and then a summary of each analysis. Ongoing research is briefly described. The chapter ends with a discussion of future research directions.

RESEARCH TO DATE

Overview

There have been twenty-one economic analyses of HIV prevention in IDUs, considering each unique combination of prevention strategy, geographic location, and modeling technique as a separate analysis. Six different prevention strategies have been examined. One, needle exchange, has been considered in depth. Analyses have been done for East Coast cities and San Francisco, for several hypothetical cities, and the US as a whole. Epidemic modeling techniques have varied from static one-year depictions of intervention recipients to dynamic five-year models portraying HIV spread in all IDUs and their partners. The following discussion provides structured summaries of the analyses.

Detailed Review of Economic Analyses

All identified economic analyses of HIV prevention in IDUs are summarized in Table 1. Each row represents a separate strategy and analytic technique. The first column specifies prevention strategy. The second indicates geographic location and also HIV incidence in IDUs because incidence is the best measure of local HIV risk. The next three columns cover program cost, epidemic modeling approach, and the reduction in HIV risk behavior or risk. Then two columns present the key findings.

Whenever possible, findings were translated into HIV infections averted per one million dollars of prevention spending. This common metric facilitates comparison among HIV prevention strategies in IDUs and in other populations. The focus on resource allocation—health benefit for a fixed amount of money—parallels a current policy debate. For comparisons with non-HIV related interventions, metrics, such as cost per quality-adjusted, life-year (QALY) and net cost would be most useful. Although only best estimates are reported, most studies included sensitivity analyses. The second findings column presents additional results or the primary results when they could not be translated into HIV infections averted per million dollars.

Pattern of Findings

Despite wide variation in quantitative findings as described later, the public health conclusion is clear. Most HIV prevention in IDUs is economically advantageous to society, often extremely so. The cost of HIV prevention is less than the cost of HIV medical care when 18 or more infections are averted per million dollars of prevention, based on the discounted lifetime cost of care calculated in the early 1990s.[10] With the recent advent of therapies that are more expensive per year and more effective in prolonging life, the break-even value for infections averted will almost certainly drop substantially.

The studies reviewed use largely comparable economic methods. For example, discounting is identical. No study discounts HIV infections averted, and financial discount rates do not affect the standardized outcome measure (HIV infections averted per $1 million) because prevention spending is assessed only for the first year of each analysis (with the exception of Kahn[11]). Prevention costing methods appear similar, relying on empirical program cost data. The year for which program cost is assessed varies little from about 1990 to 1995. As noted later on, variations in epidemic modeling methods substantially affect results.

Many factors determine cost-effectiveness. Following are some of the key factors:

Prevention strategy: The structure and effectiveness of a prevention intervention can, of course, drive cost-effectiveness. For example, extended counseling, relatively inexpensive and effective, averts an estimated 250–286 infections in two East Coast cities, whereas partner notification, costly due to the complexity of tracking partners and having limited known benefits, averts just 15–31 infections.

Program efficiency: Two needle exchange programs in similar cities, assessed using the same simplified circulation model and costing methods, avert infections in inverse relationship to the annual cost per client: 83 per million dollars when the cost is $40 per client-year and 10 when the cost is $833 per client-year. However, different costing methods can create the impression of different efficiency, so transparency and comparability are important.

Epidemic modeling technique: For the same East Coast needle exchange program, a one-year model focusing on clients estimates 83 HIV infections averted per million dollars, but a five-year model including all IDUs and their partners estimates 250 infections averted per million dollars.

Table 1. Economic Analyses of HIV Prevention in Injection Drug Users[a]

Intervention	Location (HIV Incidence)	Key Inputs and Methods			Key Findings		
		Cost	Modeling of HIV Infections Averted	Reduction in Risk Behavior (or Risk)	HIV Infections Averted per $1 Million in Prevention	Other	Ref.
HIV counseling and testing	Baltimore, Northeast city (4%, 9%)	$38–59 HIV(−); 125–160 HIV(+)	5-year epidemic evolution within group and to partners	<10% drug, < 10% sex[b] (4%)	125,77		9
Extended Counseling	Baltimore, Northeast city (4%, 9%)	79–95/multisession program	5-year epidemic evolution within group and to partners	<15% drug, <25% sex (9%)	286,250		9
Partner notification	Baltimore, Northeast city (4%, 9%)	150–180/partner identified, plus cost of HIV C&T	5-year epidemic evolution within group and to partners	<2.5% drug and sex	31,15		9
Bleach distribution	Baltimore, Northeast city (4%, 9%)	53–63/contact	5-year epidemic evolution within group and to partners	< 25% drug-bleaching rate only (1.5%)	65,34	Very sensitive to now uncertain efficacy of bleaching	9
Drug treatment	Baltimore, Northeast city (4%, 9%)	Methadone maintenance 3,000/treatment slot/year	5-year epidemic evolution within group and to partners	<80% drug (21%)	25,19	Also decreases crime and unemployment	9
Needle exchange	Northeast city (6.5%)	40/client/year	5-year epidemic evolution within group and to partners	<20% drug, <5% sex (10%)	250		20

Program	Location	Cost	Model	Behavioral risk reduction[b]	Ref.	Comments	Ref.
Needle exchange	New Haven, CT (~6%)	750/client/year in base case	Needle circulation model; clients only	Not specified (33% drug)	11	Optimal program parameters would improve cost effectiveness	21
Needle exchange	Four hypothetical US cities (1.5–6%)	40–833/client/year	Simplified needle circulation model; clients only	Not specified (17–70% drug)	10,22,74,83	Variation due to differences in incidence, cost, risk reduction	20
Needle exchange	NYC (6%)	40/client/year	1-year static; within group (five step simplified)	50% drug (50%)	333		23
Needle exchange	US (not specified)	Not specified	Percent reduction in HIV infections in IDUs, 1987–1995, based on Australian experience with needle exchange	15–33% drug	Not assessed	4,394–9,666 HIV infections averted with national NE program; medical care savings of $244–538 million	24
Programs for sterile syringe access	US (thresholds calculated)	0.15–0.97/syringe distributed	1-year static; only clients who can be provided sterile syringe for each injection	(100% drug)	Not assessed	Injection-related HIV incidence for cost neutrality = 0.3% to 1.8% for different programs	25
Unspecified-risk group targeting analysis	Northeast and San Francisco (8%, 2%)	200/person/year	Within-group 5- and 20-year epidemic evolution	10% (10%)	22–27, 12–17	Compared with < 1 in low risk populations	11

[a]The analyses listed are discussed and compared in the text.

[b]For behavioral risk reduction, use of the less than sign (<10%) means that the analysis assumes *incomplete* behavioral change in this percent of the population (e.g., of the 10% one-quarter stop sharing needles, and the remainder decrease sharing frequency. The resulting risk reduction is indicated in parentheses when appropriate.

Level of risk reduction: For needle exchange in New York City, the 50% decrease in risk behavior found in one behavioral evaluation leads to the highest estimate of infections averted (333). Smaller decreases observed in other evaluations would lead to proportionally smaller numbers of infections averted.

Variation in cost-effectiveness between cities for the same prevention strategy assessed with the same model has several causes.

HIV incidence: Higher incidence tends to yield superior cost-effectiveness because there is more risk to reduce. This is seen most clearly in a targeting model where incidence of 8% in IDUs in New York City is associated with 22–27 infections averted and incidence of 2% in IDUs in San Francisco with 12–17 infections averted. However, several phenomena blunt or reverse the advantage conferred by higher incidence, especially if the inequality in incidence is less pronounced (e.g., in the HIV Intervention Prevention Modeling Project [HIP-MP] analyses comparing Baltimore [4% incidence] with a Northeast city [9%]).

Diffusion of behavioral effects: Some models, such as HIP-MP, assume that behavioral change occurs only in HIV(−) prevention program clients. These models omit potential real-world behavioral change in HIV(+) individuals and thus do not count potential infections averted in their HIV(−) partners. In a community with high HIV incidence, HIV prevalence also will be high, so a high proportion of prevention program clients will be HIV(+), and the model will portray more prevention effort as "wasted" than in a lower incidence community.

Routes of HIV spread: Differential contributions of injection and sex-related HIV transmission can affect geographic comparisons. In Baltimore a greater proportion of the HIV infections is spread via sharing than in the Northeast city. Therefore, interventions focused on decreasing sharing have a proportionally larger benefit in Baltimore.

Primary and casual partners: Distribution of risk between partner types differs between cities, so that if intervention effectiveness varies by type of partner, one city will benefit more than the other.

Wages and prices: Variation in costs influences cost-effectiveness. The Northeast city is more expensive than Baltimore.

Nonneedle Exchange Analyses

The five nonneedle exchange prevention strategies that have undergone economic evaluation—HIV counseling and testing, extended counseling, partner notification, bleach distribution, and drug treatment—were all assessed as part of the HIV Intervention Prevention Modeling Project (HIP-MP).[9] HIP-MP focused on two East Coast cities, one in the mid-Atlantic (Baltimore; 15,000 IDUs; HIV incidence in IDUs 4%) and one in the Northeast (not identified at the request of city officials; 150,000 IDUs; HIV incidence in IDUs 9%). Since these analyses were completed, epidemic conditions have evolved and have been further studied (e.g., HIV incidence in the Northeast city is probably about 6% now), so projecting to current conditions should be done advisedly.

Prevention costs were estimated using program accounting records or resource-based costing methods. When cost data were available only for other locations, projections to the cities were done using geographic cost-of-living and wage rate indices. Modeling of HIV infections was based on a five-year dynamic model, estimating the concurrent and near future effects of a single year of prevention. HIV infections were estimated for IDU recipients of the intervention, their IDU sharing and sex partners, non-IDU sex partners, and offspring. Inputs for the model included empirical estimates of risk behavior and the risk of HIV infection per exposure. Reduction in risk behavior, including return to baseline behavior over time, was estimated from a review of the behavioral evaluation literature. Reduction in risk (i.e., decrease in incidence) was calculated from the model by entering the behavioral risk reductions. Twenty percent of IDUs in each community were assumed to receive the intervention. Outcomes were expressed as cost per HIV infection averted, which is easily translated into infections averted per million dollars of prevention spending.

HIV Counseling and Testing. HIV C&T is a relatively low-cost intervention which induces limited behavioral change. The strategy is sometimes dismissed as ineffective in IDUs.[3] However, this conclusion derives at least in part from the small sample sizes used in behavioral evaluation studies, which limit statistical power to detect small benefits. HIP-MP identified twelve behavioral evaluations, of which ten found reduction in drug risk behavior associated with HIV C&T. Similarly, five of seven found benefit for sex risk behavior. The analysis used conservative estimates of risk reduction: 90% of recipients make no change and 10% reduce but do not eliminate risky behavior. Risk reductions are maintained for a median of one year. Based on these modest changes, the best estimate of infections averted was 23 over five years in Baltimore, including 11 fewer from sharing among IDUs, 4 fewer from sex among IDUs, and 8 fewer from sex with non-IDUs. In the Northeast city, an estimated total of 247 was averted, in similar proportions. The cost-effectiveness was estimated to be better in Baltimore (125 infections averted per million dollars) than in the Northeast city (77), despite lower incidence. This occurred for the reasons described in the section Pattern of Findings, and a greater proportion of the less resource-intensive HIV($-$) C&T protocols in Baltimore, with its lower HIV prevalence.

Extended Counseling. Extended counseling is defined as education and/or support/counseling lasting 2–6 sessions, typically following after HIV counseling and testing. This intervention is also relatively low cost, if done in groups, and results in greater behavioral change than HIV C&T. HIP-MP determined that three of six studies found reduction in drug risk behavior and four of six found reduction in sex risk behavior. The analyses' estimates of risk reduction were as follows: 15% reduce (but do not eliminate) drug risk behavior, and 25% reduce sex risk behavior. Reductions are maintained for a median of two years. The best estimate of infections averted was 68 over five years in Baltimore and 698 in the Northeast city. HIV infections averted per million dollars were slightly higher in Baltimore (286) than in the Northeast city (250), for the reasons described in Pattern of Findings.

Partner Notification. Partner notification in IDUs can be very expensive as a strategy to identify at-risk individuals because of the difficulty of identifying and finding partners of infected individuals and recruiting them for HIV counseling and testing. The HIP-MP analysis assumed that all benefit derives from HIV C&T. Although it is possible that risk reduction results simply from being informed that a drug or sex partner is HIV-infected, no data exist confirming the presence or magnitude of such a benefit. HIP-MP estimated, based on published literature and data sets from the two study cities, that each IDU has 3–4 IDU partners and 1.8–2.1 non-IDU sex partners; one-third of actual partners are identified; half of identified partners are located; and half of located partners receive HIV C&T, with the same behavioral change as discussed previously. The best estimate of infections averted over five years was five in Baltimore and 29 in the Northeast city. HIV infections averted per million dollars were higher in Baltimore (31) than in the Northeast city (15), again for the reasons discussed in Pattern of Findings.

Bleach Distribution.   The analysis summarized here, like bleach distribution itself, is based on the premise that bleaching of injection equipment by IDUs reduces or eliminates HIV transmission. This premise has been called into question by epidemiological, observational, and laboratory data.[12-16] Thus, the cost-effectiveness analysis must be interpreted in the context of uncertainty about the effectiveness of bleaching. Put differently, efficacious bleaching techniques must be identified and then properly implemented by IDUs to warrant application of the following analysis. On the other hand, the HIP-MP analysis assumed no benefit from an outreach program to reach IDUs and give them bleach aside from increased bleaching, despite evidence that this outreach also led to decreased sharing.[17]

Evidence in San Francisco suggests that after wide awareness of bleach as a safety measure, active distribution and education about bleaching still resulted in doubling of bleach use from 30 to 63% (a reduction of nearly half in unbleached injections). The actual reduction is likely to vary according to preexisting practices. The HIP-MP analysis' estimates of risk reduction were conservative: 25% of bleach distribution recipients reduce risk behavior, including 25% fewer episodes without bleaching and 25% fewer episodes of bleaching done ineffectively. The reductions are maintained for a median of one year. The best estimate of infections averted over five years was 10 to Baltimore and 64 in the Northeast city. HIV infections averted per million dollars were higher in Baltimore (65) than in the Northeast city (34), for reasons reviewed in Pattern of Findings.

Drug Treatment.   Treatment of drug dependency is very effective for drug risk behavior, much more so than other interventions.[9,18,19] However, it is also much more expensive. To further complicate the assessment of its value to society via HIV prevention, drug treatment is economically justified by its salutary effects on employment and crime. The multiple benefits conferred by drug treatment create the common joint products problem. At least three approaches to this problem may be justifiable: allocate costs to each benefit by some rule; assign all costs to the employment and crime benefits (because such benefits are more socially valued) and treat HIV prevention as an added perk; and assign all costs to HIV prevention because this analysis is about HIV prevention. The strict last approach was used.

HIP-MP focused on methadone maintenance. Multiple national and local studies all found reduction in drug risk behavior, with no consistent evidence for reductions in sex risk behavior. The analysis' estimates of risk reduction were as follows: 20% of recipients make no change in risky behavior and 80% reduce the behavior. Reductions are maintained for a median of one year. The best estimate of infections averted over five years was 162 in Baltimore and 1,243 in the Northeast city. HIV infections averted per million dollars were slightly higher in Baltimore (25) than in the Northeast city (19), for the reasons described in Pattern of Findings except price, which was assumed equal for drug treatment in the two cities.

Needle Exchange Analyses

Needle exchange programs exchange used and potentially HIV-contaminated hypodermic needles/syringes for new sterile replacements, at no cost to the client. They are typically based in HIV prevention storefronts, mobile vans, or pharmacies. Most programs operate on a 1:1 exchange basis, sometimes with a limit on the number of needles one client can exchange per visit. Needle exchange programs often provide other services, such as bleach, condoms, counseling, and referral to drug treatment.

The six evaluations of needle exchange discussed following demonstrate several phenomena. First, needle exchange cost-effectiveness, which can be superior to the HIV prevention strategies discussed before, depends primarily on epidemic conditions and program design. Secondly—less importantly from a public health perspective but reassuringly for modelers—various modeling techniques yield similar results, and differences reflect explicit modeling choices (e.g., whether to count delayed effects or infections spread from IDUs to other populations).

Northeast City, Using HIP-MP Model.   The first needle exchange cost-effectiveness analysis to be discussed used a modified version of HIP-MP modeling.[20] The key change was a lowering of HIV incidence from 9% to 6.5%, to comport with newly available seroincidence data. Several aspects of the HIP-MP approach contrast with other needle exchange analyses: HIV infections were modeled over five years to portray the delayed effects of the one year of program operation; HIV infections were estimated for IDU recipients of the needle exchange and their IDU sharing and sex partners, non-IDU sex partners, and offspring; and behavioral change estimates derived from a synthesis of needle exchange evaluations.

Thirteen methodologically acceptable studies of behavioral change associated with needle exchange programs were identified. Of 12 studies examining sharing, eight found reduced sharing prevalence or frequency associated with needle exchange use and four found inconsistent or no benefit. Three of the four studies examining bleaching found a benefit. Effects on sex risk, examined in four studies, were less pronounced: two studies found reductions in the number of partners whereas one found an increase; condom use increased in one study, decreased in one, and did not change in a third. The model used intentionally low estimates of behavioral change. First, a conservative midpoint of the magnitude of change was identified from the behavioral literature. Second, this value was decreased by 50% to counteract potential overstating of needle exchange effect through oversampling of frequent attenders. Finally, as with other HIP-MP modeling, risk reductions were assumed to be concentrated in less than 20% of program clients. The most common risk reductions were cessation of sharing (62% of the 20% whose behavior changes) and decreased frequency of sharing (50% reduction among the 38% who continue to share). The changes are assumed to continue for one year after leaving needle exchange but only at 25% of original levels.

Behavioral change associated with needle exchange leads to a 15% decrease in drug-related HIV risk in clients during exchange participation and a 10% decrease in total risk. Over five years, the model estimates a total of 148 infections averted in exchange clients and their drug and sex partners in this Northeast city. There are 250 infections averted per million dollars of prevention spending, comparable to extended counseling.

New Haven, Using the Needle Circulation Model.   The needle circulation model developed by Edward Kaplan for the New Haven needle exchange is perhaps the best known mathematical model of HIV prevention effectiveness in the United States. This model estimated a 33% decrease in HIV infections in exchange clients resulting from reduced needle circulation time and thus lower HIV prevalence in needles. More recently,

Kaplan extended his analysis to incorporate economic considerations.[21] Although HIV incidence is high in New Haven IDUs (about 6%), the program is very expensive ($750 per client per year). The number of infections averted per million dollars is eleven. It is likely that substantial resources are spent on prevention services other than exchanging, such as outreach and counseling. Thus, the circulation model is conservative. It capures the benefits of needle exchange but not the benefits of these ancillary services. It is also conservative in not portraying infections averted in later years or in drug and sex partners who are not exchange clients.

The economic analysis quantifies important parameters for the New Haven exchange. The optimum annual needle exchange rate per IDU, based on maximizing net benefits, is 1,109. This yields net benefits of $750 per year per IDU, compared with $429 per year per IDU at the actual exchange rate of 168. Assuming that the marginal cost of attracting another client is proportional to the number of clients, the optimal program size is 350 clients, versus 200 in reality. The minimum HIV risk to establish a needle exchange is calculated to be 1.8 infections per 100 IDUs per year (HIV incidence = 0.05 at 64% HIV prevalence), when both fixed and marginal costs are considered. Optimal program sizes and needle exchange rates are calculated across a range of program budgets. The analysis determines the minimum budget required for the exchange to yield a net financial benefit ($164,882) and the budget where benefits are maximized ($291,664). Finally, the analysis indicates that the cost per HIV infection averted stabilizes at between $50,000 and $60,000 once the budget reaches $150,000.

Four Hypothetical Cities, Using Simplified Circulation Model. In the interest of applying the circulation model to needle exchange programs outside of New Haven, Kaplan formally derived a simplified version of the circulation model equations which was then applied by Kahn.[20,22] The simplified formula gives a minimum estimate of the proportionate decrease in HIV incidence using just two parameters: $E/(E + s)$, where E = mean number of needles exchanged per NEP client per year and s = shared injections per IDU per year. In effect, this formula reflects the probability that an exchange supplants a sharing episode or, alternatively, the probability that a used needle will be exchanged before being used again. This formula yields the same estimate of 33% reduction in HIV incidence for New Haven as does the full circulation model, given the same program inputs. The absolute number of HIV infections averted can be calculated with the percent reduction in HIV incidence, baseline sharing-related HIV incidence, and the number of HIV-negative clients. Cost-effectiveness requires, in addition, program cost.

Four hypothetical needle exchanges were modeled: an expensive (per needle) government program in the urban Northeast (HIV prevalence = 50%, incidence = 6%); a moderately costly agency-run program also in the urban Northeast; a moderately costly agency-run program in the Pacific Northwest (prevalence = 3%, incidence = 1.5%); and a low-cost activist-run program on the Pacific Coast (prevalence = 12%, incidence = 3%). The reduction in HIV incidence varied from 17 to 70%. The higher reduction was associated with more needles per client-year. The cost per HIV infection averted ranged from $12,000 in the moderate cost Northeast program (the HIP-MP Northeast city) to $98,000 in the high-cost Northeast program (New Haven). Greater efficiency was associated with low cost per needle exchanged. The analysis also suggested that for a fixed number of needles, the absolute impact is higher when the needles are spread out among a greater number of clients. This is true because the first few needles each client receives in a year are expected to have a proportionally larger impact on sharing than the last few needles. Thus, it may be more cost-effective to reach as many clients as possible rather than to provide more needles to fewer clients.

New York City, Using Simplified Behavioral Change Model.   Kahn and Sanstad proposed recently that simplified cost-effectiveness techniques can sometimes yield useful information for prevention policy.[23] They developed a method for one-year static cost-effectiveness analyses for prevention program clients, requiring four inputs: cost per HIV infection averted = program cost / [number of HIV(−) clients × HIV incidence × effectiveness]. Effectiveness is operationally defined as the percent reduction in the frequency of risk behavior (e.g., needle sharing, unprotected sex) due to an intervention. This simplified formula assumes that each risk episode confers a small and equal probability of acquiring HIV, which approximates the behavior of a binomial function in low-risk situations. The formula also assumes that adopting safer behavior (e.g., using a condom) is 100% effective. Both assumptions are often used in more complex models. However, the single-year static structure underestimates risk when HIV prevalence is rapidly rising, such as when risk behaviors are extremely frequent but HIV prevalence is still low, e.g., 1–3%.

This model found that for New York City, based on a behavioral study showing 50% reduction in sharing associated with exchange use, the cost per HIV infection averted is $2,700. Sensitivity analyses suggest that the program remains cost-effective for a range of inputs. For example, at a more conservative 30% effectiveness, as reported in other studies, the cost per HIV infection averted increases to $4,400. If the program is less efficient ($80 instead of $40 per client-year), the cost per infection averted doubles to $5,400. Finally, if drug-related incidence is assumed to be just 4% (the other 2% being sex-related), the cost per HIV infection averted is $4,000. The same modeling technique yielded estimated costs per infection averted of $12,000 for training of gay community leaders in Biloxi, MS and $195,000 for HIV testing of surgeons.

United States Needle Exchange Program 1987–1995.   Lurie and Drucker estimated the number of HIV infections in IDUs that could have been averted if the U.S. needle exchange effort had paralleled that of Australia.[24] Their analysis is conservative because it assumes relatively modest risk reductions associated with needle exchange (15–33%) and uses a low estimate of the proportion of IDU HIV infections spread from each infected IDU to sex and drug partners (0.13). Nonetheless, it found that 4,400 to 9,700 HIV infections could have been averted had U.S. needle exchange programs reached the same proportion of IDUs each year as the programs in Australia. The medical care costs associated with the preventable cases are estimated at $244 million to $538 million. The analysis concluded that if U.S. government opposition to needle exchange were dropped and the programs rapidly expanded, a similar number of HIV infections could be prevented by the year 2000.

United States Sterile Needle Access.   Lurie et al. calculated the HIV incidence required for sterile needle programs to achieve cost neutrality.[25] This analysis conservatively portrays the extreme situation that a new syringe is provided for each injection. A program that supplies a fraction of needed syringes but to a larger number of IDUs might be more efficient, as discussed in the section on four hypothetical cities. Also, infections spread to sex partners and offspring are not considered. The analysis found that the societal cost per syringe distributed is highest for needle exchange ($0.97) and lowest for syringe sale

($0.15), with intermediate values for injection kit distribution ($0.64), kit sale ($0.43), and pharmacy-based exchanging ($0.37). Program costs for kit and syringe sales are zero because the IDU pays the true resource costs. The analysis found that the injection-related annual HIV incidence needed for medical savings to equal societal resources ranged from 0.3% (for syringe sale) to 2.1% (for needle exchange). By comparison, HIV incidence in IDUs is about 2–3% in San Francisco and 6% in New York, mostly injection-related.

Targeting Analysis

This analysis compared the number of HIV infections averted by a generic prevention strategy applied in populations at different levels of HIV risk, including IDUs in two cities.[11] The analysis is built around an epidemic model that portrays new HIV infections within risk groups for five or 20 years. This model is based on simple rules about epidemic dynamics: HIV incidence at steady state is a function of HIV prevalence and exit rates; HIV incidence is proportional to the frequency of risk behaviors; and HIV prevalence changes when there are unequal numbers of exiting HIV-positives and new HIV infections. Nine target population scenarios are considered, including two that represent IDUs: "post-steady-state high risk" with HIV prevalence of 50% and incidence of 8% (similar to Northeast U.S. IDUs) and "steady-state medium risk" with HIV prevalence of 15% and incidence of 2% (similar to San Francisco IDUs). The analysis assumes that $1 million is available annually for HIV prevention at an annual cost per person of $200, a midpoint for an existing prevention program. Finally, based on reviews of prevention evaluations suggesting that most interventions reduce the frequency of risk behavior by 10–50%, the analysis conservatively assumes that prevention reduces HIV incidence by 10%.

The analysis found that in the high risk target group similar to Northeast IDUs, prevention averts 22 infections per million dollars over five years and 27 per million dollars over 20 years. In the medium-risk target group similar to San Francisco IDUs, the corresponding number of HIV infections averted is about 40% lower: 12 over five years and 22 over 20 years.

ONGOING RESEARCH

There are at least five economic evaluations of HIV prevention in IDUs currently underway. They are in various stages of development, and publications are forthcoming. Of course, there may be additional evaluations because the search for current projects was informal.

The largest project and the one with the broadest goals is a five-year HIV prevention modeling project funded by the National Institute on Drug Abuse through the Societal Institute for Mathematical Sciences. This project is multisite (Yale, Stanford, and UCSF) and has the overall goal of assessing the cost-effectiveness of HIV prevention strategies, especially in IDUs. Specific aims include improving methods to translate behavioral outcomes into epidemic outcomes, portraying production functions for changes in risky behavior, developing common measures of AIDS intervention outcomes and their value, assessing the impact and cost-effectiveness of individual prevention strategies and of groups of interventions (resource allocation), and developing approaches to better incorporate models into the policy process. The specific interventions and groups of interventions have not been selected. The analysis by Brandeau and colleagues described later is funded through this grant.

Two evaluations are furthering the assessment of needle exchange and sterile syringe availability. The author of this chapter is conducting an evaluation of the expansion of needle exchange in San Jose, California. This analysis differs from previous needle exchange cost-effectiveness analyses by being tightly integrated with a behavioral and program evaluation. For example, questions useful for modeling are added to the questionnaire administered to the study cohort, and data from needle exchange logs are used to validate IDU responses about sources of needles. Also, San Jose has very low HIV prevalence in IDUs (1–2%), so the issue of needle exchange efficiency in a low-impact area will be assessed. David Holtgrave and colleagues are currently estimating cost and infections averted for a national sterile needle campaign, including metropolitan-area specific estimates. This analysis will help inform policy debates on implementing needle exchange more widely.

One analysis (by this author) will consider a multicomponent intervention in IDUs. This "community mobilization" intervention is being designed and evaluated by Ross Gibson of the Center for AIDS Prevention Studies at UCSF and colleagues. The test community is Sacramento, and the control community is San Diego. The specific components of the intervention, still under development, may include needle exchange, street outreach, small media publicity (e.g., flyers), peer groups, brief counseling, and referral for drug treatment. The behavioral evaluation design probably has sufficient power to generate separate effectiveness (and cost-effectiveness) estimates for each intervention component. Concurrent implementation of all intervention components, however, may mean that the evaluation will estimate average effectiveness, precluding calculation of marginal cost-effectiveness ratios or individual production functions.

Margaret Brandeau and colleagues at Stanford University have developed a model of resource allocation for epidemic control of a situation faced at the Veteran's Administration Hospital in Menlo Park/Palo Alto, California.[26] This model considers the allocation of a fixed HIV prevention budget between IDU and non-IDU VA patients. The goal is to minimize the total number of new cases of HIV in the population over a specified time horizon. The analysis shows that the optimal decision for this VA population is to allocate all HIV prevention resources to IDUs. Extensive sensitivity analyses suggest that the finding is robust. The model can be applied to other populations and prevention programs.

FUTURE DIRECTIONS

Themes

Economic evaluation of HIV prevention in IDUs in the coming years will pursue three interrelated themes, modeling sophistication, program operation, and policy relevance. For some analyses these themes will intersect naturally and reinforce one another. In other instances they will conflict in subtle or overt ways. Modeling sophistication encompasses developing methods to capture more epidemic detail (e.g., intergroup HIV transmission or rapid epidemic growth), to reflect temporal shifts in epidemic dynamics (e.g., sexual transmission and evolving risk factors), or to portray complex but real-life prevention scenarios (e.g., intervention portfolios). Modeling sophistication can also mean developing and justifying simple models that include only a few key factors that drive results. A focus on program operation is the use of models to assess program mix and functioning, such as the optimal size and outreach strategy for a needle exchange program. Attention to operational issues could make HIV prevention modeling more accessible to and useful for program managers. Finally, policy relevance is developing modeling exercises to address policy decisions explicitly. Although many models have focused on policy, several factors may heighten the utility of the policy perspective: an increasing ability of models to convincingly portray epidemic trends, ongoing debate on resource allocation in HIV, and the rapidly evolving technology of HIV prevention and care.

This section is organized into discussion of selected methodological and substantive issues. It is hoped that reader will reflect on how the themes identified previously permeate the specific issues described following.

Methodological Issues

Comparability of Analyses

As HIV prevention cost-effectiveness models proliferate, it is important that methods be as comparable as possible. Such consistency will facilitate integration of results for multiple interventions and populations. Examples of methods that should be possible to standardize are intervention costing techniques, the costs of HIV care, discount rates, quality of life measures, and transmission risk for each kind of HIV exposure. Methods that may be hard to standardize but for which sensitivity analyses could be conducted to facilitate comparison with other analyses are timeframe, choice of outcome measures, proportion of risk due to sex, and inclusion in the model of HIV transmission to nonintervention clients and to other population groups.

Complexity vs. Simplicity

The most sophisticated and comprehensive models are often those that result from extended research and model design. However, complexity can make a model harder to track or may obscure the central importance of one or two factors that drive the analysis, such as change in needle sharing rates. The effort required to achieve this complexity may also delay the availability of analyses for policy decisions. An alternative is to use back-of-the-envelope simple models to provide approximate answers efficiently and quickly.[23,27] The advantages and disadvantages of complexity and simplicity must be considered and discussed for each policy problem. Systematic consideration of factors that might invalidate a simple model (e.g., extremely high HIV incidence) is critically important and can provide reassurance that the model adequately represents reality.

Intergroup HIV Transmission

HIV transmission from IDUs to other population groups, such as the non-IDU female sex partners of male IDUs, is an important aspect of epidemic spread that can quantitatively and qualitatively affect the benefits of intervening with IDUs. For example, one analysis of needle exchange found that over five years each 100 HIV infections prevented in IDUs resulted in 49 prevented in non-IDU sex partners and 12 in offspring.[20] This ratio will change according to local HIV prevalence patterns and risk behavior.

Evolving Risk Factors

The determinants of HIV risk in IDUs are complex. Risk factors for HIV infection (prevalence or incidence) have always differed somewhat by study. Some common risk factors have been needle sharing, number of sharing partners and frequency, shooting gallery use, cocaine injection, and race. Furthermore, as the epidemic evolves there has probably been an evolution in risk factor, such as an increasing importance for sex risks (e.g., number of partners and condom use) due to the decrease in needle sharing. Careful review of the most recent epidemiological studies for the relevant population is advisable.

Program Operation

Only one cost-effectiveness analysis of HIV prevention in IDUs has focused explicitly on issues of program operation, such as program start-up costs and economies or diseconomies of scale.[21] Another analysis described alternative approaches for delivering services but made no explicit link to cost-effectiveness outcomes.[28] Because more prevention programs are accepted now as effective and are being implemented in new locations, there is increasing interest in how analysis of operational efficiency can inform decisions about which program designs to fund and at what levels. A key tool for such analyses is production functions that relate program inputs to behavioral change. HIV prevention programs, however, are often difficult to portray with production functions mainly because HIV prevention outcome evaluations focus on documenting overall behavioral change, rarely considering dose-response relationships, marginal cost or benefit functions, or even costs. The challenge for modelers is to develop theoretically sound and practicable methods to document production functions in HIV prevention. Specific situations that might be addressed by such methods include relating program scale to program effectiveness (e.g., client base and behavioral change as a function of program budget); comparisons of the organizational structure of programs (e.g., adding prevention to an existing health program versus establishing a new agency); and the impact of program characteristics (e.g., fixed vs mobile needle exchange, or risk reduction counseling group size and frequency) on program effectiveness.

Substantive Issues

Protease Inhibitors

Protease inhibitors, administered in concert with nucleoside analogues like zidovudine and 3-TC, greatly depress viral burden and can yield startling reversals of clinical decline.[29] These therapies are likely to lengthen the life of HIV—infected individuals, improve health, and also sharply increase medical costs. Because of their great potential and cost, there is intensive national, state, and local discussion on how to improve access to these drugs. Protease inhibitors may also reduce the spread of HIV because they decrease viral loads by two or more orders of magnitude, often to undetectable levels. Such a benefit would add to the impetus to fund protease inhibitors. However, the relationship between viral load and ineffectivity is poorly understood. Therefore, there is a need to build models to consider a range of possible relationships between viral load and transmissibility. As empirical data become available, these models can add to their empirical base.

Budget Shifting

Few HIV prevention models have examined how prevention programs are financed or which funders accrue savings due to HIV disease averted. This makes the "costs averted" argument for HIV prevention too abstract to be compelling. Two kinds of budget shifts regularly occur. The first is organizational: investments in prevention made by one agency (e.g., the department of public health) yield financial benefits in another (e.g., Medicaid or the criminal justice system). The second is temporal: dollars spent on prevention today yield most savings at least four years in the future. Analyses of specific budget shifts can increase prevention funding by convincingly describing the location and timing of anticipated savings to individuals responsible for overall budgets (e.g., legislators).

Effects of Social Policy

Governmental social policies and programs can affect the HIV epidemic in IDUs. For example, as of January 1, 1997 the federal Supplemental Security Income program ended benefits for individuals whose drug or alcohol addiction was considered necessary to the disability determination which qualified them for SSI. This disenrollment has the potential to disrupt the lives of IDUs, perhaps leading to increased substance use, injection, and HIV risk behavior. Other social policies that can affect IDUs' risk behavior include housing and criminal justice laws and practices.

Intervention Portfolios and Resource Allocation

Assessments of individual prevention interventions do not provide guidance on the optimal prevention program "portfolio" for a specific population. The contents of such a portfolio are determined by marginal cost-effectiveness functions and how different interventions interact. A few analyses have considered issues of allocating fixed amounts of HIV prevention funds[11,26,30] but as yet none have focused on the array of prevention strategies available for IDUs. HIV prevention planners are in fact regularly faced with the challenge of selecting a mix of prevention programs. Thus, it will be extremely valuable for models to estimate the cost-effectiveness of different combinations of prevention strategies in a variety of IDU populations. Demonstrating links between optimal program mix and HIV risk characteristics (e.g., proportion of HIV transmitted via sex or risk heterogeneity) would make the results more generalizable and valuable.

Epidemics Averted

The importance of HIV prevention activities, such as needle exchange, in avoiding significant AIDS epidemics in IDUs in certain cities has been demonstrated.[31] This prevention success is thought to reflect the suppression of risky behaviors below a critical threshold. However, the precise nature of the threshold—which behaviors are critical and how much of them can be tolerated before the epidemic takes off—is not well understood nor are the costs of suppressing the risky behavior. A cost-effectiveness analysis of epidemics averted would add useful confirmation and clarification to the epidemiological associations already reported.

ACKNOWLEDGMENTS. This research was supported by the Societal Institute for the Mathematical Sciences through grant DA 09531 from the National Institute on Drug Abuse and by the Center for AIDS Prevention Studies through grant number P50 MH42459 from the National Institute of Mental Health.

REFERENCES

1. Centers for Disease Control and Prevention. *HIV/AIDS Surveillance Report* 1996; 9(no. 1): Table 3.
2. Holmberg SD. The estimated prevalence and incidence of HIV in 96 large US metropolitan areas. *Am J Public Health* 1996; 86:642–654.
3. Higgins DL, Galavotti C, O'Reilly KR, et al. Evidence for the effects of HIV antibody counseling and testing on risk behaviors. *JAMA* 1991; 266:2419–2429.
4. Auerbach JD, Wypijewska C, Brodie HKH, eds. *AIDS and Behavior: An Integrated Approach*. Institute of Medicine. Washington, DC: National Academy Press, 1994, pp. 100–109.
5. Choi KH, Coates TJ. Editorial review: Prevention of HIV infection. *AIDS* 1994; 8:1371–1389.
6. Booth RE, Watters JK. Editorial review: How effective are risk reduction interventions targeting injecting drug users? *AIDS* 1994; 8:1515–1524.
7. Des Jarlais DC, Padian N, Winkelstein W. Targeted versus generalized AIDS prevention programming in the United States (oral presentation). Presented at the *AAAS Meeting*; San Francisco, CA; February 1994.
8. Des Jarlais DC, Friedman SR, Sotheran JL, et al. Continuity and change within an HIV epidemic: Injecting drug users in New York City, 1984 through 1992. *JAMA* 1994; 271(2):121–127.
9. Kahn JG, Washington AE, Showstack JA, Berlin M, Phillips K. *Updated Estimates of the Impact and Cost of HIV Prevention in Injection Drug Users*. Report prepared for the Centers for Disease Control and Prevention. San Francisco: Institute for Health Policy Studies, University of California at San Francisco, 1992.
10. Guinan ME, Franham PG, Holtgrave DR. Estimating the value of preventing a human immunodeficiency virus infection. *Am J Preventive Med* 1993; 10:1–4.
11. Kahn JG. The cost-effectiveness of HIV prevention targeting: How much more bang for the buck? *Am J Public Health* 1996; 86:1709–1712.
12. Gleghorn AA, Doherty MC, Vlahov D, et al. Inadequate bleach contact times during syringe cleaning among injection drug users. *J Acquired Immune Defic Syndr* 1994; 7:767–772.
13. Titus S, Marmor M, Des Jarlais D, et al. Bleach use and HIV seroconversion among New York City injection drug users. *J Acquired Immune Defic Syndr* 1994; 7:700–704.
14. Vlahov D, Muñoz A, Celentano DD, et al. HIV seroconversion and disinfection of injection equipment among intravenous drug users, Baltimore, Maryland. *Epidemiology* 1991; 2:444–446.
15. Shapshak P, McCoy CB, Shah SM, et al. Preliminary laboratory studies of inactivation of HIV-1 in needles and syringes containing infected blood using undiluted household bleach. *J Acquired Immune Defic Syndr* 1994; 7:754–759.
16. Contoreggi C, Jones SW, Simpson PM, et al. A model of syringe disinfection as measured by polymerase chain reaction for human leukocyte antigen and HIV genome. *Eighth International Conference on AIDS*, Amsterdam, 1992, Abstract P.C. 4280; 2:C291.
17. Watters JK, Cheng Y-T, Segal M, et al. Epidemiology and prevention of HIV in heterosexual IV drug users in San Francisco, 1986–1989. (Oral Presentation). *Sixth International Conference on AIDS*. San Francisco, 1990. Abstract F.C. 106.
18. Office of Technology Assessment. AIDS-related Issues. The effectiveness of drug abuse treatment: Implications for controlling AIDS/HIV infection. Washington, DC: U.S. Government, 1990:1–114.
19. Hubbard RL, Marsden ME, Rachal JV, et al. *Drug Abuse Treatment: A National Study of Effectiveness*. Chapel Hill, NC: University of North Carolina Press; 1989.
20. Kahn JG. "Chapter 18: Are NEPs cost-effective in preventing HIV infection?" In Lurie P, Reingold AL, eds. *The public health impact of needle exchange programs in the United States and abroad*. Report prepared for the Centers for Disease Control and Prevention, School of Public Health, University of California, Berkeley and Institute for Health Policy Studies, University of California, San Francisco, 1993.
21. Kaplan EH. Economic analysis of needle exchange. *AIDS* 1995; 9:1113–1119.

22. Kaplan EH. Back-of-the-envelope estimates of needle exchange effectiveness (working paper), 1993.
23. Kahn JG, Haynes-Sanstad K. Meaningful standards: Making good decisions about HIV prevention. *AIDS Public Policy J* 1997; 12:21–30.
24. Lurie P, Drucker E. An opportunity lost: HIV infections associated with the lack of a national needle-exchange programme in the USA. *Lancet* 1997; 349:604–608.
25. Lurie P, Gorsky RD, Jones TS, et al. Assessing the cost-effectiveness of needle exchange and pharmacy-based programs to increase sterile syringe availability for injection drug users (IDUs). Presented at *Workshop on Sterile Needles and Syringes for Drug Users who Continue Injecting*, Baltimore, MD, February 16, 1995.
26. Richter A, Brandeau ML, Owens DK. Optimal resource allocation for HIV prevention: An application to the Menlo Park/Palo Alto VA Hospital (working paper).
27. Kaplan EH, Brandeau ML. AIDS policy modeling by example. *AIDS* 1994; 8(Suppl. 1):S333–S340.
28. Kahn JG. "Chapter 8: What do NEPs cost?". In Lurie P, Reingold AL, eds. *The public health impact of needle exchange programs in the United States and abroad*. Report prepared for the Centers for Disease Control and Prevention, School of Public Health, University of California, Berkeley and Institute for Health Policy Studies, University of California, San Francisco, 1993.
29. Deeks SG, Smith M, Holodniy M, et al. HIV-1 protease inhibitors. A review for clinicians. *JAMA* 1997; 277(2):145–153.
30. Kaplan EH. Economic evaluation and HIV prevention community planning—a policy analyst's perspective. In Holtgrave D, ed. *Handbook of Economic Evaluation of HIV Prevention Programs*, New York: Plenum Press, 1998.
31. Des Jarlais DC, Hagan H, Friedman SR, et al. Maintaining low HIV seroprevalence in populations of injecting drug users. *JAMA* 1995; 274(15):1226–1231.

Economic Evaluation of HIV Counseling and Testing Programs

The Influence of Program Goals on Evaluation

PAUL G. FARNHAM

INTRODUCTION

Human immunodeficiency virus (HIV) counseling and testing (CT) has been a major component of the interventions used to prevent HIV infection in the US during the past ten years. According to data gathered from 65 states, cities, and territories fully or partially funded by HIV prevention cooperative agreements from the Centers for Disease Control and Prevention (CDC), the number of reported HIV tests increased from more than one million in 1989 to 2.7 million in 1992, with a slight decrease to 2.4 million in 1994.[1] In 1994, the largest proportion of these publicly funded tests were performed in HIV CT sites (30.8%) and sexually transmitted disease (STD) clinics (28.0%). Approximately 12% of the tests were performed in family planning clinics, 8.5% in health departments, 5.9% in prenatal/obstetric clinics, and 4.8% in drug treatment centers.

CDC has recommended that persons at high risk for HIV undergo counseling and testing.[2] Yet, several national surveys have estimated that the majority of those at greatest risk for HIV infection have not been tested for HIV antibody.[3,4] Phillips and Coates[5] report that approximately 40% of persons with risk factors for HIV have not been tested and that many persons have not been retested after engaging in risky sexual or injection practices. One study of persons diagnosed with AIDS during 1990–1992 found that many of these persons were not tested until they were admitted to an acute-care health facility for an HIV-related disease or other illness.[6] Persons in this study were unlikely to report that their first HIV test occurred at an STD clinic or drug treatment center even though they had visited these facilities. A substantial number of persons in this sample also reported obtaining tests late in the course of illness.

To address concerns regarding this reported lack of counseling and testing among persons with the greatest need, legislation has been proposed and/or implemented for counseling and testing in many settings and for different populations: acute care settings;[7] mandatory premarital testing;[8] mandatory or voluntary testing for physicians, surgeons,

PAUL G. FARNHAM • Department of Economics, Georgia State University, Atlanta, Georgia 30303; and Division of Prevention Research and Analytic Methods, Epidemiology Program Office, Centers for Disease Control and Prevention (CDC), Atlanta, Georgia 30333.

Handbook of Economic Evaluation of HIV Prevention Programs, edited by Holtgrave. Plenum Press, New York, 1998.

dentists, and other health-care workers;[9,10] mandatory and/or voluntary testing of pregnant women and/or newborns;[11,12] employee testing in the work place;[13] testing at drug treatment centers and through street outreach programs.[14] HIV testing also continues at blood donation centers.[15] Counseling and testing in these settings may have varying effects, costs, and ethical and legal implications.

The goals of HIV counseling and testing have also changed. When the enzyme-linked immunosorbent assay (ELISA) used to detect HIV antibodies was first licensed in 1985, its primary function was to screen the blood supply so that positive or reactive units of blood could be discarded or set aside for research.[16] Because the demand for testing was expected to overburden blood donation centers and to prevent persons practicing high-risk behavior from donating blood to find out their HIV antibody status, a nationwide Alternate Test Site (ATS) Program was begun by the states with CDC guidance and federal government support. An integral part of the ATS testing process was the counseling that occurred both before and after the test (pre- and posttest counseling). This emphasis on risk reduction counseling made the ATS program a key component of the national HIV prevention effort and resulted in renaming the intervention as HIV Counseling and Testing Sites (CTS). The objectives of the intervention were to help uninfected persons initiate and sustain behavioral change to prevent them from becoming infected and to assist infected persons from transmitting the infection to others.

By the end of 1989, a further shift in the goals of the HIV CT programs occurred with the introduction of drugs, such as zidovudine (ZDV). New emphasis was placed on the early detection of infected persons so that they could be referred for medical monitoring and intervention.[16] Since then, the goals of behavioral change and early detection have been intertwined at counseling and testing sites. Early detection has become even more important during 1996, considering the research findings on the reduction of viral load through combination antiretroviral therapy.[17] Consequently, concerns have been raised regarding how the counseling and testing process impacts the dual goals of risk reduction for all persons and encouraging health-care-seeking behavior among infected persons.[18]

HIV CT programs also have been subject to numerous evaluations and economic analyses. A survey of the early literature regarding the quantitative economic evaluation of HIV-related prevention and treatment services[19] documented that 38% of the 47 references surveyed focused on some type of HIV screening program, 34% on a clinical prevention or medical service, and 13% on partner notification programs. Studies included in this survey met four criteria: (1) the study is a published abstract, chapter, or article; (2) the study contains a description of an HIV or AIDS-related prevention or treatment service; (3) the study contains a quantitative description of the costs and consequences of the intervention; and (4) the study contains a direct quantitative comparison of these costs and consequences.

In an update of this survey two years later, Holtgrave et al.[20] determined that the number of citations meeting the inclusion criteria described increased from 47 to 93. Of the 78% of the studies focusing on domestic HIV/AIDS interventions, approximately an equal number focused on behavioral change interventions and on antibody screening/testing programs only. Among behavioral change interventions, counseling, testing, referral, and partner notification interventions received the most study.

This chapter presents an update of a subset of the literature surveyed in Holtgrave et al.[20] The focus is on published articles or book chapters that analyze HIV counseling and testing interventions in different settings or populations. All of the studies included meet the basic inclusion criteria of Holtgrave et al.[19,20] The analysis is limited to studies of domestic interventions. A total of 43 articles or chapters is surveyed.

This literature survey analyzes how differences in the goals and settings for HIV CT affect both the operation and the evaluation of the interventions. Arguments concerning the effects of program goals are developed first, followed by an analysis of how the 43 economic evaluation studies viewed differences in goals and outcomes. Finally, implications for future research and public policy questions are discussed.

THE GOALS OF HIV COUNSELING AND TESTING

The previous introduction outlines how the goals of the HIV counseling and testing process have changed and how they continue to evolve. When the ELISA antibody test was first introduced and today in blood donation centers, the emphasis was and is on detecting HIV-infected blood, so that it is excluded from the nation's blood supply. Risk identification and donor deferral strategies are also employed to reduce the number of "window period" (HIV-infected but antibody negative) units.[21] The standard practice at blood donation centers is to discard the donated blood if the ELISA antibody test is positive, but to notify donors of their serostatus only if the battery of ELISA tests and confirmatory Western blot tests are positive, confirming infection.[22] Thus, the major emphasis at blood donation centers is on detecting infected persons, not on providing risk reduction or prevention messages to all persons, infected or uninfected. Posttest counseling and referral information are provided only to those who test positive on the entire series of screening and confirmatory tests.

If the primary goal of counseling and testing pregnant women is to prevent transmission of HIV to their infants, the focus of this intervention is also detecting infected persons. This goal has become important given the results of AIDS Clinical Trial Group (ACTG) Protocol 076 in 1994 documenting that treating infected pregnant women and their infants with ZDV reduces the rate of perinatal HIV transmission from 25% to 8%.[23,24] A cost-effectiveness study conducted by Gorsky et al.[25] of the current CDC guidelines, recommending universal counseling and voluntary testing of pregnant women and ZDV treatment for infected women and their infants, indicated that the medical costs saved by this intervention exceed the cost of the intervention itself, resulting in overall cost-savings for society. Because of the low prevalence of HIV among pregnant women, the cost of the intervention is driven by the cost of counseling and testing women who turn out to be uninfected. Of the estimated $65.1 million expended for counseling and voluntary testing of all pregnant women in the United States, $64.5 million (99%) is directed to the counseling and testing of uninfected women.[25] The intervention might be more cost-effective if counseling and testing could be targeted to high-risk women who are more likely to be infected. However, Landesman et al.[26] and Krasinsky et al.[27] have described problems with identifying such women, and the costs of a more targeted approach have not been identified.

Cost-effectiveness analysis becomes more complicated, however, if the goal of counseling and testing pregnant women for HIV is to provide benefits to their infants by preventing infections and also to provide benefits to their sex and needle-sharing partners by providing information on the woman's serostatus and promoting behavioral change. By screening pregnant women, other adults have reaped benefits that, it has been estimated, exceed the benefits acquired by their infants.[28] However, providing benefits to either the infants or partners of infected women indicates that the intervention should concentrate on finding *infected* pregnant women to achieve the greatest cost-effectiveness.

Multiple goals for HIV counseling and testing exist in drug treatment centers. In addition to the prevention and medical benefits of counseling and testing, another program goal pertains to the effect HIV CT has on admission of injection drug users (IDUs) into treatment and on which category of persons is most likely to enter: those already infected, those at high risk for infection, or those at low risk or uninfected.[29] Concerns in this setting thus involve benefits to both the infected and the uninfected. Furthermore, not all persons entering these centers actually receive HIV counseling and testing, given bureaucratic factors (e.g., difficulties in scheduling sessions, counselor absences, and staff vacancies)[30] and factors influencing the acceptance of HIV testing in this setting.[14]

Farnham et al.[31] confronted the issue of HIV CT program goals in their economic analysis comparing the counseling and testing procedures used at publicly funded testing sites with the more rapid screening tests now available. These authors stressed that long-term behavioral effects of the two testing procedures are unlikely to differ, so that the relevant outcome measure is the provision of correct test information to persons undergoing testing. The processes differ because all persons are required to return to the testing site to obtain test results and counseling under current guidelines, whereas only persons whose test results are positive with rapid screening would be asked to return for results of a confirmatory Western blot test. In either case, however, policy makers and researchers must address the issue of whose test results are relevant—those only of infected persons or those of both the infected and the uninfected.

Farnham et al.[31] used each outcome measure in their study, which determined that the rapid screening test was generally more cost-effective regardless of outcome measure because many clients who are uninfected can receive test results and posttest counseling in one visit. However, if the goal of the HIV CT process is to focus *only* on infected persons, the rapid screening test is more cost-effective only if decision makers consider that information received from the rapid screening test alone is as valuable as that provided by the confirmatory Western blot test. If decision makers have concerns (e.g., the occurrence of false positives) about providing preliminary information to "likely infected" persons from the rapid screening test, there is no advantage from a cost-effectiveness perspective to using this test over the standard ELISA test used in the guidelines.

Differences in outcome measures were also substantial in the sensitivity analysis of this study.[31] If policy is to focus only on HIV-infected persons, *decreasing* the number of uninfected persons tested would have made the current HIV CT procedure more cost-effective, because fewer costs would be incurred for testing the uninfected. If the goal is to focus on both infected and uninfected persons, the return rate of uninfected individuals has a greater impact on the evaluation of the two procedures. An increase from 0.40 to 0.95 in the probability that an uninfected person returns for test results or a decrease from 1.00 to 0.34 in the likelihood that an uninfected person accepts the rapid CT procedure, with all other factors constant, would have made the cost-effectiveness ratios of the two procedures equal.[31] Thus, the goal of the counseling and testing process, whether its focus is only on infected persons or on both infected and uninfected persons, is critical to the economic evaluation of the use of the current or rapid screening test in publicly funded testing sites.

Because the goals of HIV counseling and testing are likely to be vague, undefined, or intertwined from a programmatic perspective, this lack of clarity can affect the evaluation of these interventions. Counseling and testing interventions that emphasize risk reduction and prevention target both infected and high-risk uninfected persons, whereas interventions emphasizing medical treatment and referral focus more on identifying infected persons. The mix of these two approaches may be a function of institutional setting and location.

The extent of the benefits of the HIV CT process and the associated costs are influenced by the case mix of the clients in the intervention and the setting for counseling and testing. Different counseling approaches are used for infected and uninfected persons,[18] and differential effects on behavioral change are likely to result from this process.[32,33] The extent of the benefit chain can also vary. Depending on the setting for HIV CT, benefits can accrue only to the person receiving services, or benefits can extend to other associated groups (e.g., the person's sex and needle-sharing partners, children, and health-care providers).

Different costs can also be associated with a mix of clients and the emphasis of the intervention, particularly when the counseling is combined with alternative batteries of screening and confirmatory tests. Farnham et al.[31] estimated that the total cost under the HIV CT procedure currently followed in publicly funded clinics is $103 for an infected person and $33 for an uninfected person, each of whom has been correctly informed of his/her serostatus and has received posttest counseling. Higher costs for an infected person accrue from administering a battery of three ELISA screening tests, a Western blot confirmatory test, and conducting longer counseling sessions. These differential costs may have an effect on the evaluation of HIV CT in alternative settings, particularly if the prevalence of illness is similar in these settings.

Much of the existing economic evaluation literature for HIV CT has focused on HIV seroprevalence as the key factor influencing the cost-effectiveness of the intervention.[34] However, the nature of the benefit chain and the types of costs measured vary across studies. Thus, by placing a priority on seroprevalence, other factors influencing the outcomes of the studies may be overlooked. This chapter surveys the existing economic evaluation studies of HIV CT to determine how variations in the evaluation methodology affect the resulting effectiveness and cost-effectiveness measures of HIV counseling and testing used in different settings.

THE LITERATURE SURVEY

The 43 articles and chapters selected for this research were surveyed for the following characteristics: setting, type of study, perspective of study, time frame, type of intervention, behavioral change assumptions, outcome measures, extent of the benefit chain, input costs included, and output costs or benefits included. Information was compiled and analyzed using Filemaker Pro 3.0.

The HIV counseling and testing economic evaluations were classified in ten categories according to setting: sites serving pregnant women and/or newborns;[25,28,35–40] acute-care hospitals;[41–48] offices of physicians, dentists, and other health care workers;[49–55] sites for premarital testing;[56–61] blood donation screening centers;[22,62–65] public clinics[31,66] general screening sites;[34,67,68] work sites;[69] drug treatment centers;[70,71] street outreach sites.[72]

Studies were classified as cost-effectiveness analyses, in which outcome measures were simply counted, cost-utility analyses in which quality adjustments were made to basic outcome measures, or cost-benefit analyses in which societal valuations of the outcome measures were included.[73,74] The perspective for measuring costs and effects was noted. Economic evaluation studies generally use the societal perspective that measures all costs and effects regardless of their distribution among persons. However, some studies may examine costs and benefits paid and received by particular health-care providers and payers (public or private). The time frame of the analysis was recorded because some studies focus only on one year or period whereas others measure effects in a multiyear/period framework.

The type of intervention, the extent of the benefit chain, and the nature of any behavioral change assumptions were also surveyed. Coding the type of intervention (i.e., whether the goal was only testing/screening or whether the intervention included the effects of both counseling and testing) presented a particular problem for this research. Because CDC guidelines and recommendations include both pre- and posttest counseling in the testing process,[75] the economic evaluations of the interventions surveyed were likely to state that the intervention involved both counseling and testing and that the evaluation includes some measure of the costs of counseling in the analysis. However, because program goals are often vague and economic evaluations are typically model-based analyses and not surveys of client mix and costs of real-world counseling and testing programs, the evaluator often must impose a structure to define the goals of the interventions.

In this research, an intervention was coded as *testing/screening only* (even if counseling costs were included as input costs) if *no* behavioral change assumptions were included in the analysis of the intervention, which affected the rate of transmission to persons other than the person tested. In this case, the program/intervention is evaluated as if its goal is only testing/screening, even if this outcome is not the true goal of the program. For example, in the study by McCarthy et al.,[34] the authors developed models of disease progression for cohorts of persons who were and were not screened for HIV and compared costs and years of life gained between the two strategies. Although costs of counseling are included in the analysis, no assumptions were made about behavioral change. Thus, the benefits in the model are defined solely in terms of additional life years gained by the client from early medical intervention. The model is applied to cohorts with different prevalences of HIV, so that inferences can be drawn about the cost-effectiveness of screening in various subpopulations. The authors acknowledged the existence of benefits from behavioral change, but these were not included in the analysis, even though they may be the goals of real-world HIV screening programs.

Thus the type of intervention is closely related to the extent of the benefit chain and the assumptions about behavioral change. In models that measure outcomes by the number of infections prevented, the crucial issue is whose infections are averted. Are infections averted simply because of the testing process and a resulting policy (i.e., testing physicians prevents transmission to some patients if physicians restrict their practice, testing pregnant women prevents transmission to certain infants if the ZDV intervention is completed), or are they averted because some type of behavioral change resulted from the counseling and testing process? Multiple goals may occur in the counseling and testing process in any of the settings. Counseling and testing physicians may provide benefits to their patients, because the physicians know their serostatus, and to their sex partners if a behavioral change results from the CT process. Testing pregnant women provides benefits both to their infants (knowledge of the mother's serostatus combined with the ZDV treatment) and to their sex and needle-sharing partners (behavioral change from counseling and testing). The benefit chain is measured in this research by using the following categories: patient only, sex partners of patient, needle-sharing partners of patient, children of patient, clients of patient, providers for patient, and persons receiving transfusions of the patient's blood.

Further classification problems pertain to the benefits patients receive from the counseling and testing process. Patients' knowledge of their serostatus can lead to early and/or better access to medical treatment services—a stated goal of the CT process. In many of these models, early medical treatment is included as an additional cost. The effects of early knowledge of serostatus on length and quality of life (the benefits of testing to the person) depend on disease stage. Antiretroviral therapy reduces mortality for persons with advanced HIV disease. Although the effects on persons in less advanced stages are less certain, aggressive therapy with three-drug regimens is currently recommended.[76] Thus, some economic evaluations do include estimates of life-years gained as a measure of these benefits to the patient.

The defining and coding of benefits to the patient is most important in economic evaluations that measure outcomes by the number of infections *identified* or cost per infection identified. Sometimes benefits to patients are not measured even though they are assumed to exist. For this study, if no benefits to the patient were actually measured in the paper surveyed (quality/length of life, effects of early intervention), the "patient only" category under the extent of benefit chain heading was *not* checked in the coding process. This could result in cases where no categories of the benefit chain variable were recorded.

As the discussion implies, outcome measures can vary substantially among economic evaluations. Studies can simply measure the number of persons screened or the number of infections identified by a screening process. They can also make assumptions about the number of infections that will be prevented by a particular screening process, either through behavioral change on the part of the person screened or through clinical or public health policies (i.e., practice restrictions by health-care workers, acceptance of the ZDV intervention by infected pregnant women, or removal of infected donated blood from the blood supply). If infections averted are measured, they can be used as the basis for calculating the resulting number of life years saved in a cost-effectiveness analysis, the quality-adjusted, life-years saved (QALYs) in a cost-utility analysis, or the valuation that society places on life-years saved in a cost-benefit analysis.[74]

The costs of the HIV counseling and testing interventions were also surveyed in this research. Intervention costs are incurred for pretest counseling, screening and confirmatory tests, and posttest counseling. From a societal perspective, the costs of patient time, both on-site and traveling to the site, should be included. The costs of outreach may also be relevant for certain types of interventions. Intervention costs may be estimated from a disaggregated "bottom up" approach, which focuses on the individual components of the CT process, or from a "top down" approach, which uses aggregate estimates.[74,77]

Categories of output costs in cost-effectiveness and cost-utility studies and measures of economic benefits in cost-benefit studies are the final set of variables analyzed in this survey. Cost-effectiveness and cost-utility studies typically compare intervention costs with costs that are saved as a result of the intervention. These often include the medical costs saved, but may also include the indirect costs of labor market productivity.[73,74] To estimate society's willingness to pay for the outcomes of the intervention (e.g., the economic benefits), contingent valuation methods or labor market valuations are typically used.[78,79] These approaches rely on either individual responses to hypothetical questions about willingness to pay or revealed behavior about persons' willingness to take risks in the labor market.

RESULTS OF THE SURVEY

Cost-effectiveness studies are still the dominant form of economic analysis for HIV counseling and testing interventions. Thirty-three studies were coded as cost-effectiveness analyses (CEA), four as cost-utility analyses (CUA), and ten as cost-benefit analyses (CBA) (see Table 1). Two studies contained a cost-effectiveness and a cost-utility analysis, whereas two other studies contained a cost-effectiveness and a cost-benefit analysis. Cost-effectiveness analyses were used to evaluate HIV CT in all of the settings except work-site testing. Cost-utility analysis was used in four of the settings—hospitals, offices of health-care workers, sites for premarital testing, and blood donation centers. Three of the ten cost-benefit studies were used to evaluate the counseling and testing of pregnant women, and two were used to evaluate blood donation centers. The remaining cost-benefit studies covered all areas except general screening, drug treatment centers, and street outreach sites.

Although researchers generally argue that the societal perspective is the most appropriate viewpoint for economic evaluation,[74] less than one-half of the studies surveyed (20 out of 43) took this perspective. Ten studies took the health-care provider perspective, whereas only three took the perspective of public or private payers. Ten of the studies did not state what perspective was used.

Approximately 80% of the studies (35) focused on one year or period, and eight took a multiperiod approach (see Table 2). Thus, most studies did not try to estimate how the outcomes would change after the first year or period. Several studies note that the additional effects or benefits in subsequent periods would be fewer than in the first period, given that most HIV infections are detected with the first round of screening and only new infections are identified subsequently. This example describes the economic concept of the declining marginal productivity or diminishing returns of an intervention.[80] For studies including behavioral change assumptions, the results are sensitive to the nature of those assumptions. In particular, Brandeau and Owens[35] noted that the benefits of screening pregnant women would be reduced if those women returned to high-risk behavior after the initial screening.

Table 1. Number of Studies Showing HIV CT Setting by Study Type and Perspective, N = 43 Studies

Setting	Type of Study			Perspective			
	CEA	CUA	CBA	Societal	Health-Care Provider	Public/Private Payer	Not Given
Pregnant women	5	0	3	4	2	0	2
Acute-care hospital	7	1	1	4	3	1	0
Health-care worker	6	1	1	4	2	0	1
Premarital testing	5	1	1	1	3	0	2
Blood donation	3	1	2	2	0	0	3
Public clinic	1	0	1	2	0	0	0
General screening	3	0	0	0	0	1	2
Work-site testing	0	0	1	0	0	1	0
Drug treatment	2	0	0	2	0	0	0
Street outreach	1	0	0	1	0	0	0
Total studies	33	4	10	20	10	3	10

Table 2. Number of Studies Showing HIV CT Setting by Time Period, Type of Intervention, and Behavior Change Assumption, N = 43 Studies

Setting	Time Period One	Time Period Multi	Testing Only No Behavioral Change Assumptions	Counseling and Testing Behavioral Change: Infected	Counseling and Testing Behavioral Change: High-Risk, Uninfected
Pregnant women	6	2	6	2	0
Acute-care hospital	7	1	6	2	1[a]
Health-care worker	5	2	6	1	0
Premarital testing	6	0	3	3	0
Blood donation	4	1	4	1	0
Public clinic	2	0	1	1	1[a]
General screening	1	2	3	0	0
Work-site testing	1	0	1	0	0
Drug treatment	2	0	1	1	1[a]
Street outreach	1	0	1	0	0
Total studies	35	8	32	11	3

[a]Study included assumptions for both infected and high-risk uninfected groups.

The type of intervention and the behavioral change assumptions are closely intertwined. Studies that did not include any behavioral changes assumptions were classified as "testing only." Thirty-two of the 43 studies surveyed did not include any behavioral change assumptions (see Table 2). These include the 31 studies, which were coded as "testing only," and the street outreach study, which was classified as "counseling with the distribution of prevention materials." The 32 studies that did not measure behavioral change included most or all of the studies in each setting, except for premarital testing. Only one-half (3 of 6) of the premarital testing studies were classified as "testing only" with no behavioral change assumptions. The other three premarital studies did include assumptions about changes in the behavior of infected persons. Studies classified as "counseling and testing" generally included assumptions only about the behavioral change of infected persons. In addition to the three premarital studies, two studies each of counseling and testing of pregnant women and in hospitals, and one study of counseling and testing in health-care worker offices, blood donation centers, public clinics, and drug treatment centers included these types of assumptions. Only three studies in the following settings included assumptions about behavioral change in high-risk, uninfected persons: hospitals; public clinics; and drug treatment centers. None of the studies surveyed made any assumptions about behavioral change among low-risk, uninfected persons.

A total of 35 studies included one outcome measure, six studies included two measures, and two studies included three measures. The most common outcome measures were infections identified (18 studies) and infections averted (21 studies) (see Table 3). Infections identified were more likely to be used in the studies of hospital and premarital counseling and testing. Infections averted were most likely to be used as an outcome measure in the studies of pregnant women, health-care workers, and blood donation centers. Life-years saved were used in two of the studies of health-care workers and in one of the general

Table 3. Number of Studies Showing HIV CT Setting
by Type of Outcome Measure, N = 43 Studies

| | Outcome Measure | | | | |
Setting	Infections Identified	Infections Averted	Life-Years Gained	QALYS Gained	Other
Pregnant women	2	5	0	0	3[a]
Acute-care hospital	5	2	0	1	1[a]
Health-care worker	2	6	2	2	0[a]
Premarital testing	4	2	0	1	0[a]
Blood donation	1	3	0	1	1[a]
Public clinic	1	1	0	0	0
General screening	1	1	1	0	0
Work-site testing	1	0	0	0	0
Drug treatment	1	1	0	0	0
Street outreach	0	0	0	0	1
Total studies	18	21	3	5	6

[a]Studies included multiple outcome measures.

screening studies. Quality-adjusted, life-years (QALYs) were used in two studies of health-care workers and in one study in each of the following areas: hospital testing; premarital testing; and testing at blood donation centers.

A total of 13 studies did not measure benefits to any groups of individuals in regard to the extent of the HIV CT benefit chain measured. These studies focused on outcomes measured as the number of infections identified. Seven of the 13 studies occurred in the settings of hospitals and sites for premarital counseling and testing. A total of 19 studies measured benefits to one group, six studies focused on two groups, three studies on three groups, and two studies included four groups of beneficiaries. Benefits to sex partners were measured in 11 studies, primarily in the areas of premarital and hospital testing and the testing of pregnant women. Benefits to needle-sharing partners were measured in only four of the studies. Benefits to other groups were related to the relevant setting. Children's benefits were measured only in the studies of pregnant women and premarital testing. Benefits to clients and providers were associated with health-care worker testing and testing in hospitals, and transfusion recipients were the focus of the studies of blood donation centers.

Input costs of screening and confirmatory tests were the costs most likely to be measured in the studies surveyed (see Table 4). Forty-one studies measured the former and 39 studies measured the latter. Fewer studies measured the costs of counseling. Twenty-eight studies include pretest counseling costs; thirty-one studies include posttest counseling costs. Only two studies measured patient travel time and time on-site. Thus, almost all studies focus on the costs of provider inputs and not patient inputs. Furthermore, 22 of the 43 studies use aggregate figures that do not distinguish among the input cost categories. Aggregate cost figures were more likely to be used in the studies of premarital testing (all of these studies) and in the testing of pregnant women and health-care workers. Specialized costs were included in particular settings: ZDV costs in the analyses of pregnant women; the costs of discarded blood in blood donation centers; and the replacement costs or decreased productivity of health-care workers in those studies.

Table 4. Number of Studies Showing HIV CT Setting by Type of Input Cost, N = 43 Studies

Setting	Input Cost					
	Pretest Counseling	Screening Test	Confirmatory Test	Posttest Counseling	Patient Time	Aggregate Costs
Pregnant women	7	8	7	7	1	5
Acute-care hospital	4	8	8	4	0	3
Health-care worker	6	7	7	6	0	4
Premarital testing	6	6	6	6	0	6
Blood donation	0	5	4	2	0	1
Public clinic	2	2	2	2	1	1
General screening	1	2	2	2	0	2
Work-site testing	0	1	1	0	0	0
Drug treatment	2	2	2	2	0	0
Street outreach	0	0	0	0	0	0
Total studies	28	41	39	31	2	22

Regarding outcome costs and benefits, 25 studies do not include any of the categories measured. A total of 13 studies include one category, three studies include two categories, and two studies include three categories. Medical costs saved were the most likely category of outcome costs included. Six of the 14 studies including these cost-savings focus on the counseling and testing of pregnant women. Only five studies include measures of indirect costs saved. The cost-benefit analyses surveyed measured economic benefits of the interventions by using only labor market valuations. None of these studies use contingent valuation methods.

DISCUSSION AND POLICY ANALYSIS

Both the operation and the evaluation of HIV counseling and testing interventions are influenced by multiple goals adopted by these programs. Conflicts exist between the goals of prevention, which focus on persons who are infected and those who are not, and medical treatment issues, which focus on the infected. The prevention goal has several complexities owing to uncertainties over the effects of counseling and testing on behavioral change[32,33] and the value of CT for uninfected persons.[5] Furthermore, HIV CT is performed in settings where these goals are intertwined, and in addition, they also may be vague and undefined.

Healton et al.[81] illustrate this conflict between goals in their analysis of New York State's voluntary HIV CT program in women's health care settings in 1991. They argue that the goals of case finding (identifying HIV-infected women) and HIV prevention may work at cross-purposes. An agency which focuses on case finding by emphasizing the testing component of the process may achieve its results by sacrificing progress in education and prevention goals, particularly if the testing emphasis reduces the number of women who agree to pretest counseling. Programs that focus on prevention counseling may understate the benefits of early access to medical services achieved through testing and knowledge of serostatus.

Ambiguities in the definition and operation of HIV CT programs are reflected in the economic evaluation of these interventions. Substantial variation exists in the characteristics of the economic evaluation studies of HIV counseling and testing, even though this literature is relatively small. These studies do not answer all of the relevant questions about the costs and effects of these programs, given the data used and the approaches taken in the analyses.

Most of the studies of HIV CT are cost-effectiveness studies that use outcome measures, such as the number of HIV infections identified or averted. The U.S. Public Health Service Panel on Cost-Effectiveness in Health and Medicine issued guidelines that recommend the use of cost-utility analysis as the standard methodology for economic evaluation of health-care treatment and prevention studies.[82] Only four of the studies surveyed used this methodology. Although most of these studies were completed before the Panel's recommendations were issued, the direction for future research is clear. There has been only limited application of cost-benefit analysis in this area, largely because this technique is favored more by economists than health services or public health researchers. Moreover, none of the cost-benefit studies surveyed use the recently developed contingent valuation methods for benefit estimation.

Less than one-half of the studies surveyed use the societal perspective for the analysis, and 20% do not state the perspective of the study. Thus, much of this literature does not conform to the cost-effectiveness panel's guidelines that advocate a societal approach for a baseline analysis.[82] Most of the studies surveyed do not measure the opportunity cost of the intervention because patient/client costs are not included. However, these implicit costs can have substantial effects on program participation and act as important barriers for prevention activities.[83]

Almost 80% of the studies focus on only one year or time period. Thus, the subsequent effects and costs of the intervention are unknown. The additional effects of the intervention are likely to decline because of the concept of diminishing returns noted previously. Furthermore, the effects of subsequent behavioral change, either positive or negative, are rarely modeled. Approximately 75% of the studies surveyed include *no* behavioral change assumptions. Although this result may reflect the uncertainty in the literature about the effects of HIV CT on behavioral change,[32,33] it means that a key goal of HIV counseling and testing has not been well evaluated. Of the 32 studies without behavioral change assumptions in this survey, approximately one-half use the number of infections identified as the outcome measure, whereas the remaining studies use the number of infections averted. The latter studies focus on the areas of counseling and testing pregnant women and health care workers, so that infections were prevented by ZDV therapy and practice restrictions, respectively.

The authors of a majority of the studies surveyed argue that HIV seroprevalence is the most important factor influencing the cost-effectiveness of the intervention. These studies advocate the targeting of HIV counseling and testing on groups and in settings where there are likely to be greater concentrations of the infected or high-risk uninfected, as opposed to widespread screening of the general population or low-risk groups. However, because HIV seroprevalence may be similar in many of the settings analyzed in this research, the importance of other factors, which might influence the choice of setting, is not clear from these analyses.

This problem is magnified by the variation in the methodologies of estimating costs and effectiveness among the studies surveyed in this research. The costs of HIV CT differ for the infected and the uninfected and may differ by setting. In some cases costs are borne by the client (travel and wait time) and in other cases by the provider (street outreach). However, more than one-half of the studies surveyed use only aggregate cost figures with no breakdown among the categories of counseling and testing. Only two studies include any valuation of patient/client time. Outreach costs that may be incurred to find infected and high-risk persons who do not appear for counseling and testing in the various settings have not been analyzed, but may significantly affect the ability of policy makers to target counseling and testing programs on these groups. Furthermore, because most of the articles surveyed are model-based analyses and not specific studies of the actual operation of HIV CT in various settings, implementation problems and costs are typically not included. Counseling and testing costs are often modeled simply as a function of seroprevalence because these costs are higher for infected persons. This approach does not recognize that many of the costs discussed previously may also become more significant as seroprevalence increases. Thus, most of the existing studies have not included data that would allow researchers to adequately analyze the effect of variables other than seroprevalence on the effectiveness and costs of these HIV interventions in different settings.

Supplementing model-based analyses of HIV CT interventions with studies of existing counseling and testing programs in different geographic areas and institutional environments would help increase the relevance of the model-based conclusions and provide additional insights into factors that influence the operation of actual programs (i.e., goal emphasis, participation by specific sets of clients) or into new policy directions. For example, Healton et al.[81] argue for a universal approach for counseling but an approach targeted on high-risk women regarding HIV testing on the basis of their evidence of the information retained from counseling sessions and the acceptance of counseling and testing services in their study of women's clinics in New York State. Results such as this can provide better input data for the model-based analyses and verification or refutation of the insights of the more conceptual approach.

Conflicts between the prevention and medical objectives of HIV counseling and testing are likely to increase. If research continues to show that the new antiretroviral therapies reduce and maintain low viral loads,[76,84] the medical objectives of HIV CT and the benefits of early testing for influencing the course of disease will increase in importance, regardless of knowledge of the effects of counseling and testing on behavioral change. Thus, technological developments may eventually determine the goals and objectives of the HIV counseling and testing intervention. The costs of these drug therapies are considerable, however, and will influence their availability and use by different populations. Because these new drug costs are part of the total medical costs associated with a case of HIV infection, their inclusion will likely change the outcomes and conclusions about the cost-effectiveness of HIV prevention interventions. Thus, economic factors will continue to affect the implementation of HIV counseling and testing programs and the economic evaluation of HIV CT compared with other prevention interventions.

ACKNOWLEDGMENT. Dr. Farnham acknowledges the assistance of Robert L. Collins in conducting and organizing the literature search in this chapter.

REFERENCES

1. HIV counseling and testing in publicly funded sites: 1993–1994 summary report. U.S. Department of Health and Human Services. Atlanta: Centers for Disease Control and Prevention, March 1996.

2. Centers for Disease Control. Public Health Service guidelines for counseling and antibody testing to prevent HIV infection and AIDS. *MMWR* 1987; 36:509–515.

3. Anderson JE, Hardy AM, Cahill K, Aral S. HIV antibody testing and posttest counseling in the United States: Data from the 1989 National Health Interview Survey. *Am J Public Health* 1992; 82(11):1533–1535.

4. Berrios DC, Hearst N, Coates TJ, et al. HIV antibody testing among those at risk for infection. The National AIDS Behavioral Surveys. *JAMA* 1993; 270:1576–1580.

5. Phillips KA, Coates TJ. HIV counseling and testing: Research and policy issues. *AIDS Care* 1995; 7:115–124.

6. Wortley PM, Chu SY, Diaz T, et al. HIV testing patterns: Where, why, and when were persons with AIDS tested for HIV? *AIDS* 1995; 9:487–492.

7. Janssen RS, St. Louis ME, Satten GA, et al. HIV infection among patients in U.S. acute care hospitals. *N Engl J Med* 1992; 327:445–452.

8. Rowe M, Ryan C. *AIDS: A Public Health Challenge.* Washington, DC: Intergovernmental Health Policy Project, George Washington University; 1987; pp. 2–21.

9. Centers for Disease Control. Recommendations for preventing transmission of human immunodeficiency virus and hepatitis B virus to patients during exposure-prone invasive procedures. *MMWR* 1991; 40(RR-8): 1–9.

10. Bowleg L. An overview of 1992 state HIV/AIDS laws. *Intergovernmental AIDS Rep.* June 1992:1–4.

11. Minkoff H, Willoughby A. Pediatric HIV disease, zidovudine in pregnancy, and unblinding heelstick surveys. Reframing the debate on prenatal HIV testing. *JAMA* 1995; 274:1165–1168.

12. Ploughman P. Public policy versus private rights: The medical, social, ethical, and legal implications of the testing of newborns for HIV. *AIDS & Public Policy J* 1995/96; 10:182–204.

13. Farnham PG. Defining and measuring the costs of the HIV epidemic to business firms. *Public Health Rep* 1994; 109:311–318.

14. Reardon J, Warren N, Keilch R, et al. Are HIV-infected injection drug users taking HIV tests? *Am J Public Health* 1993; 83:1414–1417.

15. Petersen LR, Doll LS, White CR, et al. Heterosexually acquired human immunodeficiency virus infection and the United States blood supply: Considerations for screening of potential blood donors. *Transfusion* 1993; 33:552–557.

16. Rugg DL, MacGowan RJ, Stark KA, Swanson NM. Evaluating the CDC program for HIV counseling and testing. *Public Health Rep* 1991; 106:708–713.

17. Carpenter CCJ, Fischl MA, Hammer SM, et al. Antiretroviral therapy for HIV infection in 1996. Recommendations of an international panel. *JAMA* 1996; 276:146–154.

18. Doll LS, Kennedy MB. HIV counseling and testing: What is it and how well does it work? In Schochetman G, George JR, eds. *AID Testing: A Comprehensive Guide to Technical, Medical, Social, Legal, and Management Issues,* 2nd ed. New York: Springer-Verlag; 1994; p. 302.

19. Holtgrave DR, Valdiserri RO, West, GA. Quantitative economic evaluations of HIV-related prevention and treatment services: A review. *Risk: Health, Safety & Environment* 1994; 5:29–47.

20. Holtgrave DR, Qualls NL, Graham JD. Economic evaluation of HIV prevention programs. *Annu Rev Public Health* 1996; 17:467–488.

21. Johnson ES, Doll LS, Satten GA, et al. Direct oral questions to blood donors: The impact on screening for human immunodeficiency virus. *Transfusion* 1994; 34:769–774.

22. Gelles GM. Costs and benefits of HIV-1 antibody testing of donated blood. *J Policy Anal Manage* 1993; 12:512–531.

23. Connor EM, Sperling RS, Gelber R, et al. Reduction of maternal-infant transmission of human immunodeficiency virus type 1 with zidovudine treatment. *N Engl J Med* 1994; 331:1173–1180.

24. Recommendations of the Public Health Service Task Force on the use of zidovudine to reduce perinatal transmission of human immunodeficiency virus. *MMWR* 1994; 43(No. RR-11).

25. Gorsky RD, Farnham PG, Straus WL, et al. Preventing perinatal transmission of HIV—costs and effectiveness of a recommended intervention. *Public Health Rep* 1996; 111:335–341.

26. Landesman S, Minkoff HL, Holman S, et al. Serosurvey of human immunodeficiency virus infection in parturients: Implications for human immunodeficiency virus testing programs of pregnant women. *JAMA* 1987; 258:2701–2703.

27. Krasinsky K, Borkowsky W, Bebenroth D, et al. Failure of voluntary testing for human immunodeficiency virus to identify infected parturient women in a high-risk population. *N Engl J Med* 1988; 318:185.

28. Brandeau ML, Owens DK, Sox CH, Wachter RM. Screening women of childbearing age for human immunodeficiency virus: A model-based policy analysis. *Manage Sci* 1993; 39:72–92.

29. McCusker J, Willis G, McDonald M, et al. Admissions of injection drug users to drug abuse treatment following HIV counseling and testing. *Public Health Rep* 1994; 109:212–218.

30. Farley TA, Cartter ML, Wassell JT, Hadler JL. Predictors of outcome in methadone programs: Effect of HIV counseling and testing. *Conn Med* 1994; 58:165–171.

31. Farnham PG, Gorsky RD, Holtgrave DR, et al. Counseling and testing for HIV prevention: Costs, effects, and cost-effectiveness of more rapid screening tests. *Public Health Rep* 1996; 111:44–53.

32. Higgins DL, Galavotti C, O'Reilly KR, et al. Evidence for the effects of HIV antibody counseling and testing on risk behaviors. *JAMA* 1991; 266:2419–2429.

33. Holtgrave DR, Qualls NL, Curran JW, et al. An overview of the effectiveness and efficiency of HIV prevention programs. *Public Health Rep* 1995; 110:134–146.

34. McCarthy BD, Wong JB, Muñoz A, Sonnenberg FA. Who should be screened for HIV infection? A cost-effectiveness analysis. *Arch Intern Med* 1993; 153:1107–1116.

35. Brandeau ML, Owens DK. When women return to risk. Costs and benefits of HIV screening in the presence of relapse. In Kaplan EH, Brandeau ML, eds. *Modeling the AIDS Epidemic: Planning, Policy, and Prediction.* New York: Raven Press; 1994; p. 121.

36. Dunn DT, Nicoll A, Holland FJ, Davison CF. How much paediatric HIV infection could be prevented by antenatal HIV testing? *J Med Screen* 1995; 2:35–40.

37. Ecker JL. The cost-effectiveness of human immunodeficiency virus screening in pregnancy. *Am J Obstet Gynecol* 1996; 174:716–721.

38. Houshyar A. Screening pregnant women for HIV antibody: Cost-benefit analysis. *AIDS & Public Policy J* 1991; 6:98–103.

39. Lewis R, O'Brien JM, Ray DT, Sibai BM. The impact of initiating a human immunodeficiency virus screening program in an urban obstetric population. *Am J Obstet Gynecol* 1995; 173:1329–1333.

40. Mauskopf JA, Paul JE, Wichman DS, et al. Economic impact of treatment of HIV-positive pregnant women and their newborns with zidovudine. *JAMA* 1996; 276:132–138.

41. Harris RL, Boisaubin EV, Salyer PD, Semands DF. Evaluation of a hospital admission HIV antibody voluntary screening program. *Infect Control Hosp Epidemiol* 1990; 11:628–634.

42. Henry K, Campbell S. The potential efficiency of routine HIV testing of hospital patients—data from a CDC sentinel hospital. *Public Health Rep* 1992; 107:138–141.

43. LaCroix SJ, Russo G. A cost-benefit analysis of voluntary routine HIV-antibody testing for hospital patients. *Soc Sci Med* 1996; 42:1259–1272.

44. Lawrence VA, Gafni A, Kroenke K. Preoperative HIV testing: Is it less expensive than universal precautions? *J Clin Epidemiol* 1993; 46:1219–1227.

45. LeGales C, Moatti JP, Paris-Tours Study Group of Antenatal Transmission of HIV, Group '9 Maternites.' Cost-effectiveness of HIV screening of pregnant women in hospitals of the Paris area. *Eur J Obstet Gynecol Reprod Biol* 1990; 37:25–33.

46. Lurie P, Avins AL, Phillips KA, et al. The cost-effectiveness of voluntary counseling and testing of hospital inpatients for HIV infection. *JAMA* 1994; 272:1832–1838.

47. Mullins JR, Harrison PB. The questionable utility of mandatory screening for the human immunodeficiency virus. *Am J Surg* 1993; 166:676–679.

48. Owens DK, Nease RF, Harris RA. Cost-effectiveness of HIV screening in acute care settings. *Arch Intern Med* 1996; 156:394–404.

49. Chavey WE, Cantor SB, Clover RD, et al. Cost-effectiveness analysis of screening health care workers for HIV. *J Fam Pract* 1994; 38:249–257.

50. Gerberding JL. Expected costs of implementing a mandatory human immunodeficiency virus and hepatitis B virus testing and restriction program for healthcare workers performing invasive procedures. *Infect Control Hosp Epidemiol* 1991; 12:443–447.

51. Owens DK, Harris RA, Scott PM, Nease RF Jr. Screening surgeons for HIV infection: A cost-effectiveness analysis. *Ann Intern Med* 1995; 122:641–652.

52. Phillips KA, Lowe RA, Kahn JG, et al. The cost-effectiveness of HIV testing of physicians and dentists in the United States. *JAMA* 1994; 271:851–858.

53. Russo G, La Croix SJ. A second look at the cost of mandatory human immunodeficiency virus and hepatitis B virus testing for healthcare workers performing invasive procedures. *Infect Control Hosp Epidemiol* 1992; 13:107–110.

54. Sell RL, Jovell AJ, Siegel JE. HIV screening of surgeons and dentists—a cost-effectiveness analysis. *Infect Control Hosp Epidemiol* 1994; 15:635–645.

55. Yawn BP. Clinical decision analysis of HIV screening. *Fam Med* 1992; 24:355–361.
56. Altman R, Shahied SI, Pizzuti W, et al. Premarital HIV-1 testing in New Jersey. *J Acquired Immune Defic Syndr Hum Retrovirol* 1992; 5:7–11.
57. Cleary PD, Barry MJ, Mayer KH, et al. Compulsory premarital screening for the human immunodeficiency virus: Technical and public health considerations. *JAMA* 1989; 258:1757–1762.
58. McKay NL, Phillips KM. An economic evaluation of mandatory premarital testing for HIV. *Inquiry* 1991; 28:236–248.
59. Petersen LR, White CR. Premarital Screening Study Group. Premarital screening for antibodies to human immunodeficiency virus type 1 in the United States. *Am J Public Health* 1990; 80:1087–1090.
60. Turnock BJ, Kelly CJ. Mandatory premarital testing for human immunodeficiency virus: The Illinois experience. *JAMA* 1989; 261:3415–3418.
61. Weinstein MC, Graham JD, Siegel JE, Fineberg HV. Cost-effectiveness analysis of AIDS prevention programs: Concept, complications, and illustrations. In Turner CF, Miller JG, Moses LE, eds. *AIDS: Sexual Behavior and Intravenous Drug Use.* Washington, DC: Natl. Acad. Press; 1989; p. 471.
62. Eisenstaedt RS, Getzen TE. Screening blood donors for human immunodeficiency virus antibody: Cost-benefit analysis. *Am J Public Health* 1988; 778:450–454.
63. Etchason J, Petz L, Keeler E, et al. The cost-effectiveness of preoperative autologous blood donations. *N Engl J Med* 1995; 332:719–724.
64. Mendelson DN, Sandler SG. A model for estimating incremental benefits and costs of testing donated blood for human immunodeficiency virus antigen (HIV-AG). *Transfusion* 1990; 30:73–75.
65. Schwartz JS, Kinosian BP, Pierskalla WP, Lee H. Strategies for screening blood for human immunodeficiency virus antibody. *JAMA* 1990; 264:1704–1710.
66. Holtgrave DR, Valdiserri RO, Gerber AR, Hinman AR. Human immunodeficiency virus counseling, testing, referral, and partner notification services: A cost-benefit analysis. *Arch Intern Med* 1993; 153:1225–1230.
67. Gail MH, Preston D, Piantadosi S. Disease prevention models of voluntary confidential screening for human immunodeficiency virus (HIV). *Stat Med* 1989; 8:59–81.
68. Nahmias S, Feinstein CD. Screening strategies to inhibit the spread of AIDS. *Socio-Econ Plan Sci* 1990; 24:249–260.
69. Bloom DE, Glied S. Benefits and costs of HIV testing. *Science* 1991; 252:1798–1804.
70. Gorsky RD, MacGowan RJ, Swanson NM, DelGado BP. Prevention of HIV infection in drug users: A cost analysis. *Preventive Med* 1995; 24:3–8.
71. Kahn JG, Washington AE, Showstack JA, et al. Counseling and testing. In *Updated Estimates of the Impact and Cost of HIV Prevention in Injection Drug Users.* Report prepared for the Centers for Disease Control. San Francisco: Institute of Health Policy Studies, University of California; 1992; p. 47.
72. Wright-DeAguero LK, Gorsky RD, Seeman GM. Cost of outreach for HIV prevention among drug users and youth at risk. *Drugs Soc* 1996; 9:185–197.
73. Drummond MF, Stoddart GL, Torrance GW. *Methods for the Economic Evaluation of Health Care Programmes.* New York: Oxford University Press; 1987.
74. Haddix AC, Teutsch SM, Shaffer PA, Duñet DO, eds. *Prevention Effectiveness: A Guide to Decision Analysis and Economic Evaluation.* New York: Oxford University Press, 1996.
75. Centers for Disease Control and Prevention. Recommendations for HIV testing services for inpatients and outpatients in acute-care hospital settings; and Technical guidance on HIV counseling. *MMWR* 1993;42(No. RR-2).
76. Carpenter CCJ, Fischl MA, Hammer SM, et al. Antiretroviral therapy for HIV infection in 1997. Updated recommendations of the International AIDS Society-USA Panel. *JAMA* 1997; 277:1962–1969.
77. Gorsky RD. A method to measure the costs of counseling for HIV prevention. *Public Health Rep* 1996; 111(Suppl. 1):115–122.
78. Tolley G, Kenkel D, Fabian R, eds. *Valuing Health for Policy. An Economic Approach.* Chicago: The University of Chicago Press; 1994.
79. Fisher A, Chestnut LG, Violette DM. The value of reducing risks of death: A note on new evidence. *J Policy Anal Manage* 1989; 8:88–100.
80. Phelps CE. *Health Economics.* New York: Harper Collins; 1992.
81. Healton C, Messeri P, Abramson D, et al. A balancing act: The tension between case-finding and primary prevention strategies in New York State's voluntary HIV counseling and testing program in women's health care setting. *Am J Preventive Med* 1996; 12(Suppl. 1):53–60.

82. Gold MR, Siegel JE, Russell LB, Weinstein MC, eds. *Cost-Effectiveness in Health and Medicine*. New York: Oxford University Press; 1996.
83. Riportella-Muller R, Selby-Harrington ML, Richardson LA, et al. Barriers to the use of preventive health care services for children. *Public Health Rep* 1996; 111:71–77.
84. Deeks SG, Smith M, Holodniy M, Kahn JO. HIV-1 protease inhibitors. A review for clinicians. *JAMA* 1997; 277:145–153.

Economic Evaluation of HIV Screening Interventions

DOUGLAS K. OWENS

SCREENING FOR HIV: BACKGROUND

Screening for human immunodeficiency virus (HIV) is a potentially beneficial intervention because it enables providers to offer early medical intervention to people who have HIV and to provide counseling that may encourage these people to reduce high-risk behavior that can transmit HIV. Despite this relatively straightforward medical rationale, few topics in public health have been more controversial than screening for HIV. Certain authors have vilified targeted screening for HIV as unethical,[1] whereas other authors have considered HIV screening for certain groups to be an important preventive public-health tool.[2] Screening for HIV is controversial in part because of the social stigmatization and discrimination that may accompany disclosure that a person has HIV. Evaluation of the social and ethical concerns about HIV screening should play a central role in policy makers' decisions to implement programs. In this chapter, however, I focus on the medical and economic consequences of screening for HIV. The outcomes associated with an HIV screening program are fundamental considerations in decisions about screening because if screening is either medically ineffective or too costly, we do not need to consider the other difficult potential problems associated with screening.

I summarize economic evaluations of HIV screening for three important populations: women, patients, and health-care workers. I emphasize assessments of screening women of childbearing age (including women who are pregnant at the time of screening) because the prevalence of HIV is higher in women of this age and because detection of HIV in these women may facilitate measures to reduce perinatal HIV transmission. Because current guidelines[3] recommend screening inpatients and outpatients who are examined in acute-care settings in which the prevalence of HIV is 1% or greater, I highlight studies that examined this population. Evaluation of the cost effectiveness of general screening[4,5] or of other HIV preventive interventions[6] is beyond my scope. I do not review studies of intensive behavioral interventions. For the purposes of this chapter, I consider that screening includes testing for HIV with associated, routine, pre- and posttest counseling.

The question I seek to answer is whether HIV screening is cost-effective in women,

DOUGLAS K. OWENS • VA Palo Alto Health Care System, Palo Alto, California 94304; and Section on Medical Informatics, Department of Medicine, and Department of Health Research and Policy, Stanford University, Stanford, California 94305.

Handbook of Economic Evaluation of HIV Prevention Programs, edited by Holtgrave. Plenum Press, New York, 1998.

patients, or health-care workers. An answer to this question first requires determining whether screening is effective, that is, Does early detection through screening lead to a better medical outcome for the identified person or to reduced transmission to sexual partners, needle-sharing partners, or to newborns? In contrast to certain other interventions, such as mammography for early detection of breast cancer, HIV screening has not been evaluated in randomized, controlled trials. Thus, researchers must infer the efficacy of screening from evidence that is circumstantial, often by mathematical models. These inferences are complex and depend on evaluating the benefit of early medical therapy on length and quality of life and the effect of screening on behavior that may transmit HIV. I discuss these topics further in sections following. After assessing whether screening is effective, investigators must estimate the costs associated with the screening program to complete an economic analysis.

There are several ways to perform an economic analysis of HIV screening programs.[6] A comprehensive economic analysis should include any incremental costs associated with a screening program. Such costs include, for example, the cost of incremental medical treatment required for those persons detected with HIV. Because studies that evaluate only the costs of testing and counseling, without discussing downstream incremental costs, provide an incomplete and potentially misleading economic evaluation, I emphasize studies that performed formal analyses in either a cost-effectiveness or a cost-benefit framework.

In a cost-effectiveness analysis, the researchers evaluate the expenditures required to obtain a particular medical outcome, such as preventing an infection. Methods are available to estimate the medical costs saved from preventing an HIV infection[7] and to develop monetary thresholds that indicate whether programs evaluated in terms of HIV infections prevented are cost effective.[8] Cost-effectiveness analyses may also report outcomes as expenditures per year of life saved or if the analysis incorporates the effect of screening on quality of life, as expenditures per quality-adjusted year (QALY) of life saved. Studies that report expenditures per year of life saved or per QALY gained enable policy makers to compare HIV screening to other HIV-related interventions (for example, the cost effectiveness of prophylaxis for opportunistic infections[9]) and to interventions for non-HIV-related conditions (for example, screening for breast cancer). These analyses require a method for translating the number of infections prevented into the number of years of life saved and, if the researchers consider quality of life, an assessment of the effect of a screening intervention on quality of life. Although such analyses require additional complexity, the payoff is a more comprehensive economic evaluation that facilitates comparison of HIV screening with other interventions that policy makers and clinicians must consider.

Alternatively, researchers may report the outcome of their economic evaluation in a cost-benefit framework by valuing medical outcomes (for example, an HIV infection averted) in terms of dollars. In a cost-benefit framework, a screening program would be desirable if the benefits of screening (expressed in dollars) outweigh the costs of screening.

The choice of a cost-effectiveness threshold is inherently a value judgment and is controversial.[10–13] However, interventions commonly accepted as cost-effective usually cost between $10,000 and $150,000 per life-year saved.[14–16] Direct comparisons of the cost effectiveness of interventions should be performed cautiously because economic studies often use different assumptions, methods, or perspectives to formulate an evaluation. As a rough guideline for interpreting the cost-effectiveness of HIV screening in specific populations, I note whether the cost-effectiveness of screening is within this range.

An important component of an economic analysis of HIV screening programs is evaluating (or predicting) the effect of the screening and counseling on the behavior of the screened persons. An understanding of the person's behavioral response to screening is crucial because the benefits of screening are mediated through changes in behavior. Will people identified with HIV seek and comply with medical care? If they do not, they will not realize the potential benefit from early medical intervention. Will people identified with HIV reduce high-risk behavior, such as unprotected sex or needle sharing? If they do not, the screening program will not reduce transmission of HIV. Will women seek prenatal care less often if they believe they will be screened for HIV?[17] If women are deterred from seeking prenatal care, they (and their newborns) may experience an increase in adverse outcomes that outweighs the potential benefit from early detection of HIV. In addition to providing a brief summary of evidence about the behavioral response to screening (see later section), I note authors' assumptions about the behavioral change after screening.

The Benefit of Early Medical Intervention

Early detection of HIV benefits the people screened if they receive medical care that they would not have received in the absence of screening and if that care extends their lives or improves quality of life. Because there have been no randomized studies of HIV screening, there is no direct evidence whether early detection through screening improves length or quality of life. Rather, we must evaluate the stage of disease at which people are identified through screening and assess the evidence that medical interventions delivered at that time provide benefit.

People detected with HIV through screening are found at varying stages of disease. In the US, in states that report the occurrence of both HIV and AIDS, 70% of people are first tested for HIV within one year of developing AIDS.[18] In a national sample of people diagnosed with AIDS, approximately 50% had their first HIV test within one year of developing AIDS.[19] These data suggest that many people are unaware of their HIV infection until they have advanced disease. Our experience with voluntary screening in asymptomatic patients confirms these national data: many people identified with HIV are unaware of their infection and have advanced disease as assessed by a CD4 count. Thus, in addition to detecting people who have early HIV disease, a screening program will probably find a significant proportion of people who are at relatively advanced stages of disease and are candidates for prophylaxis for opportunistic infections or initiation of antiretroviral disease. For patients who have advanced disease, primary prophylaxis for *Pneumocystis carinii* pneumonia improves survival,[20] as does treatment with antiretroviral medication.

In addition to prophylaxis for opportunistic infections, antiretroviral therapy is the primary medical treatment that may benefit people whose HIV infection is identified through screening. The effect of antiretroviral therapy on length and quality of life is complex and depends on the stage of HIV disease. The advent of antiretroviral treatment began with the finding that such therapy reduces mortality in patients who have advanced, symptomatic HIV disease[21] compared to therapy with a placebo. There is no disagreement that antiretroviral therapy is appropriate for patients with CD4 counts less than 200 cells/ mm^3. A significant proportion of patients detected through screening would thus quality for treatment. Whether antiretroviral therapy benefits patients who do not have advanced HIV disease is less clear. Results from a number of studies are consistent with the hypothesis that, in earlier disease, zidovudine monotherapy delays progression to disease transiently by approximately 1 year[22-29] but does not influence survival. Combination therapy with zidovudine and didanosine or zalcitabine or sequential monotherapy with didanosine or zal-citabine after zidovudine alone is superior to zidovudine alone in patients with intermediate-stage disease and provides a modest survival advantage of three to six months.[30] Combination therapy with two[31,32] (lamivudine and zidovudine) or three reverse transcriptase inhibitors (nevirapine in addition to zidovudine and didanosine) improves long-term immunologic and virological effects of therapy.[33] More recently, the finding that HIV viral replication occurs at astonishing rates throughout disease has led to the hypothesis that combination antiretroviral therapy should begin early in disease.[34–37] Protease inhibitors provide further antiretroviral activity when used in addition to reverse transcriptase inhibitors, and provide a new potential option for early combination therapy.[38,39] Although the usefulness of combination antiretroviral therapy in early HIV disease requires further study, the available evidence suggests that such therapy is promising.[40]

In summary, the available studies provide evidence that screening for HIV would identify people at stages of disease when medical intervention, including antiretroviral therapy, prophylaxis for opportunistic infections, and screening for other diseases would provide a net benefit in length and quality of life for such people. The change in philosophy to provide combination antiretroviral treatment early in disease provides added urgency to identify people with HIV before they present with symptoms from advanced HIV disease. Quantification of the extent to which detection through screening may prolong life is difficult, however. I note authors' assumptions about the effects of early identification on length of life.

Effect of Screening on High-Risk Behavior

The effect of screening on subsequent risk behavior has been studied in a variety of populations.[41–46] Although the degree of behavioral change found varies in different studies, generally only modest changes in behavior have been observed. Secular trends in risk behavior (such as the observed decreased risky sex in populations of homosexual men) confound many studies, which makes it difficult to assess the degree to which knowledge of HIV status per se determines changes in risk behavior. In addition, recent evidence suggests that certain behavioral changes are short lived and relapse to risky behavior.[47] A study of counseling and testing in women found no significant change in the reported risk behavior of women who tested negative for HIV.[48] Holtgrave reviewed studies of behavioral change related to testing and counseling and concluded that the preponderance of evidence indicates no change in risk behavior in people who test negative and modest change limited to subgroups who test positive.[49] Coates and colleagues reviewed behavioral interventions and concluded that the evidence of effectiveness was most clear-cut when testing is embedded in long-term prevention programs.[46]

SCREENING OF WOMEN

The Centers for Disease Control and Prevention[50] and the U.S. Preventive Services Task Force[51] recommend voluntary HIV screening for pregnant women who have a history of high-risk behavior. The following section outlines the rationale for HIV screening programs for women of childbearing age. The section after highlights behavioral questions with respect to these screening programs. The subsequent section reviews economic analyses of screening programs for women. The next section summarizes these findings, highlights gaps in current knowledge, and discusses policy questions related to screening women.

Rationale for Screening

In addition to conferring potential benefits from early medical intervention and counseling-induced reductions in risk behavior, detection of HIV in women of childbearing age enables screened HIV-positive women to take steps to reduce the chance of transmission to their newborns. Zidovudine given to women during pregnancy reduces transmission of HIV to newborns (in a randomized trial, mother-to-infant transmission of HIV occurred in 25% of women who received a placebo, compared with 8% of women who received zido-vudine).[52,53] Many providers also counsel women who have HIV infection to avoid breast feeding because breast feeding can transmit HIV.[54] In addition, HIV transmission to newborns increases when fetal membranes rupture more than four hours before deliv-ery.[55,56] Whether clinical interventions that aim to reduce the time between rupture of membranes and delivery would reduce HIV transmission is unknown but is under investiga-tion.[55] A woman can choose to institute interventions to reduce transmission only if she is aware of her HIV infection status during pregnancy.

Behavioral Effects of Screening

The effects of an HIV screening program for women depend on whether identification with HIV changes women's decisions with respect to childbearing, reduces high-risk behavior, and does not discourage enrollment in prenatal-care programs. Evidence regard-ing these factors is mixed. In an urban population of injecting-drug users (IDU), knowledge of HIV status did not significantly affect women's decisions regarding childbearing,[57] although pregnancy-termination rates were slightly higher in women infected with HIV than in those who were not (50% compared with 44%, respectively, a difference that was not statistically significant). A similar study of IDUs in Britain also found no statistically significant difference in pregnancy-termination rates, but rates were high in women who were HIV infected (45% termination rate) and women who were not infected with HIV (35% termination rate).[58] Other populations have not been well studied. As I noted pre-viously, the effect of testing and counseling on high-risk behavior is modest, and women who test negative for HIV do not reduce high-risk behavior substantially.[48] Finally, a preliminary analysis indicates that small changes in rates of women who obtain prenatal care could outweigh the benefit of early detection of HIV infection.[17]

Economic Analyses

There are relatively few analyses of the cost-effectiveness of HIV screening of women (see Table 1). Brandeau and colleagues performed a cost-benefit analysis of voluntary screening of women of childbearing age.[59,60] The authors used a dynamic model of the HIV epidemic that assesses the effect of changes in behavior on the course of the epidemic. The study was performed before the effect of zidovudine on perinatal HIV transmission was known and therefore did not consider reduction in perinatal HIV transmission as a potential benefit from detecting HIV in women of childbearing age. The study defines women at high risk as those who inject drugs; women at medium risk as those who had many sex partners

Table 1. Selected Economic Evaluations of HIV Screening

Population/ Reference	Quantitative Outcome[a]	Conclusion	Comment
Women			
Brandeu[59,60]	Net savings = $431 to $12,132 per high-risk woman screened	Screening is cost-beneficial in medium-and high risk groups	Benefit from reduced transmission due to zidovudine not evaluated; quality of life not considered
Lewis[62]	Screening would reduce cost by $175,500 per year	Reduction in treatment costs for newborns outweighs the costs screening and treatment	Assumed that no HIV-positive women would be identified prior to screening, and that all would accept treatment with zidovudine
Wilfert[2]	Save $320 million per year worldwide	Screening and treatment with zidovudine are cost saving	Did not include all incremental costs associated with medical care for women with HIV; overestimated the lifetime cost of treatment of an HIV infected child
Mauskopf[64]	Screening pregnant women is cost saving if prevalence ≥ 0.46%	Offering zidovudine to women known to be HIV-positive reduces health-care expenditures; cost effectiveness of screening varies according to HIV prevalence	A comprehensive evaluation of screening and treatment with zidovudine in U.S.
Mansergh[6%]	$1115 to $3748 per HIV infection averted	Program is inexpensive by standards of developed countries, but costs may exceed available resources in certain sub-Saharan countries	Evaluates screening and short-course treatment with zidovudine in sub-Saharan Africa; efficacy of short-course treatment not demonstrated but under study
Patients			
Lurie[66]	Detection of HIV in inpatients costs $16,104 per case identified	Screening to prevent transmission to HCW costs $753 million per case averted; nonmedical factors (e.g., discrimination) should be resolved before screening implemented	Estimated specificity for HIV tests lower than that in other analyses (see text)
Henry[71]	$4,530 to $9,060 per case identified	Costs vary according to HIV seroprevalence	Included only test costs
Harris[72]	$14,550 per case identified	Hospitals are an efficient and practical setting for HIV testing	Excluded treatment costs

Study	Cost estimate	Conclusion	Comments/assumptions
McCarthy[67]	$11,000 to $29,000 per life-year gained	Screening should be offered routinely to all persons in defined populations where the seroprevalence is 0.5%	Assumed benefit of early medical therapy of 2.3 years; used 1990 Medicaid reimbursements as cost estimates, which are lower than certain other estimates
Owens[68]	$47,200 per year of life saved when prevalence = 1%; see Tables 2 and 3	Effect of screening on quality of life and risk behavior is important determinant of cost effectiveness	Evidence about the effect of screening on quality of life and on frequency of risk behaviors is limited
Physicians			
Gerberding[90]	$287,000 per health-care worker identified in first year	No definitive recommendation	Included only direct cost to the hospital
Russo[91]	Expected annual costs $780,000 outweighed by expected annual benefit ($58,080–$83,635)	Hospital screening program would be wasteful expenditure	Extensions of analysis by Gerberding
Chavey[92]	Cost of $9.2 million per transmission prevented	Screening to prevent transmission to patients is an expensive use of health-care resources	Benefit to screened surgeons or their sexual partners was not examined; only direct costs were included
Yawn[93]	$50 million per HIV infection prevented	Policy depends on HIV seroprevalence, sensitivity and specificity of tests, and public policy	Did not consider induced costs of practice restriction
Sell[94]	$139,571 (dentists) to $899,336 per transmission prevented (surgeons)	Neither voluntary nor mandatory screening is cost-effective	Did not consider induced cost of screening; assumed that 90% of infected physicians would volunteer for screening and that 90% of the physicians identified would restrict their practice accordingly
Phillips[95]	$81,000 cost savings to $29.8 million expenditures per patient infection averted	Results sensitive to seroprevalence and transmission risk; study neither justified nor precluded mandatory testing	Medium-risk scenario ($1,208,000 per HIV infection averted) may be most representative; high-risk scenario assumes HIV prevalence of 1%
Schulman[96]	Reduction of 0.05 to 3.1 transmissions per year	Screening surgeons would be costly	Did not perform formal cost-effectiveness analysis
Owens[76]	$458,000 per year of life saved (one-time screening); $1,098,000 (annual screening)	Cost per year of life saved exceeds that for commonly accepted interventions	Included benefit to patients, surgeons, and sexual partners of surgeons; included costs from loss of productivity of surgeons

[a]See individual studies for range of estimates and assumptions underlying the estimates. Estimates from different studies are not directly comparable because of differences in methods, populations, and assumptions.

or who were sexual partners of men who were bisexual or injected drugs; and women at low risk of infection as any who were not at high or medium risk. The authors evaluated screening under a variety of assumptions about behavioral response to screening. In the most pessimistic scenario, they assumed that women reduced childbearing by 12% and sexual and needle-sharing contacts by 5%. The most optimistic scenario assumed corresponding values of 50% and 70%, respectively. The authors found that screening produced net savings per woman screened from $431 (pessimistic scenario) to $12,132 (optimistic scenario) in high-risk groups; from $37 (pessimistic scenario) to $2718 (optimistic scenario) in medium- and high-risk groups; and −$35 (pessimistic scenario) to $152 (optimistic scenario) in all risk groups.

This study has several important findings. First, the benefits of screening outweigh the costs in medium- and high-risk groups, even with modest changes in behavior. Second, the importance of the behavioral response to screening is highlighted by the variation by a factor of 30 in the quantitative results, based on varying assumptions about changes in behavior. In a subsequent analysis that further highlighted the importance of screening-induced changes in behavior, the authors showed that relapse to high-risk behavior attenuated the benefits of a screening program.[47] Finally, the authors find that the primary benefit of a screening program for women comes not from reduction in perinatal transmission but rather from reduced transmission to sexual and needle-sharing partners. Whether this finding would still hold given the efficacy of zidovudine in reducing perinatal transmission is not known. The study did not include an analysis of the effect of screening on quality of life. In addition, the risk groups, as defined, may be difficult to use clinically because women may not report or be aware of their risk behavior.[61] However, the study found that screening was cost beneficial if the prevalence of HIV was 0.14% or greater and if women reduced their sexual contacts by 13% or greater. Thus, identification of women with specific high-risk behavior may not be necessary to justify screening and counseling in populations in which the prevalence of HIV is sufficiently high.

Subsequent to the finding that zidovudine reduces perinatal transmission, several investigators have examined the costs and benefits of HIV screening of women. Two studies that performed limited economic analyses provided preliminary evidence that screening and treatment with zidovudine could reduce health-care costs. A cost analysis of a voluntary screening program in an urban obstetric practice in which the prevalence of HIV was approximately 0.3% found that the savings from prevention of transmission of HIV to newborns outweigh the costs of a screening and treatment program.[62] However, the authors assumed that none of the women with HIV would be identified prior to screening and that all would accept treatment with zidovudine. These assumptions result in a favorable estimate of the benefit of screening. The authors do not indicate whether screening would save money if less than 100% of women accept zidovudine treatment. In a second study, Wilfert indicated that screening and treatment of pregnant women with zidovudine would be cost saving (test expenditures would be offset by savings in treatment expenditures), but the analysis does not include all incremental costs associated with medical care for women identified with HIV and estimates the lifetime cost of treatment of an HIV infected child as $280,000.[2] This cost estimate is over two times as high as recently published estimates.[63,64] Therefore, this study may underestimate the cost of a screening program and substantially overestimate the monetary savings from preventing HIV transmission. Although each of these studies suggest that screening is cost saving, neither provide a definitive analysis.

Two studies that comprehensively evaluate the costs and benefits of screening and

treatment of HIV-positive pregnant women highlight important differences in those programs in industrialized countries compared with developing countries. Mauskopf and colleagues evaluated a hypothetical program to screen and treat HIV-positive pregnant women
in the United States.[64] Their study considers screening costs, treatment costs, willingness to
be tested for HIV, willingness to be treated with HIV, and pregnancy-termination rates. They
found that an HIV screening and treatment program would reduce health-care expenditures
if the prevalence of HIV in the screened population were 0.46% or greater. This finding is
striking because the study does not include an economic valuation of the benefit from
reduced transmission (i.e., infections averted) a factor that would make the program even
more favorable. Screening and comprehensive counseling of all pregnant women (estimated prevalence 0.17%) would cost $154,461 to $184,423 per HIV infection averted.
However, if all women were screened but only those women in high-risk populations or
those whose HIV test was positive received counseling, the program would result in net
savings of $18 million to $31 million. A study of HIV screening and short-course zidovudine
treatment for HIV-positive pregnant women in sub-Saharan Africa estimated that the
program would cost $1115 to $3748 per HIV infection prevented.[65] The estimated cost per
HIV infection averted was lower than the corresponding estimate for a program in the
United States, in part, because the short-course of zidovudine is less expensive and because
the prevalence of HIV infection among pregnant women was estimated as 12.5%. Although
such a program would be inexpensive by the standards of a developed country, the costs
may exceed the resources available in developing countries.[65]

Summary and Implications

Analyses performed before the finding that zidovudine therapy reduces perinatal
transmission indicate that screening women of childbearing age is cost beneficial, at least
for women whose behavior puts them at medium to high risk for HIV. Analyses performed
subsequently provide further evidence that screening and treatment with zidovudine is cost-
effective or cost-saving in pregnant women. No current studies have evaluated both the
benefit from counseling-induced reduction in HIV transmission to sexual partners and the
benefit from reduced HIV transmission to newborns. Thus, an HIV screening program may
be more economically favorable than these individual studies suggest. None of the available
studies evaluated the effect of early detection on quality of life, a potentially important
determinant of the cost effectiveness of screening (see later sections). Finally, each of the
analyses depend on assumptions about women's behavioral response to screening. The
available empiric evidence is limited. Rigorously designed studies of the behavioral response to screening and counseling would provide a foundation for further assessing the
cost-effectiveness of screening in women of childbearing age. Given this caveat, the
available evidence suggests that an intervention that engenders substantial reductions in
high-risk behavior or facilitates treatment of HIV-positive pregnant women with zidovudine would profoundly improve health outcomes and reduce health-related expenditures.

SCREENING OF PATIENTS

The CDC currently recommends that acute-care hospitals and associated clinics offer
voluntary HIV screening to inpatients and outpatients aged 15 to 54 years, if the prevalence

of HIV in the patient population is 1% or greater.[3] The rationale for this CDC guideline is that early detection of HIV would allow early medical intervention and counseling about high-risk behavior that transmits HIV. A second reason to screen has been offered by several authors: to protect health-care workers from exposure to HIV. We examine studies that evaluate both reasons to screen. The behavioral questions with respect to screening of patients are similar to those discussed previously.

Economic Analyses

Several analyses estimate the expenditures per case of HIV infection identified for hospital-based HIV screening programs (Table 1). Lurie and colleagues estimated that screening inpatients would result in identifying 168,874 infections and expenditures of $16,104 per case per year identified, when the prevalence of HIV is 1.0%.[66] Appropriately, this estimate includes the cost of early medical therapy for people identified with HIV. The authors calculated that if screening were limited to populations in which the HIV prevalence is 1% or greater, that 5400 people per year would be falsely identified with HIV, based on an assumption that the specificity of the sequence of HIV diagnostic tests is 0.999. Other authors[67,68] have assumed substantially higher specificity for the sequence of tests, as reflected in high-quality screening programs,[69,70] and therefore have calculated much lower rates of false-positive tests. Lurie and colleagues[66] identified HIV prevalence among the screened population as one of the most important determinants of the efficiency of screening, as have other analyses.[67,68] A cost analysis at a hospital whose population had an HIV prevalence of approximately 1% estimated the cost of identifying a new HIV infection at $4,530 to $9,060, exclusive of counseling or treatment costs.[71] A similar study estimated expenditures of $14,550 per case identified, exclusive of treatment costs.[72] Because treatment costs should be included in analyzing the economic implications of a screening program, the estimates by Lurie and colleagues are more representative of actual economic costs of screening.

Lurie and colleagues also evaluated the cost effectiveness of screening inpatients for the purpose of preventing HIV transmission to health-care workers. They estimated that such a program would prevent 3.6 HIV infections per year at a cost of $2.7 billion, or $753 million per infection averted.[66] Therefore, they concluded that screening inpatients for HIV should not be undertaken to prevent transmission to health-care workers.

Other analyses have evaluated the cost of screening inpatients in terms of life-years saved, or QALYs gained.[67,68] These analyses used Markov models to estimate the number of years of life saved by screening (in contrast to other approaches that estimate the number of HIV infections averted). In a Markov model, a cohort of patients is tracked over time in a mathematical simulation.[73–76] These models estimate the health outcomes in and expenditures for the cohort; incorporate progression of disease from asymptomatic infection to AIDS to death; and can incorporate adjustments for quality of life for health states associated with morbidity. By estimating the health outcomes and costs with and without screening, investigators can use such models to calculate the marginal cost-effectiveness of HIV screening programs. McCarthy and colleagues evaluated HIV screening in the general population and concluded that HIV screening cost approximately $19,000 per life-year saved (inflated to 1993 dollars) in populations in which the prevalence of HIV is 0.5%.[67] Although their analysis did not specifically address inpatient screening, it implies that screening would be cost-effective in hospitals whose patients have a prevalence of HIV of

0.5% or greater. Of note, these investigators assumed that early medical intervention extended life by 2.3 years, an estimate that may be optimistic given current evidence. Their analysis did not address the effect of screening on the rate of transmitting HIV.

Our group of investigators used a Markov model to evaluate two additional factors not addressed in previous studies of HIV screening in acute-care settings: the effect of screening on quality of life and the benefit from reduced transmission of HIV to sexual partners of patients identified with HIV.[68] To assess the effect of screening on quality of life, we used quality adjustment for HIV health states based on the time-trade-off technique.[77,78] The time-trade-off technique converts a decrement in quality of life into a decrement in length of life. Therefore, if identification with HIV lowers quality of life, then the benefit of longer life expectancy due to early medical intervention is attenuated. Because assessments by patients of quality of life based on the time-trade-off technique were not available, our assessments of quality of life were based on a survey of 128 physicians.[78] To assess the benefit from reduced transmission of HIV, we assumed that testing and counseling reduce sexual transmission of HIV by 15%, and we examined a range of values in sensitivity analyses.[68]

We estimated that an HIV screening program, implemented according to the CDC guidelines, would identify 110,000 case of HIV infection (based on estimates by Janssen and colleagues[79]) during the first year of screening, and would prevent another 565 HIV infections in sexual partners of HIV-positive patients identified through screening if all eligible patients participate in screening (see Table 2). Incremental treatment costs for patients identified through screening were $2 billion for patients identified during the first year of implementing the screening program. The substantial cost of additional treatment illustrates the importance of including such costs in an analysis of screening. If, as is likely, less than 100% of eligible patients participate in a screening program, the number of cases identified and the costs would be reduced proportionally. For example, if 50% of eligible patients participate in screening, both the number of people identified and the costs of the program would be reduced by 50%, if the prevalence of HIV in the group that declined was equal to that in the group that accepted screening.

The cost effectiveness of screening varies with the prevalence of HIV in the screened

Table 2. Health and Economic Outcomes of HIV Screening in Acute-Care Settings[a]

Outcome	
Health outcomes	
Number of people screened[b]	2,998,000
Number of people identified with HIV infection[b]	110,000
Number of infections prevented for sexual partners	565
Life-years gained by patients[c]	50,500
Life-years gained for sexual parters of patients by preventing HIV infection	13,500
Economic outcomes ($)	
Total cost of screening[d]	170,886,000
Cost of early treatment for people identified with HIV infections[e]	2,000,000,000
Total costs saved by preventing infection of sexual partners	15,700,000

[a]Modified with permission from Ref. 68; copyright 1996, American Medical Association.
[b]As estimated by Janssen and colleagues.[79]
[c]Life years are discounted at 5%.
[d]First-year costs are based on testing and counseling costs of $57 per person.
[e]Net present value of incremental lifetime medical costs for people identified during the first year of the program. Calculated with the assumption that 80% of people identified are asymptomatic, and 20% are symptomatic.

Table 3. Cost Effectiveness of HIV Screening in Acute-Care Settings[a,b]

	Benefit Only to Persons Screened		Benefit to Persons Screened and to Their Sexual Partners[c]	
Prevalence (%)	Cost per Year of Life Saved ($)	Cost per Quality-Adjusted Year of Life Saved[d] ($)	Cost per Year of Life Saved ($)	Cost per Quality-Adjusted Year of Life Saved[c] ($)
0.5	59,700	117,300	46,400	70,700
1.0	47,200	92,400	36,600	55,500
4.0	37,800	73,800	29,200	44,200

[a]Modified with permission from Ref. 68; copyright 1996, American Medical Association.
[b]Assumes that all people identified with human immunodeficiency virus (HIV) receive care.
[c]Calculated assuming that one sexual partner is at risk for HIV infection at any given time.
[d]The quality adjustments needed to calculate quality-adjusted life-years saved were based on a survey of 128 physicians.[78] Quality adjustments for the health states: asymptomatic HIV infection, 0.9; symptomatic HIV infection, 0.42; and acquired immunodeficiency syndrome (AIDS), 0.17.

population (see Table 3). In a population with an HIV prevalence of 1%, screening required expenditures of $47,200 per year of life saved. As noted in Table 3, screening is less cost-effective if the analysis includes the effect of screening on quality of life and is more cost effective if the analysis includes the benefit from reduced transmission of HIV. The effect of screening on quality of life is an important determinant of the cost-effectiveness of screening (see Figure 1).

Our estimate of the cost effectiveness of screening (without considering quality of life or reduced transmission) was higher than that of McCarthy and colleagues (for example, $59,700 compared with $19,000 per year of life saved at a prevalence of 0.5%). The primary explanation for the difference is that our analysis assumes that early medical intervention prolongs life by approximately 1 year, rather than by 2.3 years, and that McCarthy and colleagues use Medicaid treatment costs, which were lower than our estimated costs.

Summary and Implications

Is HIV screening of patients cared for in acute-care settings cost-effective? From a policy perspective, it is difficult to interpret studies that calculate only the cost per case of HIV detected. We cannot compare these studies to evaluations of other health interventions. For example, how does the cost effectiveness of a screening program that costs $16,104 per case of HIV identified compare with a breast cancer screening program that costs, say, $45,000 per quality-adjusted, life-year saved?[15] Because the metrics of the evaluations are different, the cost-effectiveness of the programs are difficult to compare. Of the studies that use estimated expenditures per case of HIV identified, Lurie and colleagues provide the most complete analysis. McCarthy and colleagues use an estimate for the effectiveness of early medical intervention that may overstate the benefit from screening, but as anti-retroviral therapy improves, their estimate may become more realistic. Our analysis indicates that, without considering quality of life or reduced HIV transmission, the cost-effectiveness of inpatient screening in populations with a prevalence of 1% or greater falls within the realm of interventions that clinicians often consider cost-effective. Our study raises questions about the effect of screening on quality of life and about the benefit from

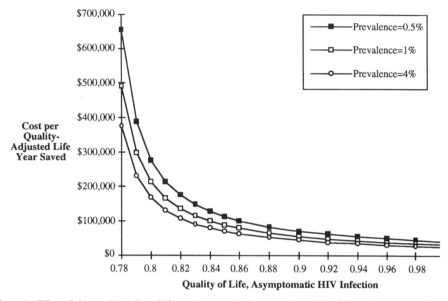

Figure 1. Effect of changes in quality of life on the cost-effectiveness of screening. Effect of the quality of life on the cost-effectiveness of an HIV screening program. The horizontal axis shows the quality adjustment for the health state asymptomatic HIV-infection. A quality adjustment of 0 indicates that the health state was judged equivalent to death. A quality adjustment of 1 indicates that the health state was judged equivalent to normal health. Estimates of the cost-effectiveness are shown for three different prevalences of HIV in the screened population and include both the benefit to individuals who have HIV infection and the benefit to their sexual partners. Reprinted with permission from Ref. 68; copyright 1996, American Medical Association.

reduced transmission of HIV but does not provide definitive answers. How identifying people with HIV affects their quality of life has not been studied adequately. If detecting HIV through screening reduces quality of life, the cost-effectiveness of screening declines substantially. The quality-of-life adjustments we used were based on assessments by physicians.[78] A study of the experiences of patients identified through screening would be helpful. In addition, our analysis indicate that even modest reductions in high-risk behavior could provide a significant improvement in the cost-effectiveness of a screening program. The degree to which such reductions occur requires further documentation. Thus, we can tentatively assert that the cost-effectiveness of HIV screening in acute-care settings is comparable to that of other frequently performed interventions, but a definitive answer awaits further study of screening-induced changes in quality of life and in risk behavior.

SCREENING OF HEALTH-CARE WORKERS

In 1991, a young woman who was dying from AIDS presented an impassioned plea during a hearing before Congress. She asked the legislators to take steps to prevent transmission of HIV from health-care workers to patients.[80] This remarkable Congressional hearing occurred because investigators at the CDC had concluded that the woman had been infected with HIV during an invasive dental procedure.[81] After further study, the CDC concluded that the same dentist had transmitted HIV to five additional people.[82–86] These cases led to several proposals to reduce the risk of transmission of HIV to patients, including, at one extreme, proposals for mandatory screening of physicians and jail terms for physicians who infected patients.[87,88] The current CDC guidelines are substantially more moderate and recommend that medical organizations identify exposure-prone procedures; that physicians who perform such procedures determine whether they are infected with HIV; and that physicians who are infected with HIV refrain from performing exposure-prone procedures, unless they have explicit permission of local authorities.[89] Although current guidelines do not call for mandatory HIV screening of physicians, these proposals have led investigators to evaluate whether screening providers for HIV would be an effective and cost-effective policy to reduce HIV transmission from provider to patient.

Economic Analyses

Investigators have evaluated the costs and benefits of screening providers in various populations and have used different analytic approaches (Table 1). Gerberding evaluated a program to screen physicians, dentists, nurses, and paramedics and to prohibit HIV-infected providers from performing invasive procedures.[90] She estimated that the program would cost $287,000 per health-care worker identified with HIV. This analysis included costs associated with restricting the practices of HIV-infected providers and direct costs to the hospital. An extension of this analysis to a cost-benefit framework concluded that the expected annual costs of screening ($780,000) far outweighed the expected annual benefit ($58,080 to $83,635), and therefore that screening would waste scarce resources.[91] Chavey and colleagues used a mathematical model to evaluate a hypothetical program to test all health-care workers in their university-based teaching hospital and concluded that each case of HIV transmission averted would cost $9,177,615.[92] Their analysis did not assess the benefits to health-care workers from detecting their HIV or other potential benefits, such as reduced transmission to the health-care workers' sexual partners. Another analysis of a mandatory screening program calculated costs of $50 million per HIV infection averted.[93] That analysis, however, includes costs of testing both patients and all health-care workers. Sell and colleagues evaluated theoretical voluntary and mandatory screening of programs and concluded that neither were "convincingly" cost effective.[94]

Phillips and colleagues comprehensively assessed a program to screen all physicians and dentists. They concluded that a mandatory program should not be implemented unless further evidence of cost-effectiveness was gathered.[95] These authors found that costs and benefits of HIV screening vary substantially based on model assumptions, particularly about seroprevalence of HIV among physicians and about the rate of transmission. However, they estimate that the value of a prevented HIV infection would have to exceed $20 million if the benefits of screening were to outweigh the costs. This calculation includes as a cost of the program the losses of productivity associated with restricting the practice of providers. Schulman and colleagues use a mathematical simulation model to estimate that, in the absence of a screening program, surgeons would transmit HIV between 0.5 and 36.9 times per year in the US, depending on assumptions about HIV prevalence among surgeons and rates of transmission.[96] They concluded that the cost of a surgeon-screening program would be high, but they did not perform a formal cost-effectiveness analysis.

Although none of these studies suggest that screening health-care workers would provide an efficient method for reducing HIV transmission to patients, several questions remain unanswered. First, because individual studies often emphasize a specific aspect of the screening program, such as the perspective of a particular hospital, the studies do not include all the potential benefit from an HIV screening program for health-care workers. Such a program could have three potential benefits: reduced transmission of HIV to patients, early medical therapy for health-care worker whose HIV infection is detected through the screening program, and reduced transmission of HIV to sexual partners of the health-care workers. Studies that omit these potential benefits from an economic analysis could underestimate the cost effectiveness of screening. Secondly, the studies do not consider the effect of screening on quality of life. As we noted previously, the effect of screening on quality of life is an important determinant of the cost-effectiveness of screening. However, because inclusion of quality of life probably would result in a less favorable economic evaluation, it is unlikely that considering quality of life would change the conclusions of the studies (even without assessing the effect of screening on quality of life, the studies indicate that screening health-care workers is economically inefficient). Finally, none of the studies estimate the cost-effectiveness of screening in terms of dollars spent per year of life saved. Thus, policy makers and clinicians could not easily compare the cost-effectiveness of a screening program for health-care workers to that of other interventions.

To address these questions, our group used a Markov-based analysis to evaluate the cost-effectiveness of a mandatory HIV screening program for surgeons.[76] Because surgeons perform more invasive procedures than other health-care workers, screening for HIV to prevent transmission to patients probably would be more cost-effective in this group than in any other. We included the benefit to patients (reduced transmission), the benefit to surgeons (early medical therapy), and the benefit to surgeons' sexual partners (reduced transmission). We had previously estimated the probability of HIV transmission during an invasive procedure and the associated loss of life expectancy for the patient.[75] The analysis assumes that surgeons identified with HIV would no longer be able to perform invasive procedures but could continue medical practice.

We estimated that a one-time, national screening program for surgeons would identify 137 surgeons with HIV, prevent 4.3 infections in patients, and 0.9 infections in sexual partners of the identified surgeons. Preventing these infections would result in gains of 21.2 years for all patients, 69.4 years for the identified surgeons, and 28.3 years for the sexual partners of surgeons (all health outcomes were discounted at 5%). We estimated the direct medical costs of screening at $8,074,000, the cost of treatment for the surgeons identified with HIV at $2,976,000, and the cost of lost wages to the surgeons at $43,638,000. Of note, the largest benefit from screening surgeons for HIV resulted from early medical intervention for the surgeons (69.4 life-years saved), rather than from preventing transmission of HIV to patients (21.2 life-years saved) or to sexual partners (28.3 life-years saved).

We calculated that the cost-effectiveness of a mandatory HIV screening program for surgeons as $458,000 per life-year saved for a program that screens each surgeon once and is $597,000 or $1,098,000 per life-year saved for a program that screens surgeons every 10 years or every year, respectively. When we included the effect of screening on quality of life, the program cost more than $1,400,000 per quality-adjusted year of life saved, regardless of the screening frequency.

An important factor in evaluating the cost-effectiveness of an HIV screening program for health-care workers is the induced cost from lost productivity of health-care workers who are restricted from performing invasive procedures. We believe, as do other investigators,[91] that these are legitimate economic costs of a policy that prevents health-care workers from delivering care commensurate with their training. We estimated the loss of productivity from HIV-infected surgeons as the change in income after restriction of their practice. We assumed that the surgeons' salaries would decrease from the average salary of a surgeon to the average salary of an internist.[76] However, because certain analysts would exclude such costs, we recalculated the cost-effectiveness of a program to screen surgeons by assuming no induced costs from lost productivity. Given this assumption, a one-time screening program costs $91,000 per life-year saved, a program that screens every 10 years costs $122,000 per life-year saved, and an annual screening program costs $539,000 per life-year saved. Thus, even after we excluded the surgeon's lost wages, the screening program remains expensive.

Summary and Implications

Although there is widespread agreement that providers should take all reasonable precautions to prevent transmission of HIV to patients, economic evaluations of programs to identify HIV-infected providers and to restrict these workers from performing invasive procedures consistently indicate that such programs would realize small benefits at a high price. The studies that we reviewed used different methods and examined different populations, but none found that screening providers for HIV would be cost-effective, given the information currently available about provider-to-patient transmission rates. On the contrary, the studies suggested that such screening programs would result in expenditures per year of life saved that substantially exceed those of commonly accepted interventions. These studies were based on the best available estimates of the rates of transmission of HIV to patients during invasive procedures. Continued surveillance to ensure that future transmission rates do not exceed those observed to date appears warranted. Unless such surveillance reveals higher transmission rates than observed previously, we can conclude that implementing screening programs for health-care workers to prevent HIV transmission to patients would be an inefficient use of public resources.

CONCLUSIONS

In this chapter, I sought to evaluate critically the published economic evaluations of HIV screening in women, patients, and health-care workers. The review of the published studies of screening of women suggests that such programs are likely to be cost-effective or cost saving in women whose behavior places them at medium or high risk of acquiring HIV. The question of whether to screen women has assumed new urgency since the finding that use of zidovudine during pregnancy reduces transmission of HIV to newborns. Economic evaluations of HIV screening of pregnant women suggest that such programs would be economically favorable, particularly if counseling could be performed inexpensively. However, recent evidence indicates that even in women who are known to have HIV, not all receive zidovudine.[97] This finding highlights a priority for future research: study of interventions, including behavioral interventions, to ensure that women identified with HIV receive care that improves their health and reduces transmission. Substantial questions also remain about the effectiveness of screening in inducing reductions in risk behavior and how detecting HIV will affect women's decisions regarding childbearing. There is a dearth of rigorously controlled studies of these important behaviors. Randomized trials in situations where they are appropriate, ethical, and feasible would be helpful.[98]

The cost-effectiveness of HIV screening of inpatients and outpatients in acute-care settings, as recommended by the CDC, depends on the prevalence of HIV in the population screened, on whether screened HIV-positive patients reduce behavior likely to transmit HIV, and on how detecting HIV affects quality of life. Exclusive of the effect of screening on quality of life and of the public-health benefit of screening, the cost effectiveness of screening at the CDC-designated threshold seroprevalence of 1% falls within the range of other medical interventions commonly performed. Unanswered questions include how screening affects quality of life and to what extent testing and counseling reduce high-risk behavior in this population. Screening patients to reduce HIV transmission to providers is not warranted, based on current data.[66]

We found that screening surgeons to reduce transmission of HIV to patients requires expenditures of $458,000 to $1,098,000 per year of life saved, depending on the frequency of screening, when we considered the losses of productivity associated with restricting surgeons' practices. Screening other health-care workers would likely be less cost-effective than screening surgeons. The economic evaluations that we reviewed suggest that the costs of screening programs for health-care workers to prevent transmission to patients substantially exceeds the range of commonly accepted screening interventions.

ACKNOWLEDGMENT. Dr. Owens is supported by a Career Development Award from the VA Health Services Research and Development Service.

REFERENCES

1. Working Group on HIV Testing of Pregnant Women and Newborns. HIV infection, pregnant women, and newborns. *JAMA* 1990; 264:2416–2420.
2. Wilfert CM. Mandatory screening of pregnant women for the human immunodeficiency virus. *Clin Infect Dis* 1994; 19:664–666.
3. CDC. Recommendations for HIV testing services for inpatients and outpatients in acute-care hospital settings and technical guidance on HIV counseling, *MMWR* 1993; 42:1–6.
4. Holtgrave DR, Valdiserri RO, Gerber AR, Hinman AR. Human immunodeficiency virus counseling, testing, referral, and partner notification services: A cost-benefit analysis. *Arch Intern Med* 1993; 153:1225–1230.
5. Farnham PG, Gorsky RD, Holtgrave DR, Jones WK, Guinan ME. Counseling and testing for HIV prevention: Costs, effects, and cost-effectiveness of more rapid screening tests. *Public Health Rep* 1996; 111:44–53.
6. Holtgrave DR, Valdiserri RO, West, GA. Quantitative economic evaluations of HIV-related prevention and treatment services: A review. *Risk: Health, Safety & Environment* 1994; 5:29–47.
7. Guinan ME, Farnham PG, Holtgrave DR. Estimating the value of preventing a human immunodeficiency virus infection. *Am J Preventive Med* 1994; 10:1–4.
8. Holtgrave DR, Qualls NL. Threshold analysis and programs for prevention of HIV infection. *Med Decision Making* 1995; 15:311–317.
9. Freedberg KA, Alpher JL, Seage GR, et al. The cost effectiveness of preventing AIDS complications [abstract]. *J Gen Intern Med* 1996;11(Suppl. 1):58.
10. Laupacis A, Feeny D, Detsky A, Tugwell P. How attractive does a new technology have to be to warrant adoption and utilization? Tentative guidelines for using clinical and economic evaluations. *Can Med Assoc J* 1992; 146:473–481.
11. Laupacis A, Feeny D, Detsky A, Tugwell P. Tentative guidelines for using clinical and economic evaluations revisited. *Can Med Assoc J* 1993; 148:927–929.

12. Naylor C, Williams J, Basinski A, Goel V. Technology assessment and cost-effectiveness analysis: Misguided guidelines? *Can Med Assoc J* 1993; 1 48:921–924.
13. Gafni A, Brich S. Guidelines for the adoption of new technologies: A prescription for uncontrolled growth in expenditures and how to avoid the problem. *Can Med Assoc J* 1993; 148:913–917.
14. Russell L. Some of the tough decisions required by a national health plan. *Science* 1989; 246:892–896.
15. Eddy D. Screening for breast cancer. *Ann Intern Med* 1989; 111:389–399.
16. Eddy D. Screening for cervical cancer. *Ann Intern Med* 1990; 113:214–226.
17. Nakchbandi IA, Longenecker JC, Ricksecker MA, Latta RA, Day HJ, Smith DG. Should HIV testing be mandatory for pregnant women? [abstract]. *J Gen Intern Med* 1996; 11(Suppl. 1):53.
18. Fleming PL, Ward JW, Morgan MW, Buckler JW, Hu D, et al. Mandatory HIV reporting: Characteristics of adults reported with HIV compared to AIDS in the United States. *Proceedings of the Ninth Annual International Conference on AIDS/IV STD World Congress, June 1993*. Berlin: International AIDS Society and the World Health Organization. 1993;1:[abstract WS-C17-2].
19. Wortley PM, Chu SY, Diaz T, et al. HIV testing patterns: Where, why, and when were persons with AIDS tested for HIV. *AIDS* 1995; 9:487–492.
20. Fischl MA, Dickinson GM, La Voie L. Safety and efficacy of sulfamethoxazole and trimethoprim chemoprophylaxis for *pneumocystis carinii* pneumonia in AIDS. *JAMA* 1988;259: 1185–1189.
21. Fischl MA, Richman DD, Grieco MH, et al. The efficacy of azidothymidine (AZT) in the treatment of patients with AIDS and AIDS-related complex. *N Engl J Med* 1987; 317:185–191.
22. Fischl MA, Richman DD, Hansen N. The safety and efficacy of zidovudine (AZT) in the treatment of subjects with mildly symptomatic human immunodeficiency virus type 1 (HIV) infection. *Ann Intern Med* 1990;112: 727–737.
23. Volberding PA, Lagakos SW, Koch MA, et al. Zidovudine in asymptomatic human immunodeficiency virus infection: A controlled trial in persons with fewer than 500 CD4-positive cells per cubic millimeter. *N Engl J Med* 1990; 322:941–949.
24. Hamilton JD, Hartigan PM, Simberkoff MS, et al. A controlled trial of early versus late treatment with zidovudine in symptomatic human immunodeficiency virus infection. Results of the Veterans Affairs Cooperative Study. *N Engl J Med* 1992; 326:437–443.
25. Cooper D, Gatell J, Kroon S, et al. Zidovudine in persons with asymptomatic HIV infection and CD4+ cell counts greater than 400 per cub millimeter. *N Engl J Med* 1993; 329:297–303.
26. Concorde Coordinating Committee, Concorde: MRC/ANRS randomised double-blind controlled trial of immediate and deferred zidovudine in symptom-free HIV infection. *Lancet* 1994; 343:871–881.
27. Volberding P, Lagakos S, Grimes J, et al. The duration of zidovudine benefit in persons with asymptomatic HIV infections. *JAMA* 1994; 272:437–442.
28. Graham NMH, Zeger SL, Park LP, et al. The effects on survival of early treatment of human immunodeficiency virus infection. *N Engl J Med* 1992; 326:1037–1042.
29. Vella S, Giuliano M, Dally S, et al. Long-term follow-up of zidovudine therapy in asymptomatic HIV infection: Results of a multicenter cohort study. *JAIDS* 1994; 7:31–38.
30. Graham NMH, Hoover DR, Park LP, et al. Survival in HIV-infected patients who have received zidovudine: Comparison of combination therapy with sequential monotherapy and continued zidovudine monotherapy. *Ann Intern Med* 1996; 124:1031–1038.
31. Staszewski S, Loveday C, Picazo JJ, et al. Safety and efficacy of lamivudine-zidovudine combination therapy in zidovudine-experienced patients. A randomized controlled comparison with zidovudine monotherapy. *JAMA* 1996; 276:111–117.
32. Katlama C, Ingrand D, Loveday C, et al. Safety and efficacy of lamivudine-zidovudine combination therapy in antiretroviral-naive patients. A randomized controlled comparison with zidovudine montherapy. *JAMA* 1996; 276:118–125.
33. D'Aquila RT, Hughes MD, Johnson VA, et al. Nevirapine, zidovudine, and didanosine compared with zidovudine and didanosine in patients with HIV-1 infection. *Ann Intern Med* 1996;124:1019–1030.
34. Ho DD, Neuman AU, Perelson AS, et al. Rapid turnover of plasma virions and CD4 lymphocytes in HIV-1 infection. *Nature* 1995;373:123–126.
35. Wei X, Ghozh SK, Taylor ME, et al. Viral dynamics in human immunodeficiency virus type 1 infection. *Nature* 1995;373: 117–122.
36. Havlir DV, Richman DD. Viral dynamics of HIV: Implications for drug development and therapeutic strategies. *Ann Intern Med* 1996;124:984–994.
37. Richman DD. HIV therapeutics. *Science* 1996; 272:1886–1888.

38. Collier AC, Coombs RW, Schoenfeld DA, et al. Treatment of human immunodeficiency virus infection virus with saquinavir, zidovudine, and zalcitabine. *N Engl J Med* 1996; 334:1011–1017.

39. Schapiro JM, Winters MA, Stewart F, et al. The effect of high dose saquinavir on viral load and CD4⁺ T-cell counts in HIV-infected patients. *Ann Intern Med* 1996; 124:1039–1050.

40. Carpenter CCJ, Fishl MA, Hammer SM, et al. Antiretroviral therapy for HIV infection in 1996. Recommendation of an international panel. *JAMA* 1996; 276:146–154.

41. Higgins DL, Galavotti C, O'Reilly KR, et al. Evidence for the effects of HIV antibody counseling and testing on risk behaviors. *JAMA* 1991; 266:2419–2429.

42. Wenger NS, Linn LS, Epstein M, Shapiro MF. Reduction of high-risk sexual behavior among heterosexuals undergoing HIV antibody testing: A randomized clinical trial. *Am J Public Health* 1991; 81:1580–1585.

43. Wenger NS, Greenberg JM, Hilborne LH, Kusseling F, Mangotich M, Shapiro MF. Effect of HIV antibody testing and AIDS education on communication about HIV risk and sexual behavior: A randomized, controlled trial in college students. *Ann Intern Med* 1992; 117:905–911.

44. Calsyn DA, Saxon AJ, Freeman G, Whittaker S. Ineffectiveness of AIDS education and HIV antibody testing in reducing high-risk behaviors among injection drug users. *Am J Public Health* 1992; 82:573–575.

45. Vanichseni S, Choopanya K, Des Jarlais DC, et al. HIV testing and sexual behavior among intravenous drug users in Bangkok, Thailand. *J Acquired Immune Defic Syndr* 1992; 5:1119–1123.

46. Stryker J, Coates T, DeCarlo P, Haynes-Sanstad K, Shriver M, Makadon H. Prevention of HIV infection. *JAMA* 1995; 273:1143–1148.

47. Brandeau ML, Owens DK. When women return to risk: Costs and benefits of HIV screening in the presence of relapse. In Kaplan E, Brandeau ML, eds. *Modeling the AIDS Epidemic: Planning, Policy and Prediction.* New York: Raven Press; 1994: pp. 121–136.

48. Ickovics J, Morrill A, Beren S, Walsh U, Rodin J. Limited effects of HIV counseling and testing for women. *JAMA* 1994; 272:443–448.

49. Holtgrave DR, Qualls NL, Curran JW, Valdiserri RO, Guinan ME, Parra WC. An overview of the effectiveness and efficiency of HIV prevention programs. *Public Health Rep* 1995; 110:134–146.

50. CDC. U.S. Public Health Service recommendations for human immunodeficiency virus counseling and voluntary testing for pregnant women. *MMWR* 1995;44:1–15.

51. U.S. Preventive Services Task Force. *Guide to Clinical Preventive Services*, 2nd ed. Baltimore: Williams & Wilkins; 1996: pp. 303–323.

52. Connor E, Sperling R, Gelber R, et al. Reduction of maternal-infant transmission of human immunodeficiency virus type 1 with zidovudine treatment. Pediatric AIDS Clinical Trials Group Protocol 076 Study Group. *N Engl J Med* 1994; 331:1173–1180.

53. CDC. Recommendations of the U.S. Public Health Service task Force on the use of zidovudine to reduce perinatal transmission of human immunodeficiency virus. *MMWR* 1994; 43(RR-11):1–20.

54. Dunn DT, Newell ML, Ades AE, Peckham CS. Risk of human immunodeficiency virus type 1 transmission through breastfeeding. *Lancet* 1992; 340:585–588.

55. Landesman SH, Kalish LA, Burns DN, et al. Obstetrical factors and the transmission of human immunodeficiency virus type 1 from mother to child. *N Engl J Med* 1996; 334:1617–1623.

56. Landers DV, Sweet RL. Reducing mother-to-infant transmission of HIV—the door remains open. *N Engl J Med* 1996; 334:1664–1665.

57. Selwyn PA, Carter RJ, Schoenbaum EE, Robertson VJ, Klein RS, Rogers MF. Knowledge of HIV antibody status and decisions to continue or terminate pregnancy among intravenous drug users. *JAMA* 1989; 261:3567–3571.

58. Johnstone FD, Brettle RP, MacCallum LR, Mok J, Peuthever JF, Burns S. Women's knowledge of their HIV antibody state: Its effect on their decision whether to continue the pregnancy. *Br Med J* 1990;300: v23–24.

59. Brandeau ML, Owens DK, Sox CH, Wachter RW. Screening women of childbearing age for human immunodeficiency virus: A cost-benefit analysis. *Arch Intern Med* 1992; 152:2229–2237.

60. Brandeau ML, Owens DK, Sox CH, Wachter RW. Screening women of childbearing age for human immunodeficiency virus infection: A model-based policy analysis. *Manage Sci* 1993; 39:72–92.

61. Brunswick AF, Aidala A, Dobkin J, Howard J, Titus SP, Banaszak-Holl J. HIV-1 seroprevalence and risk behaviors in urban African-American community cohort. *Am J Public Health* 1993; 83:1390–1394.

62. Lewis R, O'Brien JM, Ray DT, Sibai BM. The impact of initiating a human immunodeficiency virus screening program in an urban obstetric population. *Am J Obstet Gynecol* 1995; 173:1329–1333.

63. Hsia DC, Fleishman JA, East JA, Hellinger FJ. Pediatric human immunodeficiency virus infection. Recent evidence on the utilization and costs of health services. *Arch Pediatr Adolescent Med* 1995; 149:489–496.

64. Mauskopf JA, Paul JE, Wichman DS, White AD, Tilson HH. Economic impact of treatment of HIV-positive pregnant women and their newborns with zidovudine. Implications for screening. *JAMA* 1996; 276:132–138.
65. Mansergh G, Haddix AC, Steketee RW, et al. Cost-effectiveness of short-course zidovudine to prevent perinatal HIV type 1 infection in a sub-Saharan African developing county setting. *JAMA* 1996; 276:139–145.
66. Lurie P, Avins AL, Phillips KA, Kahn JG, Kowe RA, Ciccarone D. The cost-effectiveness of voluntary counseling and testing of hospital inpatients for HIV infection. *JAMA* 1994; 272:1832–1838.
67. McCarthy B, Wong J, Muñoz A, Sonnenberg F. Who should be screened for HIV infection? A cost-effectiveness analysis. *Arch Intern Med* 1993; 153:1107–1116.
68. Owens DK, Nease RF, Harris RA. Cost-effectiveness of HIV screening in acute care settings. *Arch Intern Med* 1996; 156:394–404.
69. Burke DS, Brundage JF, Redfield RR, et al. Measurement of the false positive rate in a screening program for human immunodeficiency virus infections. *N Engl J Med* 1988; 319:961–964.
70. MacDonald KL, Jackson B, Bowman RJ, et al. Performance characteristics of serologic tests for human immunodeficiency virus type-1 (HIV-1) antibody among Minnesota blood donors. *Ann Intern Med* 1989; 110:617–621.
71. Henry K, Campbell S. The potential efficiency of routine HIV testing of hospital patients—data from a CDC sentinel hospital. *Public Health Rep* 1992; 107:138–141.
72. Harris R, Boisaubin E, Salyer P, Semands D. Evaluation of a hospital admission HIV antibody voluntary screening program. *Infect Control Hosp Epidemiol* 1990; 11:628–634.
73. Beck JR, Pauker SG. The Markov process in medical prognosis. *Med Decision Making* 1983; 3:419–458.
74. Sonnenberg FA, Beck JR. Markov models in medical decision making: A practical guide. *Med Decision Making* 1993; 13:322–338.
75. Owens DK, Nease RF. Transmission of human immunodeficiency virus (HIV) infection between physicians and patients: A model-based analysis of risk. In Kaplan E, Brandeau ML, eds. *Modeling the AIDS Epidemic: Planning, Policy and Prediction.* New York: Raven Press; 1994: pp. 153–177.
76. Owens DK, Harris RA, Scott PM, Nease RF. Screening surgeons for human immunodeficiency virus (HIV): A cost-effectiveness analysis. *Ann Intern Med* 1995; 9:641–652.
77. Owens DK, Sox HC. Medical decision making: Probabilistic medical reasoning. In Shortliffe EH, Perreault LE, Fagan LM, Wiederhold G, eds. *Medical Informatics: Computer Applications in Medicine.* Reading MA: Addison-Wesley; 1990; pp. 70–116.
78. Owens DK, Nease RF. Physician beliefs about occupational risk and severity of health states associated with HIV and hepatitis infection. *Proceedings and Abstracts of the Sixth International Conference on AIDS, June 1990.* San Francisco: University of California San Francisco and the World Health Organization 1990; 3:308.
79. Janssen R, St. Louis M, Satten G, et al. HIV infection among patients in U.S. acute care hospitals. Strategies for the counseling and testing of the hospital patients. *N Engl J Med* 1992; 327:445–452.
80. Hilts PJ. AIDS victim urges Congress to enact testing bill. *New York Times.* New York; September 27, 1991:A8.
81. CDC. Possible transmission of human immunodeficiency virus to a patient during an invasive dental procedure. *MMWR* 1990; 39:489–493.
82. CDC. Update: Transmission of HIV infection during an invasive dental procedure—Florida. *MMWR* 1991; 40:21–33.
83. CDC. Update: Investigations of patients who have been treated by HIV-infected health-care workers. *MMWR* 1992; 41:344–346.
84. Ciesielski C, Marianos D, Ou C, et al. Transmission of human immunodeficiency virus in a dental practice. *Ann Intern Med* 1992; 116:798–805.
85. Ou CY, Ciesielski CA, Myers G, et al. Molecular epidemiology of HIV transmission in a dental practice. *Science* 1992; 256:1165–1171.
86. CDC. Update: Investigations of persons treated by HIV-infected health-care workers—United States. *MMWR* 1993; 42:329–331.
87. Hilts PJ. Congress urges AIDS tests for doctors. *New York Times.* New York; October 4, 1991:A9.
88. Rosenthal E. Angry doctors condemn plans to test them for AIDS. *New York Times.* New York; October 20, 1991:B5,7.
89. CDC. Recommendations for preventing transmission of human immunodeficiency virus and hepatitis B virus to patients during exposure-prone invasive procedures. *MMWR* 1991;40(No. RR-8):1–9.
90. Gerberding JL. Expected costs of implementing a mandatory human immunodeficiency virus and hepatitis B virus testing and restriction program for healthcare workers performing invasive procedures. *Infect Control Hosp Epidemiol* 1991; 12:443–447.

91. Russo G, La Croix SJ. A second look at the cost of mandatory human immunodeficiency virus and hepatitis B virus testing for healthcare workers performing invasive procedures. *Infect Control Hosp Epidemiol* 1992; 13:107–110.

92. Chavey W, Cantor S, Clover R, Reinarz J, Spann S. Cost-effectiveness analysis of screening health care workers for HIV. *J Fam Pract* 1994; 38:249–257.

93. Yawn BP. Clinical decision analysis of HIV screening. *Fam Med* 1992; 24:355–361.

94. Sell R, Jovell A, Siegel J. HIV screening of surgeons and dentists: A cost-effectiveness analysis. *Infect Control Hosp Epidemiol.* 1994; 15:635–645.

95. Phillips KA, Lowe RA, Kahn JG, Lurie P, Avins AL, Ciccarone D. The cost-effectiveness of HIV testing of physicians and dentists in the United States. *JAMA* 1994; 271:851–858.

96. Schulman KA, McDonald RC, Lynn LA, Frank I, Christakis NA, Schwartz JS. Screening surgeons for HIV infection: Assessment of a potential public health program. *Infect Control Hosp Epidemiol.* 1994; 15:147–155.

97. Fiscus SA, Adimora AA, Schoenbach VJ, et al. Perinatal HIV infection and the effect of zidovudine therapy on transmission in rural and urban counties. *JAMA* 1996; 275:1483–1488.

98. Gerber AR, Campbell CH, Dillon BA, Holtgrave DR. Evaluating behavioral interventions: Need for randomized trials [letter]. *JAMA* 1994; 271:1317–1318.

Changing Public Policy to Prevent HIV Transmission
The Role of Structural and Environmental Interventions

MICHAEL D. SWEAT and JULIE DENISON

INTRODUCTION

Why is it that interventions at the individual level, such as health education and counseling, have become so dominant in the effort to slow the transmission of HIV and AIDS? Are interventions that include a focus on environmental changes perhaps more cost-effective than those that rely only on individual persuasion? Moreover, what can be done to facilitate greater attention to imaginative environmental interventions and the policy changes necessary to implement and sustain such interventions? In this chapter we attempt to answer these questions. First we examine some of the reasons why individually oriented intervention approaches have become so dominant. Next we review theories that have incorporated the role of environmental factors in the promotion of disease. Then we take a closer look at the role of the environment in the transmission of HIV and discuss interventions that can affect change at the environmental level. Finally, we examine the role of public policy in shaping environmental outcomes to stem HIV transmission and look at some of the ways policy advocacy has been conducted with regard to HIV and AIDS issues in rich and poor countries.

BACKGROUND

HIV prevention efforts have become so dominated by individual psychological models of behavior change that structural and environmental interventions are not often even considered an option. In fact, many people have a difficult time conceptualizing environmental interventions. This is ironic because the historical foundations of epidemiology and public health are grounded in environmental interventions, and some of the most significant

Tables 1 and 2 and passages of text describing the tables are reprinted from "Reducing HIV Incidence in Developing Countries with Structural and Environmental Interventions," by M. D. Sweat and J. A. Denison, *AIDS* 1995; **9**(Suppl. A):S251–257, by permission of the publisher.

MICHAEL D. SWEAT and JULIE DENISON • School of Hygiene and Public Health, Johns Hopkins University, Baltimore, Maryland 21205.

Handbook of Economic Evaluation of HIV Prevention Programs, edited by Holtgrave. Plenum Press, New York, 1998.

reductions in morbidity and mortality worldwide have resulted from basic changes in environment (sewers, water treatment, food inspection, nonsmoking areas, passive seat belts, cigarette taxes, etc.). Environmental interventions could result in significant reductions in new HIV infections beyond those realized from health education efforts alone. However, the AIDS epidemic is typically viewed as a medical problem caused by the risk behavior of individuals who do not know how to change, do not want to change, or do not have the means to change behavior. Therefore interventions are primarily oriented toward individuals at risk and are designed to promote changes in behavior through efforts to modify psychological processes. As a result, most theories of AIDS prevention utilized in intervention programs are designed to affect individual psychology. As such, prevention programs attempt to motivate people to reduce risk behavior or maintain low-risk behavior, primarily through persuasion. For example, education, information, counseling, HIV testing, and other such services are provided to influence individual psychological processes to change behavior. In fact, most of the major theories of AIDS risk reduction and health promotion in general are primarily psychological theories. These include *The AIDS Risk Reduction Model*,[1] theories of self-efficacy, the *Stages of Change Model*,[2] *The Theory of Reasoned Action*,[3] the *Common Sense Model of Illness Danger*,[4] the *PRECEDE Model*,[5] the *Health Belief Model*,[6–9] the *Social Learning Theory*,[10–12] and others.

This emphasis on the primacy of the individual also reflects the important historical role that *individual* freedom and liberty has played within Western institutions and cultural systems.[13] However, individualism, so prevalent in North America and western Europe, is not so pervasive in other places, including many developing countries hit hardest by AIDS. In most of Africa and Asia, community rights historically prevail over individual rights, legal protection and cultural acceptance of individual freedoms are much more limited than in industrialized countries of Europe and North America, and the role of the state, community, and family in daily discourse are sometimes much stronger than in the West. Yet interventions at the individual level often adopted from and funded by Western countries, still prevail as the dominant intervention approach even in developing countries.

Another factor that has fostered individual orientations toward AIDS prevention is that it is often much easier to carefully evaluate individual level programs than those on the environmental level. Attribution of causation for environmental interventions can sometimes be difficult to establish, and affecting change at the environmental level can be difficult to achieve. In planning intervention programs few program managers likely opt for setting goals to make substantive changes in the environment which can require policy commitment and cultural change and which may involve sensitive issues of equity, fairness, and social justice. Moreover, establishing the efficacy of societal level changes is difficult given the myriad of causal interactions present in complex social systems.

THEORETICAL CONSIDERATIONS

The impact of social structure and environment on health outcomes has been addressed from a variety of theoretical perspectives by such disciplines as sociology, epidemiology, anthropology, and public health. Each of these disciplines has incorporated the role of environmental factors somewhat differently.

Epidemiology

Historically, the role of environment in determining health has been a theoretical foundation of epidemiology. The classic tale of pioneering British epidemiologist John

Snow who determined that water from the Broad Street pump was contaminated with cholera is an excellent example of the role of environmental determinants of disease.[14] In response to this public health threat, Snow did not educate the public of the importance of avoiding certain pumps, nor did he provide counseling to enhance the public's perception of risk for cholera and self-efficacy to avoid contaminated pumps. The intervention he implemented was structural and environmental—regulations requiring filtration of the water being pumped and breaking off the handles of the contaminated pumps.[14] This classic tale of the early days of epidemiology points to the historical importance of environmental interventions.

The emphasis on environment in disease etiology has since been codified in epidemiological theory. Epidemiology recognizes three primary factors in the study of epidemics, agent, host, and environmental factors.[15] Agent factors relate to etiological causes of disease, such as lack of nutrients, poisons, and infectious agents. Host (or intrinsic) factors include individual characteristics of the disease's host, such as age, gender, ethnicity, physiological state, immunologic state, preexisting disease, and human behavior. Environmental factors include such things as climate, food density, exposure to chemical agents, urban crowding, social tensions, and socioeconomic factors, such as poverty and war. Clearly, with the AIDS epidemic aspects of the agent (viral type), the human host (STD ulcerations, behavior, status of immune system, etc.), and the environment (access to condoms) all come together to determine the severity of a given epidemic.

Medical Anthropology and Sociology

Ecological perspectives in medical anthropology and sociology also strongly recognize the relationship between environment and health. Ecological theory views humans as unique because of their ability to adapt culturally to disease and environment.[16] Diseases act as agents of natural selection and therefore affect human evolution, both biological and cultural. Adaptation implies that the environment creates certain challenges for humans to overcome and that natural selection is the process by which solutions are discovered.[17] Because environments and ecological relationships change over time, adaptation is a continual process. Moreover, there are different types of adaptive mechanisms, genetic, physiological, and cultural,[18] all of which interact with the environment.

Public Health—Enabling Approaches and Levels of Causation

A recent paper by Tawil, Verster, and O'Reilly[19] presents a theoretical perspective in which individuals are believed to take rational and appropriate decisions regarding their individual behavior. Such decisions, however, are believed to be strongly influenced by environmental factors. They also distinguish between factors which 'persuade' decisions and those which 'enable' change to occur. Enabling factors are described as "social and environmental determinants that facilitate or impede behavioral choice"[19] and are divided into economic and policy approaches. Economic enabling factors include such things as poverty, taxation on harmful products, reduced taxation on medical commodities (such as condoms), and economic forces which disrupt families, such as migration for work. Policy approaches include such factors as national laws limiting access to harmful products, policies on harm reduction interventions (such as needle exchange), distribution of condoms in schools, and decriminalization of prostitution.

In earlier writings we have also addressed the role of environmental interventions for

HIV prevention from a similar public health perspective but with specific application to the AIDS epidemic in developing countries.[20] Our theoretical view is that the causes of most health and social problems occur at multiple levels and that each level has associated change mechanisms with unique natural limits in their ability to affect change. We identify a typology of four levels of causation including (1) superstructural, (2) structural, (3) environmental, and (4) individual. Table 1 is a summary of each causal level for the discussion that follows.

Superstructural factors encompass dominant values about macro social and political arrangements, often developed over long periods of time, and physical and resource characteristics that result in advantages or disadvantages. Example of superstructural factors include economic underdevelopment, sexism, racism, and homophobia. Mechanisms of change for the superstructural level include such actions as national and international social movements, revolution, land redistribution, and war.

Structural factors include laws, policies, and standard operational procedures. For example, unregulated commercial sex and few laws to protect worker rights likely enhance

Table 1.   Levels of Causation for HIV Incidence

Causal Level	Definition	Examples	Change Mechanism
Superstructural	Macro social and political arrangements and resources and power differences that result in unequal advantages	Economic underdevelopment, declining agricultural economy, poverty, sexism, homophobia, Western domination, imperialism	National and international social movements, revolution, land redistribution, war, empowerment of disenfranchised populations
Structural	Laws, policies, and standard operating procedures	Unregulated commerical sex, bachelor wage system, no family housing required at work sites, lack of human rights laws, no financial support for social services	Legislative lobbying, civil and human rights activism, boycotts, constitutional and legal reform, voting, political pressure, structural adjustment policies by international donors
Environmental	Living conditions, resources, and opportunities, the recognition of individual, structural, and superstructural factors	Work camps with many single men and few women, few condoms, high prevalence of HIV/STD, family far away, few job opportunities, few social services, failing agricultural economy, industrialization and urbanization	Community organization, provision of social services, legal action, unionization, enforcement of laws
Individual	How the environment is experienced and acted upon by individuals	Loneliness, boredom, lack of knowledge, low risk perception, sexual urges, moral values, perceived self-efficacy, perceived locus of control	Education, provision of information, enhanced self-efficacy, rewards and punishment, counseling

HIV epidemics. Mechanisms of change at the structural level include legislative lobbying, civil and human rights activism, boycotts, constitutional and legal reform, and voting.

Environmental factors includes living conditions, resources, social pressure, and opportunities available to individuals. Examples include work camps with many men isolated from their families, poor social services, and ready access to commercial sex workers. In essence, the environmental level is the realization of individual, structural, superstructural, and other factors in the real world. Change at the environmental level is best realized through such processes as policy advocacy, community organization, legal action, and civil disobedience.

The *individual* level encompasses how the environment is experienced and acted upon by individuals. Examples include such factors as perceptions of risk, self-efficacy, loneliness, boredom, and knowledge of risk. Changes on the individual level are realized through such factors as education, provision of information, reward and punishment, enhanced self-efficacy, and counseling.

STRUCTURAL AND ENVIRONMENTAL INTERVENTIONS

As mentioned earlier, it is well documented that HIV transmission is facilitated by certain social, structural, cultural, and environmental factors. Next, we present some examples of interventions that function on these levels. First we examine examples of interventions for a variety of health issues. Then we focus on examples of structural and environment interventions for HIV transmission.

Many significant large scale changes in risk reduction and individual self-protective behavior have been wide-scale, nearly universal, and sustained over long periods of time as a result of structural and environmental interventions. Some of the many structural and environmental public health interventions that have been successfully implemented include (1) enriching foods with micronutrients (such as vitamins A and D) to assure adequate diet, (2) enhancing educational opportunities for women, which also reduces fertility rates, (3) taxing cigarettes to reduce consumption level, (4) conducting syphilis screening on all hospital admissions, (5) requiring helmets for motorcycle riders, (6) fluoridating water supplies to reduce cavities, and (7) banning smoking in public.

For example, during the past 20 years massive efforts have been made to reinforce reduction of cigarette smoking in the United States through educational programs on the dangers of smoking. Such individual approaches to smoking secession encouraged many to stop smoking. Not until smoking was banned in many public spaces, however, did the prevalence of smoking significantly decline.[21,22] These structural and environmental changes have had the effect of forcing smokers to smoke near the entrances of work sites exposed to the elements and in special sections in restaurants and airplanes. Perhaps more importantly, this also had the effect of casting smokers as social outcasts and deviants. Thus, by enhancing the individual approach to smoking secession with structural (antismoking laws) and environmental pressures (social isolation and stigma), the impact of prevention programs was significantly enhanced far beyond that which could be realized through only individualistic approaches.

Seat belt usage programs are another example of an individual level intervention that was significantly enhanced through the addition of structural and environmental interventions. Early efforts at stimulating seat belt usage were based on education campaigns at the individual level. Not until structural level seat belt use laws were passed did their use become widespread in the US. This effect was significantly enhanced when environmental level interventions were developed in the form of passive seat belts that were required in all new vehicles. Again, the expansion to structural and environmental level interventions generated behavioral change and risk reduction on a level that would be extremely difficult to achieve with interventions at the individual level alone.

Structural and environmental HIV intervention programs have advantages over those based solely on individual approaches. Social norms are most likely to change at the environmental and structural levels, and when social norms change, so too does associated behavior. Norms and values are developed primarily through socialization, which occurs through social interaction at the environmental level.[23] What is more, norms are influenced by structural changes, such as laws and policies that require adherence to proscribed behavior. Over time the new behavior can become habit, and social norm and expectations 'catch up.' For example, as mentioned earlier, seat belt usage significantly increased when their use was mandated by law. Eventually, many people, who began to use seat belts initially to avoid traffic tickets, became so accustomed to them that they now use them without thinking.

STRUCTURAL AND ENVIRONMENTAL DETERMINANTS OF HIV TRANSMISSION

There are many structural and environmental factors associated with the promotion of HIV epidemics. Here we review a few of the most salient examples of factors that are now well documented in facilitating HIV transmission, including (1) economic factors, (2) migration, urbanization, and family disruption, and (3) war, violence, and civil disturbances.

Economic Factors

The economics of AIDS has been addressed mostly from the perspective of providing medical care and the macroeconomic impact of AIDS. The role of economic factors in promoting HIV transmission has received somewhat less attention. The relationship between economics and AIDS is most apparent cross-nationally. Those countries with the lowest standards of living are also the ones with the most serious AIDS epidemics in terms of the rate of HIV incidence.[24–26] Likewise, AIDS exacerbates poverty in poor countries hit hard by the epidemic, contributing to a cycle of underdevelopment and AIDS-related mortality.[6,27] Analysis within countries also indicates that poverty in both poor and rich countries is often associated with high HIV incidence[24,28,29] and that those with fewer economic resources are likely to die more quickly from AIDS than those with greater wealth.[30,31]

Several factors directly resulting from economic underdevelopment and poverty operate on the structural, environmental, and individual levels to enhance the potential for HIV infection. On the structural level, few significant laws or policies regarding AIDS prevention are in place in developing countries. In general, in less economically developed countries the poor often find other health and social issues more important and immediate compared to AIDS, and there are few AIDS activists to encourage legal and policy reform. Moreover, most developing countries have few legal restrictions on management practices, and work environments often foster HIV risk behavior through substandard pay, few entertainment opportunities, isolation from the family, and little access to health care, especially STD care and treatment.

Structural adjustment programs and economic stagnation have also amplified the effects of poverty on the AIDS epidemic in many countries. The reduction in basic social services, infrastructure, and educational opportunities, together with enhanced unemployment, landlessness, and poverty brought on by economic decline has left Africa especially vulnerable to AIDS because these economic forces promote migration, family separation, and sex work.[32]

Migration, Urbanization, and Family Disruption

Migration is significantly associated with the development of AIDS epidemics.[33-37] Migration facilitates HIV transmission through several processes. Because of declining agricultural production in rural areas[38] and the lure of cash employment in cities,[39,40] many men migrate to cities in search of work. This process generates large populations of un- and underemployed men in urban areas, separates men from their families, and promotes urbanization.[41] Many women also migrate to urban areas and work camps in search of employment, often turning to prostitution to survive when other employment opportunities are unavailable.[42]

Many rural men who find urban employment frequently use their wages to purchase sex from commercial sex workers to satisfy their sexual desires, loneliness, boredom, and lack of entertainment.[43] HIV infection through sexual contact between sex workers and clients in developing countries has been well documented.[44-47] Most migrants return home regularly and carry HIV into the rural areas.[37] Many migrants have low levels of knowledge of HIV and AIDS and of ways to protect themselves from infection. Moreover, they frequently do not identify themselves as being at risk for infection.[34]

Significant urbanization has occurred in many developing countries during the past 30 years.[48] Economic dependency is related to the rate of urbanization, fueled largely through growth of the tertiary and informal economic sectors and inhibited growth in the industrial labor sector.[49] The increasing urbanization of developing countries has significantly facilitated HIV transmission on multiple levels. Urbanization brings people closer together in time and space, thus facilitating the potential for the rapid spread of HIV. Urbanization of traditional societies has brought many people, often young and with little knowledge of AIDS, into social environments with fewer social control mechanisms than they are accustomed to. Rapid urbanization has also promoted changes in the perceptions of responsibility to the community and family,[50] leading many to experience loneliness, isolation, and depression,[51,52] factors that are likely to promote risk taking.

War, Civil Disturbances, and Violence

A growing factor to be considered in AIDS prevention is the role of war, civil disturbances, and violence. War and civil disturbances have become significant facilitators of HIV epidemics in recent years in many countries. Military populations are often at very high risk of HIV infection.[53] Moreover, the effects of war, and preparation for war, facilitate the spread of HIV through several processes, including (1) generation of refugees, (2) disruption of prevention programs, (3) separation of military men from their families, and (4) sometimes, promotion of a disregard for individual human rights. AIDS epidemics in Africa have been especially affected by war. Rwanda is a case in point, where thousands of people fleeing brutality in their home country have ended up in camps in Tanzania, Uganda, and Zaire.[54] Conditions in these refugee camps raise the specter of large-scale AIDS epidemics due to poor social services, high population density, separation of families, poor condom availability, and little attention paid to AIDS education and prevention by health workers.

War and civil disturbances also result in disrupting AIDS prevention programs. AIDS prevention efforts in Haiti, Rwanda, Nigeria, Zaire, Uganda, Ethiopia, Myanmar, Mozambique, South Africa, Angola, and other countries with significant HIV incidence, have been significantly hampered because of political and military conflict. A climate of political repression and fear is not conducive to innovative AIDS prevention, and funding for prevention is often affected by donor embargoes on foreign aid, making both prevention and medical care for those infected with HIV difficult to obtain.[55]

Military life also has structural and environmental features that often promote HIV risk taking. Military populations, mostly men, are often separated from their families for long periods, leading to loneliness and sexual frustration. In many countries in the developing world, cash income is more readily available to members of the military than to the general population, thus providing the economic capacity to purchase commercial sex. Boredom during peacetime is also a factor that promotes frequent sex with prostitutes.[56] Moreover, the culture of some military institutions is highly sexist, and it tends to foster a group consciousness that leads to peer pressure to engage in risky behavior with little regard for the potential for HIV transmission. Military culture is based more on deference to authority than individualism and innovative behavior. Taken together, these factors have promoted high levels of HIV incidence among members of the military in many developing countries.[54] Prevention efforts that attempt to mitigate these factors without significant changes in the social structure and environment are not likely to be effective.

Violence is also a factor that promotes HIV risk, directly and indirectly. Directly, violence in the form of rape and sexual abuse result in HIV transmission to victims.[57–61] Indirectly, some studies have shown that persons who have suffered childhood sexual abuse are also more likely to become infected with HIV as adults.[57–59,62–65]

STRUCTURAL AND ENVIRONMENTAL INTERVENTIONS FOR AIDS PREVENTION

Despite the clear relationship between structural and environmental factors and HIV epidemics, there have been few attempts to intervene on the structural and environmental levels, and when they have bene attempted, such interventions have rarely been evaluated for their effectiveness. A few examples of attempts at structural and environmental interventions are found in both economically rich and poor countries.

For example, in 1984 the director of the San Francisco Public Health Department issued an order banning high-risk sex in gay bathhouses. The bathhouses were to be regulated by "monitors" who were responsible for ejecting any patron seen engaging in high-risk sexual behavior. Later that year, bathhouses were ordered closed.[56] A similar chain of events occurred in New York City in 1985 when the New York Public Health Counsel ordered the closing of gay bathhouses. In 1987 Commissioner of Health for New

York City, Stephen Joseph, expanded the closing to heterosexual sex clubs and later advocated needle exchange and condoms in prisons.[66]

There are some important lessons to be learned from these experiences. First, the initial reactions of many in the targeted community were hostile. Many saw the closing of gay bathhouses as an affront to their civil rights of free association and sexual liberation,[67] and others in the community viewed distribution of needles and condoms as advocating drug use and promiscuity.[66] Soon after the regulation of behavior in the bathhouses was initiated, however, few in the gay community continued to raise these concerns. The impact of the bathhouse closing also sent the signal that social acceptability of unprotected sex was no longer the norm. The impact that such actions has had on risk reduction remains largely unmeasured, and needle exchange and condom distribution continue to provoke public debate.

A unique structural/environmental intervention for HIV prevention known as the "100% condom program" was pioneered in northern Thailand, an area with very high incidence of HIV infection.[68–70] The "100% condom program" has several key components, including (1) the requirement that commercial sex workers use condoms with all clients, (2) the requirement that brothel owners enforce condom use by assisting commercial sex workers with uncooperative clients, (3) monitoring condom use in brothels, (4) monitoring compliance through the regular review of gonorrhea rates among commercial sex workers, and (5) graduated sanctions for noncompliance by targeting brothel owners, including closing of the establishment for repeated violations.

Initial reports indicate that the 100% condom program has had a profound effect on the level of unprotected sex and STD and HIV incidence in Thailand.[71] The program was recently expanded nationally, and impressive results have ensued with a dramatic reduction in STD incidence since the law was established.[68] Moreover, social norms toward unprotected sex with prostitutes have dramatically changed.[72] Studies indicate that it is becoming less acceptable and more difficult to have sex with a commercial sex worker without a condom in Thailand.[68–70]

Interventions based on the Thai 100% condom intervention are also being implemented in Nepal,[73] and in the Dominican Republic the authors of this chapter are conducting formative research for a 100% condom program.[74] A recent report from the Philippines showed a significant relationship between condom use and structural changes (manager/supervisor support of condom use) in brothel settings over a two-year period using a controlled longitudinal research design with comparisons made between a control site and (1) health education, (2) structural (manager education/support), and (3) combined structural and health education sites.[75] It remains to be seen whether these effects can be sustained and whether such a program would be effective outside of the Thai and Philippine context.

One controversial structural/environmental intervention for AIDS prevention was implemented in Cuba. Until recently, Cuba's AIDS control program was composed of five key components[76] including (1) blood screening for HIV, (2) widespread HIV testing of the population, (3) educational programs to reduce HIV risk behavior, (4) isolation of HIV-infected individuals in "sanatoria" with health care and living conditions better than those afforded by the average Cuban, and (5) clinical research to identify the best treatment protocols for those with HIV and AIDS.[77] The impact of this intervention approach, based largely on structural changes, has to yet be fully evaluated. More recently, many of the sanatoria have been closed, and community-based care is becoming more common.

These examples of structural/environmental HIV intervention programs point out several important issues for consideration. First, like other intervention approaches, structural and environmental interventions have a significant potential to violate individual civil rights. They especially pit the rights of individuals against the concept of collective 'community rights.' Second, community support and coordination across social institutions facilitates the success of such interventions. When the community accepts and supports changes in the social structure and environment, the intervention is more likely to succeed. Third, evaluation of such interventions needs to be conducted to identify the impact on risk behavior. Often, when a structural or environmental approach has been taken, there has been little coordinated attempt to evaluate the impact on HIV incidence. For example, in the Dominican Republic the author currently is conducting research on the effects of an intervention to monitor condom usage in selected brothels using a control design at the community level. The intervention is being jointly implemented by the government, an associated of brothel owners, and a community-based organization that provides AIDS prevention programs to sex workers. Results of the project will be used to examine the estimated impact of the policy change on HIV and STD transmission and on the cost-effectiveness of the intervention.

Examples of other possible structural and environmental interventions for consideration are provided in Table 2. Intervention efforts such as these should be investigated, and a clear research agenda needs to be defined to establish the most appropriate and effective programs. Moreover, interventions need to be developed that are as models for emulation

Table 2. Examples of Potential Structural Changes

Aids impact assessments required for large development projects, especially those funded by international donors
Laws and policies that require 100% condom usage in brothels
Laws requiring family housing at migrant labor camps
Requiring that hotels stock condoms in each room
Reduction of taxes on condoms
Changes in government policies that permit nationwide marketing of condoms and explicit AIDS prevention by mass media
Decriminalzation of needle sales
Prenatal HIV screening
Partner notification of HIV-discordant test results
Better recreational facilities at military bases to reduce boredom and the desire to go to brothels
Changes in truck routes to allow truck drivers more time with families
Employing entire families for migratory labor rather than just men to keep families intact; building housing for migrant families at work sites
Staggering paydays to dissuade group brothel attendance
Provision of check cashing facilities to dissuade payday alcohol use and risk behavior in settings where saloons are the only place available to cash checks
100% condom use programs that sanction brothel owners when condom use is lacking
Access to AIDS prevention and STD care at work sites, schools, and prisons
Mentoring programs at work sites with large numbers of migrant workers to facilitate social integration of new arrivals
Availability of condoms in both traditional and especially nontraditional outlets, such as bars, hotels, flower shops, truck stops
Improved STD care, such as use of syndromic management for STD treatment and availability of STD drugs
Needle Exchange for drug users
Distribution of condoms in schools and prisons

and that allow clear measurement of the impact of the programs on concrete changes in behavior.

STIMULATING POLICY CHANGE

To achieve structural or environmental change, one must be effective at the policy level. There are various perspectives on how policy change can be achieved. Three of the most common approaches to achieving policy change with regard to the AIDS epidemic have included (1) constituency-based lobbying, (2) grass-roots activism, and (3) scientific research. There have also been many hybrid approaches, as these are not mutually exclusive.

Constituency-based lobbying refers to efforts to achieve a specific policy objective by institutions or representatives of political interest,[78] for example, when a national hospital association presses the government to provide more funds to support medical care for persons with HIV and AIDS. AIDS is now a big business, and many groups, from health care providers and pharmaceutical companies to professional associations of nurses and physicians, have dedicated lobbyists working on AIDS-related public policy. Other groups, such as the Lambda Legal Defense Fund, the Human Rights Campaign, which lobby for gay interests, the National Educational Association, and the National Organization for Women also lobby for the interests of their constituencies. Such groups typically have professional lobbyists at the local and national level, and they also frequently develop and disseminate positions on issues through reports and press releases.

Policy change related to the AIDS epidemic has also been affected by grass-roots activism.[79] Groups like The AIDS Coalition to Unleash Power (ACT-UP) have staged public demonstrations to achieve policy change, and they have been highly effective in many instances in stimulating changes in such policies as lowering the cost of drugs to treat AIDS, speeding access to and approval of new drug therapies, and inclusion of minorities and women in clinical trials. In poorer countries and in countries with less tolerance of political dissent, as in much of Africa and Asia, grass-roots activism has been less important in stimulating policy change. Unfortunately, because few grass-roots activist groups exist in the developing world, little attention is paid to the specific needs of these countries at the international level, where many of the decisions are made concerning funding for HIV and AIDS prevention and care in developing countries, and the local level.

Scientific research has also brought about policy change as findings regarding the efficacy of treatment and prevention programs have been studied and disseminated.[80,81] This process, however, can be very slow because the rigor of scientific research requires carefully designed research projects which can take years to yield definitive results. Interestingly, some in the activist community have been highly critical of research activities, and activists have been effective in stimulating policy changes within science. The marriage of activism and science is a particularly interesting outcome of the AIDS epidemic, evidenced by the growing scientific sophistication of many grass-roots activists and the increased sensitivity to ethics in research among many in the scientific community. It is not uncommon to witness complex discussions of biological and behavioral science between activists and scientists at the International AIDS Conference, and the increased attention to ethical issues among AIDS scientists, such as inclusion in clinical trials and informed consent, clearly, directly result from pressure of activists.

Obviously there are a myriad of factors that come together in the development of policy, and the confluence of constituency groups, activists, and scientists represents perhaps the most obvious of factors in shaping public policy on AIDS issues. One important and perhaps unmeasured influence on policy is the impact of highly committed individuals who work to shape policy.

DISCUSSION AND RECOMMENDATIONS

As the worldwide AIDS pandemic matures and changes, so too must our approach to prevention. AIDS prevention programs need to incorporate more than just individualistic, psychological approaches to risk reduction. We need to learn more about how social, cultural, political, and economic factors facilitate HIV risk behavior and how to develop creative, culturally appropriate, and community-sponsored prevention programs that make substantive changes on multiple levels. Moreover, we need to recognize that although changes in superstructural factors, such as poverty, economic underdevelopment, sexism, and homophobia are pervasive and difficult and slow to change, there are still many opportunities to make changes in the social structure and environment that can lead to significant reduction in HIV incidence. Individual, psychological intervention approaches do not promote optimum changes in behavior when structural and environmental constraints are not addressed.

The role of communities in shaping and implementing structural and environmental HIV interventions is also a crucial factor in the success of such interventions, and this is an area that needs to be understood better. As discussed earlier, experience has shown that when communities get involved in a prevention program, they are much more likely to succeed. We need to look closely at the process of community mobilization, however, to understand better what processes best promote sustainable community participation and to ensure that ethical outcomes are realized. Making changes in the social structure and environment to address social and health problems carries a risk of unethical outcomes, thus carefully shaping the process of change is important. A research agenda for addressing these issues needs to be developed and undertaken.

Protection of individual liberty is important. But when does the emphasis on individualism overcome a reasonable role, and perhaps ethical obligation, for public health institutions to protect people through changes in the environment? Is it ethical for public health practitioners and institutions to operate consistently on the individual level when it is so clear that structural and environmental factors lead to risk of transmission among so many? And finally, is it more cost-effective to take a more holistic approach to AIDS prevention? These are important questions that need to be researched, debated, and resolved among public health practitioners.

In addressing these questions we must be aware that many intervention efforts that function on the structural and environmental level do not necessarily obviate individual freedoms—they often enhance them. For example, as seen with the 100% condom program in Thailand,[82,83] policies that sanction brothel owners when sex workers in the brothel become infected with sexually transmitted infections press brothel owners to support sex workers in self-protection with clients. Thus, the policy of sanctions for not using condoms targeted at brothel managers actually allows sex workers to have greater negotiation power.

In sum, we propose that those charged with developing and implementing AIDS control efforts go beyond only individualistic approaches and examine the potential for structural and environmental interventions to maximize the sustainability and cost-effectiveness of prevention programs. Moreover, such an approach would likely result in significant reductions in new HIV infections beyond those achieved only through approaches at the individual level.

REFERENCES

1. Coates T, Stall R, Cantania J, Kegeles S. Behavioral factors in the spread of HIV infection. *AIDS* 1988; 2: s239–s246.
2. Prochaska J, DiClemente C, Norcross J. In search of how people change. *Am Psychol* 1992; 47:1102–1114.
3. Ajen I, Fishbein M. *Understanding Attitudes and Predicting Behavior*. Englewood Cliffs, NJ: Prentice-Hall; 1980.
4. Leventhal H, Meyer D, Nerenz D. The common sense: Representation of illness danger. In Rachman S, ed. *Medical Psychology*. New York: Pergamon Press; 1980; pp. 7–30.
5. Green L, Kreuter M, Deeds S, K.P. *Health Education Today and the PRECEDE Framework*. Palo Alto: Medfield; 1979.
6. Becker CM. The demo-economic impact of the AIDS pandemic in sub-Saharan Africa. *World Dev* 1990; 18:1599–1619.
7. Becker M, Janz N. On the effectiveness and utility of health/hazard risk appraisal in clinical and nonclinical settings. *Health Serv Res* 1987; 22:537–551.
8. Emmons C, Joseph J, Kessler R, Wortman C, Montgomery S, D.O. Psychosocial predictors of reported behavior change in homosexual men at risk for AIDS. *Health Educ Q* 1986; 13:331–345.
9. Montgomery SJJ, Becker M, Ostrow D, Kessler R, Kirscht J. The health belief model in understanding compliance with preventative recommendations for AIDS: How useful? *AIDS Educ Prev* 1989; 1:303–323.
10. Bandura A. *Social Learning Theory*. Edgewood, NJ: Prentice-Hall; 1977.
11. Botvin G, Baker E, Botvin E, Filazzola B, Millman R. Prevention of alcohol misuse through development of personal and social competence. *J Studies of Alcohol* 1984; 45:550–552.
12. Des Jarlais D, Freidman S. The psychology of preventing AIDS among intravenous drug users. *Am Psychol* 1988; 43:865–870.
13. Chirot D. *Social Change in the Modern Era*. San Diego, CA: Harcourt Brace Jovanovich; 1986.
14. Snow J. On the mode of communication of cholera. In *Snow on Cholera*. New York: The Commonwealth Fund; 1936; pp. 1–175.
15. Lilienfeld A, Lilienfeld D. *Foundations of Epidemiology*, 2nd ed. New York: Oxford University Press, 1980.
16. Alland A, McCay B. The concept of adaptation in biological and cultural evolution. In Honigmann J, ed. *Handbook of Social and Cultural Anthropology*. Chicago: Rand McNally; 1973.
17. Brown P, Inhorn M. Disease, ecology, and human behavior. In *Medical Anthropology: Contemporary Theory and Method*. New York: Praeger; 1990; pp. 187–214.
18. McElroy A, Townsend P. *Medical Anthropology in Ecological Perspective*, 2nd ed. Boulder, CO: Westview Press; 1989.
19. Tawil O, Verster A, O'Reilly K. Enabling approaches for HIV/AIDS prevention: Can we modify the environment and minimize the risk? *AIDS* 1995; 9:1299–1306.
20. Sweat M, Denison J. Reducing HIV incidence in developing countries with structural and environmental interventions. *AIDS* 1995; 9:S251–S257.
21. Sorensen G, Pechacek T. Implementing nonsmoking policies in the private sector and assessing their effects. *NY State J Med* 1989:11–15.
22. Rigotto N. Trends in the adoption of smoking restrictions in public places and worksites. *NY State J Med* 1989:19–26.
23. Becker M, Joseph J. AIDS and behavioral change to reduce risk: A review. *Am J Pub Health* 1988; 78: 394–410.
24. Anonymous. Poor man's plague. *The Economist* 1991; 21:21–24.
25. Krueger L, Wood R, Diehr P, Maxwell C. Poverty and HIV seropositivity: The poor are more likely to be infected. *AIDS* 1990; 4:811–814.

26. Carovano K. AIDS and poverty in the developing world. *Policy Focus* 1987; 7:1–11.
27. Ainsworth M, Over M. The economic impact of AIDS on Africa. In *AIDS in Africa*. Essex M, Mboup S, Kanki P, Kalengayi M, eds. New York: Raven Press; 1994; pp. 559–587.
28. Singer M. AIDS and the health crisis of the urban poor; the perspective of critical medical anthropology. *Soc Sci Med* 1994; 39(7):931–948.
29. Wallace R. US Apartheid and the spread of AIDS to the suburbs: A multi-city analysis of spatial epidemic threshold. *Soc Sci Med* 1995; 41:333–345.
30. Mulder D, Nunn A, Wagner H, Kamali A, Kengeya Kayondo J. HIV-1 incidence and HIV-1 associated mortality in a rural Ugandan population cohort. *AIDS* 1994; 8:87–92.
31. Wagner H, Kamali A, Nunn A, Kengeya Kayondo J, Mulder D. General and HIV-1 associated morbidity in a rural Ugandan community. *AIDS* 1993; 7:1461–1467.
32. Lurie R, Hintzen P. The impact of International Monetary Fund and World Bank policies on HIV transmission in developing countries. *International Conference on AIDS*. Yokohama, August 1994.
33. Hawkes S, Hart G. Travel, migration and HIV. *AIDS Care* 1993; 5:207–214.
34. Romero-Daza N. Multiple sexual partners, migrant labor, and the makings for an epidemic: Knowledge and beliefs about AIDS among women in Highland Lesotho. *Hum Org* 1994; 53:192–205.
35. Jochelson K, Mothibeli M, Leger J. Human immunodeficiency virus and migrant labor in South Africa. *Int J Health Serv* 1991; 21:157–173.
36. Hunt C. Migrant labor and sexually transmitted disease. *J Health Soc Behavior* 1989; 30:353–373.
37. Anarfi J. Sexuality, migration and AIDS in Ghana—a socio-behavioral study. *Health Transition Rev* 1993; 3:45–67.
38. Stichter S. *Migrant Laborers*. New York: Cambridge University Press; 1985.
39. Loewenson R. Labour insecurity and health: An epidemiological study in Zimbabwe. *Soc Sci Med* 1988; 27:733–741.
40. Sanders D, Davies R. The economy, the health sector and child health in Zimbabwe since independence. *Soc Sci Med* 1988; 27:723–731.
41. Byerlee D. Rural-urban migration in Africa: Theory, policy and research implications. *Int Migration Rev* 1974; 8:543–566.
42. Padian N. Prostitute women and AIDS: Epidemiology. *AIDS* 1988;2:413–419.
43. Hunt C. Africa and AIDS: Dependent development, sexism and racism. *Mon Rev* 1988; 39:10–22.
44. Mann J, Chin J, Piot P, Quinn T. The international epidemiology of AIDS. *Sci Am* 1988; 259:82–89.
45. Carael M, Van de Perre P, Lepage H, et al. Human immunodeficiency virus transmission among heterosexual couples in central Africa. *AIDS* 1988; 2:201–205.
46. Day S. Prostitute women and AIDS. *AIDS* 1988; 2:421–428.
47. Hudson C, Anselm J, Hennis P, et al. Risk factors for the spread of AIDS in rural Africa: Evidence from a comparative epidemiological survey of AIDS, hepatitis B and syphilis in southwest Uganda. *AIDS* 1988; 2:255–260.
48. Mitchell-Weaver C. Urban systems theory and Third World development: A review. *J Urban Aff* 1991; 13: 419–441.
49. Kentor J. Structural determinants of peripheral urbanization: The effects of international dependence. *Am Sociol Rev* 1981; 46:201–211.
50. Edwards S, Borsten G, Nene L, Kunene S. Urbanization and changing perceptions of responsibilities among African fathers. *J Psychol* 1986; 120:433–438.
51. Kadushin C. Mental health and interpersonal environment: A reexamination of some effects of social structure on mental health. *Am Sociol Rev* 1983; 48:20188–20198.
52. Amato P. The effects of urbanization on interpersonal behavior: Field studies in Papua, New Guinea. *J Cross Cult Psychol* 1983; 14:353–367.
53. Torrey B, Boyle B, Way P. Seroprevalence of HIV in Africa. *US Bureau Census, CIR Staff paper: Winter*; 1990:7–9.
54. Rweymamu C. Refugee AIDS tragedy? *Panos World AIDS* 1994; 35:1–2.
55. Kellett J. The impact of prolonged war and epidemic AIDS on medical care. *CMAJ* 1989; 140:699–701.
56. Moodie D. Mine culture and miners' identity on the South African gold mines. In Bozzoli B, ed. *Town and Countryside in the Transvaal*. Johannesburg: Raven Press; 1983.
57. Burgess AW, Baker T. AIDS and victims of sexual assault. *Hosp Community Psychiatry* 1992; 43:447–448.
58. Cunningham RM, Stiffman AR, Dore P, Earls F. The association of physical and sexual abuse with HIV risk behaviors in adolescence and young adulthood: Implications for public health. *Child Abuse & Neglect* 1994; 18:233–245.

59. Zierler S, Feingold L, Laufer D, Velentgas P, Kantrowitz-Gordon I, Mayer K. Adult survivors of childhood sexual abuse and subsequent risk of HIV infection. *Am J Public Health* 1991; 81:572–575.
60. Benson JD. Abuse and HIV-related risk. *Focus* 1995; 10:5–6.
61. Baribwira C, Muteganya D, Ndihokubwayo JB, Moreno JL, Nduwimana M, Rufyikiri T. Aspects of sexually transmissible diseases in young children in Burundi: Gonorrhea caused by sexual abuse. *Medecine Tropicale* 1994; 54:231–233.
62. Carballo-Dieguez A, Dolezal C. Association between history of childhood sexual abuse and adult HIV-risk sexual behavior in Puerto Rican men who have sex with men. *Child Abuse Neglect* 1995; 19:595–605.
63. Lodico MA, DiClemente RJ. The association between childhood sexual abuse and prevalence of HIV-related risk behaviors. *Clin Pediatr* 1994; 33:498–502.
64. Lyon ME, Richmond D, LJ DA. Is sexual abuse in childhood or adolescence a predisposition factor for HIV infection during adolescence? *Pediatr AIDS HIV Infect* 1995; 6:271–275.
65. Bartholow BN, Doll LS, Joy D, et al. Emotional, behavioral, and HIV risks associated with sexual abuse among adult homosexual and bisexual men. *Child Abuse & Neglect* 1994; 18:747–761.
66. Joseph S. *Dragon at the Gates: The Once and Future AIDS Epidemic.* New York: Carroll & Graf; 1992.
67. Shilts R. *And the Band Played On.* New York: St. Martin's Press; 1987.
68. Hanenberg R, Rojanapithaykorn W, Kunasol P, Sokal D. Impact of Thailand's HIV-control programme as indicated by the decline of sexually transmitted diseases. *Lancet* 1993; 344:243–245.
69. Nelson KE, Beyrer C, Eiumtrakol S, Khamboonruang C, Celentano D. HIV prevalence and changes in risk behavior among young men in northern Thailand between 1991 and 1993. *Natl Conf Hum Retroviruses Relat Infect 2nd* 1995; 2:164.
70. Nelson K, Celentano D, Eiumtrakol S, et al. Changes in sexual behavior and a decline in HIV infection among young men in Thailand. *N Engl J Med* 1996; 335:297–303.
71. Rojanapithaykorn W. The one-hundred percent condom programme in Thailand: An update. *Int Conf on AIDS. Yokohama,* August 1994.
72. Kelly J, Sikkema K, Wintt R, et al. Outcomes of a 16-city randomized field trial of a community-level HIV risk reduction intervention. *Int Conf on AIDS,* June 1992, Amsterdam, Netherlands.
73. Bhatt P, Baltes R. "100% condom" use for Badii sex workers in Nepal. *Int Conf AIDS* 1994;10:13 (abstract no. 345D); Yokohama, Japan.
74. Sweat M. Personal communication with Martha Butler, Resident Advisor AIDSCAP Dominican Republic; 1996.
75. Morisky D, Detels R, Tiglao T, et al. Innovative behavioral interventions targeting environmental and socio-structural determinants for HIV/AIDS prevention in the Philippines (Abstract # Mo.D.1795). *XI International Conference on AIDS.* Vancouver, BC; 1996.
76. Santana S, Faas L, K. W. Human immunodeficiency Virus in Cuba: The public health response of a Third World country. *Int J Health Serv* 1991; 21:511–537.
77. Perez-Stable EJ. Cuba's response to the HIV epidemic [see comments]. *Am J Public Health* 1991; 81:563–567.
78. Marconi K, Weissman G, Van Ness P, Bowen GS, Schneider D, McClain M. Creating an agenda for research and evaluation: HIV service delivery, the Ryan White Care Act and beyond. *Int Conf AIDS* 1993; 9:947 (abstract no. PO-D36-4375), Berlin, Germany.
79. Bayer R. AIDS, ethics, and activism: Institutional encounters in the epidemic's first decade. In Bulger RE, ed. *Society's Choices: Social and Ethical Decision Making in Biomedicine.* Washington, DC: National Academy Press; 1995: pp. 458–476.
80. Arbaje M, Butler de Lister M, Gomez E, Sweat M. Lessons learned from an AIDS policy program in the Dominican Republic. *Int Conf AIDS* 1994; 10:312 (abstract no. PD0426), Yokohama, Japan.
81. Cwikel JG. After epidemiological research: What next? Community action for health promotion. *Public Health Rev* 1994; 22:375–394.
82. Rojanapithaykorn W. One hundred percent condom programme. *Int Conf AIDS* 1992:D498 (abstract no. PoD 5654), Amsterdam, Netherlands.
83. Ford N, Koetsawang S. Factors influencing condom use in a Thai massage parlour. *Int Conf AIDS;* 1992:D492 (abstract no. PoD 5622), Amsterdam, Netherlands.

8

The Cost-Effectiveness of Small Group and Community-Level Interventions

DAVID R. HOLTGRAVE and STEVEN D. PINKERTON

In February 1997, the National Institutes of Health (NIH) convened a consensus development conference on interventions to prevent HIV infection. At this conference, a panel composed of AIDS activists and esteemed scientists, who work in areas other than HIV prevention, reviewed the evidence on the effectiveness of HIV prevention interventions. The panel identified several types of HIV prevention interventions that have been rigorously assessed and found effective at reducing HIV-related risk behaviors.[1]

Foremost among the interventions deemed effective were small group and community-level interventions. Small group interventions typically consist of multiple HIV risk reduction sessions offered to six to ten clients at a time.[2] The sessions cover such topics as basic information about HIV transmission and ways to prevent infection, personal risk assessment and plans for reducing risky behavior, practice in negotiating safer behavior with sex and drug injection partners, broader discussions about personal relationships, and group reinforcement of positive steps towards enactment of safer behavior. Group sessions are typically led by a trained facilitator, but the success of the group relies on personally involving the clients in a highly interactive dialog and individually relevant skills practice exercises.

Small group interventions have been evaluated in a number of carefully conducted randomized, controlled trials. These studies have involved various populations, including at-risk women, men who have sex with men, and adolescents.[3–9] The studies have typically found statistically significant reductions in HIV-related risk behavior (examples of the effect sizes from these studies follow).

Because the restricted size of small group interventions limits their overall impact, some researchers and community-based organizations have begun to explore community-level interventions as a means of reaching larger populations of at-risk individuals.[10] Community-level interventions typically focus on altering the underlying social norms that influence risky behavior for an entire community of persons and attempting to change the risky behavior of individual community members. By modifying social norms, it is hoped that such interventions can engender widespread and durable behavioral changes within the target population.

DAVID R. HOLTGRAVE and STEVEN D. PINKERTON • Department of Psychiatry and Behavioral Medicine, Center for AIDS Intervention Research (CAIR), Medical College of Wisconsin, Milwaukee, Wisconsin 53202.

Handbook of Economic Evaluation of HIV Prevention Programs, edited by Holtgrave. Plenum Press, New York, 1998.

A small number of community-level intervention have been carefully evaluated.[7,11–16] One especially promising community-level HIV prevention model that has received considerable attention is based on Rogers' Diffusion of Innovations theory.[17] This model hypothesizes that social norms propagate through a population starting with influential members of the community. These "opinion leaders," in turn, convince others through word and action ("modeling") to adopt the desired attitudes and behaviors. By first targeting key opinion leaders, community-level interventions of limited scale can effect extensive, community-wide behavioral changes. Thus, a relatively small intervention can have a disproportional impact on behavior. Consequently, such interventions have enormous potential to reduce HIV risk behavior in a cost-effective manner.

Although these interventions have been effective, program planners and resource allocation decision makers also need information about the cost and cost-effectiveness of these interventions. The purpose of this chapter is to review all available economic evaluations of HIV prevention small group and community-level interventions.

ECONOMIC EVALUATIONS OF SMALL GROUP AND COMMUNITY-LEVEL INTERVENTIONS

Table 1 summarizes the results from each of the four available studies in this area. All of these studies were conducted by one research team at the Medical College of Wisconsin's Center for AIDS Intervention Research (CAIR). Although a common methodological framework was employed (described in Chapter 3 by Pinkerton and Holtgrave in this volume), historical changes in parameters, such as medical costs saved each time an HIV infection is prevented, result in slight methodological differences among the studies.[18] These minor methodological differences, however, do not alter any of the conclusions reached in this chapter.

Table 1. Economic Evaluation Studies of Small Group and Community-Level Interventions[a]

Investigator (Source)	Intervention	Population	Base Case Results	
			Cost-per-Client	Cost-Effectiveness
Holtgrave (19)	Group, 5-session, behavioral risk reduction	At-risk women	$269	$2,024 per QALY[b]
Holtgrave (20)	Group, 12-session, behavioral risk reduction	Gay men	$470	Cost-saving[c]
Pinkerton (21)	Group, 1-session, behavioral skills training	Gay men	$40[d]	Cost-saving
Pinkerton (26)	Community-level, peer-opinion leader, behavioral risk reduction	Gay men	$38	Cost-saving

[a]Table adapted from Holtgrave and Pinkerton, "The Economics of HIV Primary Prevention," in Peterson & DiClemente, eds., *Handbook of HIV Prevention*, with permission, Plenum Press.
[b]"QALY" indicates "quality-adjusted life years" saved by the intervention.
[c]"Cost saving" indicates that the present value of the HIV-related medical costs saved by the intervention is greater than that costs of the intervention itself.
[d]This $40 cost is the incremental cost of the skills training intervention relative to a group lecture intervention.

Small Group Intervention for At-Risk Women

A recent study evaluated the effectiveness of a five-session, cognitive-behavioral, small group intervention for increasing condom use among women attending an urban primary health-care clinic and at risk for HIV infection.[3] The study employed a randomized, controlled trial design to compare the HIV prevention intervention to a nutrition education ("control") condition. One hundred ninety-seven women participated in the study. One average, they were 29 years of age with 11 years of education. More than 97% were unemployed. Approximately 87% were African-American. All were at behavioral risk of HIV infection.

The five-session small group intervention provided basic information about HIV transmission and prevention; skills training in condom use; problem solving, negotiation, and assertiveness in sexual situations; self-management; and peer support of attempts to engage in safer behavior. A key aspect of the group was the highly interactive nature of the sessions, which brought together women to help support each others' successively safer behavior. Women were paid for group attendance and for participation in the scientific study.

Self-reported condom use at the three-month follow-up period was 56% (of vaginal intercourse acts) for the HIV prevention condition, compared to only 32% for the control condition. Both groups reported equivalent condom use at baseline measurement. Hence, the intervention was successful in achieving a statistically significant increase in condom use.

Holtgrave and Kelly[19] preformed a retrospective cost and cost-utility analysis of this intervention from the societal perspective. They included costs related to group facilitators' wages; costs of senior staff to conduct intervention tailoring, training, and quality assurance; fringe benefits; materials costs; indirect costs (shared with other programs); child care; client incentive for session attendance (but not for completing surveys); and client transportation. They attempted to estimate the cost of fielding the intervention but not the cost of scientific study. Under base-case assumptions, they estimated that the intervention cost $269 per client.

Holtgrave and Kelly used a mathematical model of HIV transmission to convert the behavioral measures collected in the original study into an estimate of HIV infections prevented by the intervention. Estimates of the amount of medical care costs saved each time an HIV infection is prevented and the number of quality-adjusted life years saved with each HIV infection averted were taken from the published literature. Holtgrave and Kelly estimated that the five-session, small group intervention cost $2,024 per quality-adjusted life year (QALY) saved. this figure compares favorably to amounts spent to "purchase" a quality-adjusted life year in other health-care arenas.

The authors performed extensive sensitivity analyses to assess the robustness of the base-case results for uncertainty in the input parameter values. The results were moderately sensitive to changes in assumptions regarding per-act transmission probabilities and to assumptions about the sex partner's HIV seroprevalence level. Under most of the many conditions considered in the sensitivity analyses, however, the results indicated that the intervention is cost-effective compared with other health-service programs.

Twelve-Session Small Group Intervention for Gay Men

Another important study assessed the effectiveness of an even more intensive, twelve-session cognitive-behavioral, small group, HIV prevention intervention for gay men.[6] The original study was a randomized, controlled trial with 104 participants. The majority of the clients (87%) were white, and their average age was 31 years. Fifty-five percent had not finished college. The participants were recruited from health department clinics, gay bars, and other community settings in a metropolitan area with approximately 400,000 residents.

The HIV prevention intervention consisted of twelve sessions focused on risk behavior education, sexual assertiveness training, self-management training, and the development of positive social support networks. The sessions were highly interactive. The comparison condition in the study was a wait-list control group. Self-reported condom use among participants immediately receiving the intervention was 23% at baseline, 65% at 4-month follow-up assessment, and 77% at 8-month follow-up assessment. The wait-list comparison condition showed a decrease in condom use before initiation of the intervention.

Holtgrave and Kelly[20] conducted a retrospective cost and cost-utility analysis of this HIV prevention intervention for gay men. They used economic evaluation techniques similar to those employed in their study of an intervention for urban women (see the previous section for details). They found that this intensive intervention for gay men cost about $470 per client. Further, they found that the medical costs saved by the HIV infections prevented by this intervention were greater than the costs of the program. Hence, the intervention is cost-saving to society. Further, extensive sensitivity analyses found that this result was robust to changes in a number of input parameter assumptions.

HIV Prevention Skills Training for Men Who Have Sex with Men

The small group interventions described above demonstrate that this intervention format induces significant reductions in participants' HIV-risk behavior and in a cost-effective manner. However, these interventions, which typically require multiple sessions are relatively costly. Conceivably, a less intensive and less expensive intervention might be more cost-effective, even if it is slightly less effective overall.

To date, only a single study has been published that addresses this particular issue.[21] This study, which reports the results of a retrospective cost-utility analysis of an intervention for men who have sex with men that was conducted in the late 1980s, directly compared the cost-effectiveness of a lecture providing basic HIV information with a more intensive (and costly) cognitive-behavioral intervention. This *incremental analysis* (see the Phillips et al. chapter in this volume[22]) answers the important question whether the additional benefits derived from including a skills training component in the intervention outweigh the extra costs. This question is especially relevant to policy makers and program managers who must decide how to allocate resources among relatively brief and more intensive HIV prevention interventions.

In the original intervention study, 584 homosexual and bisexual men were recruited from the Pittsburgh area to participate in an "AIDS prevention project."[5] All participants attended a 60- to 90-minute lecture that provided information on HIV transmission, safer sex, and the proper use of condoms. A randomly selected subset of these men (N = 319) also participated in an additional 80-minute safer sex skills building session, during which the men discussed, rehearsed, and role-played safer sex negotiation strategies.

The principal benefit derived from the addition of the skills training component to the intervention was a significant increase, relative to the lecture-only condition, in the use of condoms during anal intercourse.[5] At 6-month follow-up, condom use had increased to 62% among men in the skills training group, compared to 49% for the men who received only the safer sex lecture (the condom use figures refer to the proportion of partners with whom condoms were used). At 12-month follow-up even more substantial differences (85% vs. 56%) were reported. In the Pinkerton et al. analysis, the 6 and 12-month follow-up data were averaged, and it was estimated conservatively that the behavioral effects of the skills training intervention last only for the twelve months preceding the second follow-up assessment.[21] Thus, the question addressed by this analysis was whether it is worth the additional cost of the skills training component for a relatively small, (presumably) one-year increase in condom usage from 52% to 73%.

The cost of the skills training intervention component, over and above the cost of the safer sex lecture, was $12,657, or just under $40 per client.[21] The number of additional HIV infections averted was 3.05, at an incremental cost of approximately $4,150 per averted infection. The intervention saved a total of 21.29 QALYs (discounted at a 5% annual rate) and over $170,000 in direct medical care costs (also discounted at 5%). In the base-case analysis—indeed, under all reasonable value assignments to key parameters—the incremental cost per discounted QALY saved was negative, which suggests that the skills training component was a cost-saving addition to the overall intervention program.

Safer Sex Diffusion within a Community of Gay Men

Although community-level interventions have demonstrated great promise in research trials as an effective means of reaching large networks of at-risk individuals, only a single such intervention has thus far been subjected to rigorous economic valuation.[14] This highly influential "popular opinion leader" intervention has subsequently served as a model for several adaptations to diverse at-risk populations.[23]

In the original popular opinion leader intervention, Kelly and colleagues first enlisted the assistance of staff at several small gay bars to help them identify popular, well-connected, and socially respected members ("popular opinion leaders") of the gay community.[24] Then these men (N = 32) were recruited into the next phase of the intervention, which consisted of four weekly, 90- to 120-minute training/discussion sessions led by two to four facilitators. During these sessions the popular opinion leaders were instructed in effective communication techniques for conversing with peers about the importance of safer sex to reduce HIV risk. The leaders were encouraged to actively engage friends and other bar patrons in conversations about behavioral risk reduction and to visibly endorse safer sex norms over a period of at least two weeks. These conversations constituted the "real" intervention, which, it was hoped, would lead to reductions in risky sex practices by the population opinion leaders and the men with whom they discussed safer sex and also to community-wide reductions in risky behavior as safer sex norms diffused throughout the gay community.

Kelly and colleagues administered sexual behavior surveys to all men entering the bars on several successive nights, before initiation and several months after the completion of the intervention. (To control for potential temporal confounds, bar patrons in two comparison cities were also given the sexual behavior survey. These cities subsequently received the intervention as part of a lagged analytic design, see Kelly et al.[7]) The popular opinion leader intervention produced statistically significant reductions in the proportion of men who engaged in any unprotected anal intercourse or who had multiple sexual partners and a significant increase in condom use during anal intercourse.[14] These findings indicate that it is possible to "produce generalized changes in sexual risk behavior within an entire community population—men patronizing gay bars in a city—by enlisting the efforts of popular opinion leaders to visibly and demonstratively recommend, endorse, and support the behavioral change efforts of their friends and acquaintances" (Kelly, 1994, p. 312).[24]

Recently, Pinkerton and colleagues conducted a cost-utility analysis of the popular opinion leader intervention which indicated that, in addition to being highly effective, this HIV prevention strategy is actually cost-saving to society.[25] The overall cost of delivering the intervention was about $17,000. Salary for intervention and bar staff and incentives for the popular opinion leaders accounted for more than 70% of total expenditures. Based on the sexual behavior reported by the 449 men who completed the surveys, the intervention prevented about one-quarter of an infection in the very short two-month period following completion of the intervention. This translated into savings of about 3 QALYs and nearly $24,000 in potential HIV/AIDS-related medical care costs (all savings discounted at a 3% annual rate). Therefore the intervention is cost-saving, even under the very conservative assumptions of the analysis about the duration of intervention effects (2 months) and the overall reach of the intervention (only the 449 men who were surveyed were included in the analysis, despite the expectation that safer sex norms would diffuse throughout the gay community).

SUMMARY

In summary, several empirical studies indicate that small group and community-level interventions are effective in changing risky sexual behavior. The results of these studies further suggest that these types of interventions could be key components of a comprehensive HIV prevention program. However, program planners and resource allocation decision makers need information on the effectiveness of different interventions and also on their costs and cost-effectiveness. This chapter is a summary of the available economic evaluation literature on small group and community-level HIV prevention interventions (see Table 1).

For each intervention, the cost-per client and the basic analytic findings are summarized. As indicated, all of the analyzed interventions were either cost-saving or cost-effective. This was true even though some of the interventions were especially intensive (as many as twelve sessions per client) and the cost-per-client was measured in hundreds of dollars. These results indicate that although interventions for preventing HIV infection may at first blush seem "expensive," they are well worth the expenditure. HIV prevention is an investment in the future. Money spent now on prevention can avert substantial future medical costs associated with the care and treatment of HIV disease and AIDS.

All of the four studies involve some inherent uncertainty. Therefore, these studies all included extensive sensitivity analyses in which input parameter values were varied across plausible ranges to assess the robustness of base-care results to changes in these parameters. In general, the results of the studies were quite robust to changes in estimates of program cost, number of quality-adjusted life years saved each time an infection is averted, and the medical care and treatment costs averted by each prevented infection. However, the results are rather sensitive to the estimated number of HIV infections prevented. In turn, this estimate depends on several parameters, including behavioral outcome variables from the original randomized, controlled trials; estimates of HIV seroprevalence among intervention clients' sexual partners; estimates of the per-contact probability of sexual transmission of

HIV; and estimates of the effectiveness of condoms at reducing this probability (see Pinkerton and Abramson, chapter 2, this volume, for a thorough treatment of this topic).[26]

In particular, study results are somewhat sensitive to variations in HIV seroprevalence. Sensitivity analyses indicate that the cost-effectiveness ratios appear less favorable if assumptions of very low, local HIV seroprevalence are made in the analyses. Hence, the cost-effectiveness of intensive behavioral interventions may be questioned for populations of extremely low HIV seroprevalence. Therefore, intensive interventions may not be fiscally appropriate for low-risk areas.

Although the results of these four studies are extremely promising, more research is needed in this area. Small group interventions have been found effective when employed with adolescent populations. However, the economic evaluation of these interventions for youth remains to be completed. Research is also needed in the form of economic evaluation adjuncts to on-going and future effectiveness studies of community-level interventions.

Because of the effectiveness of small group and community-level interventions, a number of health department and nongovernmental service organizations are incorporating such interventions in their comprehensive HIV prevention programs. An important health services research question is how much it costs these service delivery organizations to field such interventions. The retrospective cost analyses described above provide initial answers to this question. However, prospective studies in this area are urgently needed.

Although the economic evaluation of small group and community-level HIV prevention interventions is a field that will continue to grow and mature, it is not too early to use the findings from these initial studies. They provide very strong evidence that such interventions are effective, also cost-effective, and, in many cases, actually cost-saving to employ. The findings are sufficiently strong that they should already begin to inform and influence the HIV prevention decision making of public health program mangers, policy makers, and community planning groups.

ACKNOWLEDGMENT.   Preparation of this chapter was supported by grants R01-MH55440 and P30-MH52776 from the National Institute of Mental Health.

REFERENCES

1. NIH Consensus Development Conference Consensus Statement. *Interventions to Prevent HIV Risk Behaviors.* Washington DC: Government Printing Office; 1997.
2. Holtgrave DR Effectiveness of behavioral interventions to prevent sexual transmission of human immunodeficiency virus infection. In V. T. DeVita, S. Hellman, S. Rosenberg, I. Curran, M. Essex, and A. S. Fauci, eds. *AIDS: Biology, Diagnosis, Treatment and Prevention*, 4th ed. Philadelphia: J. B. Lippincott; 1996: pp. 577–582.
3. Kelly JA, Murphy DA, Washington CD, et al. The effect of HIV/AIDS intervention groups for high-risk women in urban clinics. *Am J Public Health* 1994; 84:1918–1922.
4. Hobfoll SE, Jackson AP, Lavin J, et al. Reducing inner-city women's AIDS risk activities: A study of single, pregnant women. *Health Psychol* 1994; 13:397–403.
5. Valdiserri RO, Lyter DW, Leviton LC, et al. AIDS prevention in homosexual and bisexual men: Results of a randomized trial evaluating two risk reduction interventions. *AIDS* 1989; 3:21–26.
6. Kelly JA, St. Lawrence JS, Hood HV, et al. Behavioral intervention to reduce AIDS risk activities. *J Consulting Clin Psychol* 1989; 57:60–67.
7. Kelly JA, St. Lawrence JS, Stevenson LY, et al. Community AIDS/HIV risk reduction: The effect of endorsement by popular people in three cities. *Am J Public Health* 1992; 82:1483–1489.

8. Jemmott JB, Jemmott LS, Fong GT. Reductions in HIV risk-associated sexual behaviors among black male adolescents. *Am J Public Health* 1992; 82:372–377.

9. Rotheram-Borus MJ, Koopmen C, Haignere C, et al. Reducing HIV sexual risk behaviors among runaway adolescents. *JAMA* 1991; 266:1237–1241.

10. Kelly JA, Murphy DA, Sikkema KJ, et al. Psychological interventions to prevent HIV infection are urgently needed: New priorities for behavioral research in the second decade of AIDS. *Am Psychol* 1993; 48:1023–1034.

11. Choi KH, Coates TJ. Prevention of HIV infection. *AIDS* 1994; 8:1371–1389.

12. Centers for Disease Control and Prevention. Community-level prevention of human immunodeficiency virus among high-risk populations: The AIDS Community Demonstration Projects. *MMWR* 1996; 45(RR-6):1–24.

13. Kegeles SM, Hays RB, Coates TJ. The Mpowerment project: A community-level HIV prevention intervention for young gay men. *Am J Public Health* 1996; 86:1129–1136.

14. Kelly JA, St. Lawrence JS, Diaz YE, Stevenson LY, Hauth AC, Brasfield TL, Kalichman SC, Smith JE, Andrew ME. HIV risk behavior reduction following intervention with key opinion leaders of population: An experimental analysis. *Am J Public Health* 1991; 81:168–171.

15. Rietmeijer CA, Kane MS, Simons PZ, Corby NH, Wolitski RJ, Higgins DL, Judson FN, Cohn DL. Increasing the use of bleach and condoms among injecting drug users in Denver: Outcomes of a targeted, community-level HIV prevention program. *AIDS* 1996; 10:291–298.

16. Holtgrave DR, Qualls NL, Curran JW, et al. An overview of the effectiveness and efficiency of HIV prevention programs. *Public Health Rep* 1995; 110:134–146.

17. Rogers EM. *Diffusion of Innovations*. New York: Free Press; 1983.

18. Holtgrave DR, Pinkerton SD. Updates of cost of illness and quality of life estimates for use in economic evaluations of HIV prevention programs. *J Acquired Immune Defic Syndr Hum Retrovirol*, in press.

19. Holtgrave DR, Kelly JA. Preventing HIV/AIDS among high-risk urban women: The cost-effectiveness of a behavioral group intervention. *Am J Public Health* 1996; 86:1442–1445.

20. Holtgrave DR, Kelly JA. The cost-effectiveness of an HIV/AIDS prevention intervention for gay men. *AIDS and Behavior*, in press.

21. Pinkerton SD, Holtgrave DR, Valdiserri RO. Cost-effectiveness of HIV prevention skills training for men who have sex with men. *AIDS* 1997; 11:347–357.

22. Phillips K, Haddix A, Holtgrave DR. Chapter 1 in this volume.

23. Sikkema KJ, Kelly J, Heckman T, et al. Effects of community-level behavior change intervention for women in low-income housing developments. Presented at the *XI International Conference on AIDS*, Vancouver, Canada, July 7–12, 1996, Abstract TuD454.

24. Kelly JA. HIV prevention among gay and bisexual men in small cities. In DiClemente RJ, Peterson JL, eds. *Preventing AIDS: Theories and Methods of Behavioral Interventions*. New York: Plenum Press; 1994: 297–317.

25. Pinkerton SD, Holtgrave DR, Kelly JA, et al. Cost-effectiveness of a community-level HIV risk reduction intervention. To be presented at the *1997 Annual Meeting of the American Public Health Association* (abstract).

26. Pinkerton SD, Abramson P. Chapter 2 in this volume.

9

The Cost-Effectiveness
of the Components of a Comprehensive
HIV Prevention Program
A Road Map of the Literature

DAVID R. HOLTGRAVE

No locale in the United States has an HIV prevention program that consists of just one type of service. The citizens of any geographic area have a wide variety of HIV prevention needs, and an array of services must be delivered to meet those diverse needs. It is the job of HIV prevention community planning groups and other public health decision makers to craft an appropriate service array for their jurisdiction.

There is no one generally agreed upon set of services that comprises a truly comprehensive program. However, in its guidance for state health department grantees, the Centers for Disease Control and Prevention (CDC) have identified several key components that at least should be considered for inclusion.[1] These components include HIV counseling, testing, referral and partner notification; health education and risk reduction; and public information.[1,2]

An updated version of this taxonomy is displayed in Table 1. The service categories are reasonably self-explanatory. They include some categories for which the effectiveness has been empirically established (e.g., small-group interventions). Some categories rest on a foundation of theory, plausibility, and promise, but not unequivocal data (e.g., postexposure prophylaxis in nonoccupational settings).

Ideally, decision makers responsible for HIV prevention programming and resource allocation would have access to economic evaluative information on all of these types of services. They would know how many resources each intervention type consumes (via cost analysis); the most efficient form of delivering each service category (via cost minimization analysis); the relative cost-effectiveness of each category relative to other HIV prevention service types (via cost-effectiveness analysis); and the relative cost-effectiveness of each category relative to interventions in other disease areas (via cost-utility analysis). Cost and cost-minimization analyses are feasible for each service category displayed in Table 1 and should be available (eventually) to decision makers. Cost-utility analyses may be more useful than cost-effectiveness analyses that utilize outcome measures, such as "cost per

DAVID R. HOLTGRAVE • Department of Psychiatry and Behavioral Medicine, Center for AIDS Intervention Research (CAIR), Medical College of Wisconsin, Milwaukee, Wisconsin 53202.

Handbook of Economic Evaluation of HIV Prevention Programs, edited by Holtgrave. Plenum Press, New York, 1998.

Table 1. Possible Interventions
in a Comprehensive HIV Prevention Program

HIV counseling and testing, referral and partner notification
Health education and risk reduction
Individual and couples counseling (sans testing)
Small-group interventions
Organizational and community-level interventions
Public information, mass media, and social marketing
Syringe exchange
Referral to drug treatment
Street and community outreach
STD and HIV treatment
Post-exposure prophylaxis
Occupational
Nonoccupational
Perinatal transmission prevention
Societal, policy, and legal interventions
Prevention case management

HIV infection averted." Using "cost per quality-adjusted life-year saved" as an outcome (in cost-utility analysis) allows comparing HIV prevention interventions to each other *and* to interventions in other disease areas. Further, some HIV prevention interventions have intended outcomes that may effect quality of life but not necessarily mortality (e.g., a reduction in discriminatory actions in the workplace). A cost-utility framework allows, at least theoretically, inclusion of such benefits in the analysis.

A cost-utility analysis on each intervention type would allow for the construction of a league table of HIV prevention interventions (however, all of the methodological cautions noted by Paltiel and colleagues in this volume should be duly noted when considering league tables). A carefully constructed league table would contain cost-utility ratios for various types of HIV prevention interventions and foster comparison of the intervention types on the basis of relative cost-effectiveness. However, now the literature does not contain such comprehensive information.

In this brief chapter, we note the available sources of economic evaluation studies for each intervention category. The purpose of this chapter is to provide a road map to the extant economic evaluative information for each category—not to reiterate or summarize all available findings. Rather, the goal is to highlight access points to such information.

For intervention categories which have not yet been subjected to economic evaluation, we provide some thoughts to shape the research agenda. In particular, we note whether cost-utility analysis of an intervention type appears feasible and whether or not attention might be better limited to cost and cost minimization analyses.

HIV COUNSELING, TESTING, REFERRAL, AND PARTNER NOTIFICATION

In this book, Farnham provides a detailed review of the available economic evaluative studies on HIV counseling and testing.[3] Also in this volume, Owens describes economic evaluations of HIV testing used for screening (especially in health care workers, health care patients, and pregnant women).[4] Therefore, the economic evaluations on HIV counseling and testing have been identified and are readily accessible.

Referral systems that link counseling and testing sites and other related services (e.g., early medical care for HIV-seropositive persons or intensive prevention services for HIV-seronegative persons at continued risk of infection) have been the subject of almost no attention in the economic evaluative literature. These referral systems are crucial links between important HIV-related services, and they are found nearly everywhere HIV counseling and testing services are provided. Because they have important consequences and consume (perhaps) significant resources, they are important candidates for economic evaluative study. However, economic evaluative studies of referral systems are hampered by the difficulty of expressing the impact of referrals systems in some unit like "HIV infections averted" or "quality-adjusted life years saved." Although it is possible, for instance, to ascertain the "cost per HIV+ client successfully referred to early intervention medical services," such an outcome measure would permit comparison of various referral systems to each other but not to other HIV-related prevention services or programs in other disease areas. Hence, economic evaluative studies of referral systems might most effectively concentrate on cost and cost-minimization analysis. In particular, it would be useful to identify the most efficient of several referral systems for achieving comparable outcomes in terms of patients successfully referred to important, other services.

Holtgrave et al.[6] identified six economic valuative studies of *partner notification services*. Five of the six studies were cost-effectiveness analyses that employed an outcome measure of "cost per HIV-seropositive partner identified" (values ranged roughly between $800 and $3200). As with referral systems, such an outcome measure permits comparing partner notification systems to each other but not to other HIV prevention interventions or services in other disease areas. Unlike referral systems, however, economic evaluations of partner services do not seem necessarily limited to cost-minimization studies. It is possible to develop mathematical models that link the number of HIV-seropositive persons identified by partner notification services with the number of HIV infections averted when such notified clients receive HIV counseling and testing (as well as other related) services.[6] Such models can be based on the effectiveness of HIV counseling and testing services in changing HIV-related risk behavior.[5,7] Refinement and applications of such models are important next steps in the economic evaluation literature on partner notification. Ultimately, cost-utility analyses of partner notification systems appear feasible.

HEALTH EDUCATION AND RISK REDUCTION

Earlier in this volume, Holtgrave and Pinkerton reviewed the literature on small-group and community-level health education and risk reduction interventions.[8] The extant information from this literature is readily accessible and includes a number of cost-utility analyses.

Missing from this literature, however, is attention to the health education and risk reduction interventions delivered in organizational settings, such as schools, businesses, labor organizations, and faith communities. Such economic evaluative work should begin with careful cost analyses so that the true resources consumed by the programs are identified. Going further to, say, full scale cost-utility analyses may be difficult because some of these programs have intended outcomes other than quantifiable changes in HIV-related risk behavior or infections averted. For example, these programs attempt to achieve changes in parents' attitudes towards children receiving HIV-related information in schools, modify managers' and labor leaders' attitudes towards workers living with HIV infection, reduce discrimination in workplace policies, and increase volunteerism among members of the workforce and faith communities (among other goals). Such outcomes are extremely important for structuring an environment that enables HIV prevention programs to be established and allows persons living with HIV infection to be supported by co-workers and neighbors rather than being discriminated against. Although these outcomes are important, they are not easily cast into a cost-utility analytic framework. Hence, economic evaluative work in this area might focus on cost and cost-minimization analyses along with methodological work to explore the feasibility of linking attitudinal outcomes and improvements in quality of life. For instance, if discrimination is reduced, quality of life theoretically increases. What remains to be done, however, is a detailed explication and possible *quantification* of such a linkage between reduction in discrimination and improvement in the quality of life.

PUBLIC INFORMATION, MASS MEDIA, AND SOCIAL MARKETING

Holtgrave[9] reviewed all published studies that evaluated the effects of public information, mass media, and social marketing efforts related to HIV prevention. He found two studies that examined the economic value of airtime donated by U.S. broadcasters to HIV-related public service messages.[9-11] One additional study examined the cost of media efforts in developing countries.[9,12] To our knowledge, no other economic evaluative work has been done in this particular area.

Identifying the costs of media efforts and assessing the airtime donated to them are excellent beginnings in developing an economic evaluative effort in this area. However, much more remains to be done. Media campaigns take a tremendous amount of resources to develop and roll out. Cost information about campaign planning, development, and implementation are key for decision makers attempting to determine if they can afford such a program in their locale.

Even if a campaign is already developed (e.g., by a national agency) and can be implemented in a given locale, assessing airtime eventually donated to the campaign is important for program evaluative purposes. If no funding is available to pay for broadcasting, then donated airtime is the only means of making the campaign's messages available. Practical techniques for monitoring donated airtime should be available to all governmental and nongovernmental agencies implementing HIV prevention media efforts.

Conducting a cost-utility analysis of a public information, mass media, or social marketing intervention is more or less feasible depending on the outcome measure employed in the efficacy or effectiveness evaluation of the intervention. A few mass media evaluative studies have used biological outcome measures, and several have used HIV-related behavioral change as an outcome measure.[9] HIV-related risk behavioral outcome measures can often be converted via mathematical modeling into estimates of HIV infections averted and quality-adjusted life years saved (as described in the chapters by Pinkerton and colleagues).[13,14] Therefore, media campaigns, about which the behavioral or biological effects are known, are reasonable candidates for cost-utility analyses.

However, mass media intervention evaluations of efficacy or effectiveness also have employed any of a number of other outcome measures including condom sales, perceived risk, anxiety about HIV, homophobic attitudes, and discriminatory hiring practices in the work place.[9] As noted above with some other types of interventions, these outcome measures are important in fighting the HIV epidemic. However, casting them into a cost-utility analytic framework is problematic. Carefully theoretical and methodological work is needed to consider the appropriate way to link these outcome measures with improvement in quality of life if cost-utility analyses are to be possible. In the meantime, cost, cost-minimization, and donated airtime analyses are important starting points.

Syringe Exchange, Referral to Drug Treatment, and Street and Community Outreach

These interventions are largely related to HIV transmission via drug injection practices. The economic evaluative studies in these areas are reviewed by Kahn in this volume and are not summarized again here.[15]

STD and HIV Treatment

Some recent studies have found that treating sexually transmitted diseases (STDs) is an effective means of preventing HIV transmission.[16] This is especially true in geographical areas where HIV transmission is spread primarily via heterosexual behavior.[16] A study unveiled at the 1996 International Conference on AIDS in Vancouver found that treatment of STDs is effective and also cost-effective in such settings.[17] Research remains to be done to determine the effectiveness and cost-effectiveness of STD treatment as a means of HIV prevention in areas where HIV transmission is primarily via injected drug use and homosexual behavior.

Although not yet empirically established, there is much current speculation that treatment of HIV disease with new, advanced therapies (including protease inhibitors) can reduce the infectiousness of HIV-seropositive persons. As more data become available to support (or refute) this hypothesis, it will be important to conduct cost-utility analyses of HIV treatment (as a means of prevention) via-à-vis other types of HIV prevention interventions. Recent economic analysis of HIV disease treatments have focused on the relative cost-effectiveness of new triple combination therapies compared with older forms of single and dual therapies.[18] This type of analysis is important for comparing HIV treatments to each other, but not necessarily for comparing HIV treatment (as a type of prevention) to other forms of HIV prevention.

Postexposure Prophylaxis

After exposure to blood products possibly infected with HIV, it may be effective to take a short course of treatment for HIV disease so as to potentially block establishment of HIV disease. Such postexposure prophylaxis may occur after occupational exposures or nonoccupational (the latter might occur via sexual or drug injecting behavior or sexual assault). Cost-utility analyses have been conducted for both occupational and nonoccupational postexposure prophylaxis.[19,20] However, the effectiveness of postexposure prophylaxis for nonoccupational settings is a parameter with considerable uncertainty. Current estimates of its effectiveness rest on a case-control study of postexposure prophylaxis for health-care workers.[21] As better estimates of effectiveness become available, the available cost-utility analytic work must also be updated.

Perinatal Transmission Prevention

In his chapter in this volume, Owens reviews the economic evaluations (including cost-effectiveness analyses) of screening pregnant women for HIV infection so that they may be given therapies effective at reducing the rate of perinatal HIV transmission.[4] Farnham provides additional, relevant information on counseling and testing issues.[3] We do not reiterate this overview here.

Societal, Policy, and Legal Interventions

In his chapter, Sweat reviews the economic evaluation issues related to societal, policy and legal interventions, and the data are readily available.[22] He notes the need for much further economic evaluative work in this area.

Prevention Case Management

Prevention case management is the client-centered assessment of HIV prevention service needs, identification of relevant service organizations, and successful coordination of referrals and service delivery. Without HIV prevention case management, clients might receive no (or inappropriate) services or get lost in the service delivery system and become disenchanted. Prevention case management is central to a comprehensive HIV prevention program.

Clearly, prevention case-management systems are excellent candidates for cost and cost-minimization analysis (so that the affordability of the systems can be assessed and the systems compared to each other). However, cost-utility analyses requires thoughtful linkage between prevention case-management service delivery and quality-adjusted life years saved by the case-management system. This linkage is possible if a causal chain is established between the case-management system, access of other HIV prevention interventions (such as small group interventions), the effectiveness of these other interventions, and the quality-adjusted life years saved by these other interventions. Of course, this causal chain is long, and its explication and quantification may be quite difficult. An important next step in the area is a very careful exegesis of this causal chain. Even if cost-utility analysis is not possible, cost and cost-minimization studies still provide useful information to answer a limited set of policy questions about affordability and the best way to achieve a certain level of success in service coordination for a given resource level.

Other Programmatic Components

Previously we discussed various types of interventions possible in a comprehensive HIV prevention program. Of course, a comprehensive program has other elements that are not interventions themselves. These important elements include program planning and evaluation, research, surveillance, infrastructure maintenance, program administration, and capacity building. When considering the economic evaluation of a comprehensive program, these elements are best considered part of the overhead cost of the overall program.

CONCLUSIONS

Persons who allocate HIV prevention resources to assemble elements and interventions into a comprehensive, meaningful program would benefit from a league table of cost-utility analyses for each major intervention type. (Of course, cost and cost-minimization information is helpful, too, but for answering a more limited range of policy questions.) In this chapter we have seen that several types of interventions have been subjected to full scale cost-utility analyses, yet other categories remain to be addressed. Most of the categories that have not been subjected to cost-utility analyses have intervention goals that are not directly expressed in behavioral or epidemiological terms. For such interventions, important conceptual and methodological work remains to be done to link outcomes, such as discrimination reduction, to improvements in quality of life. Also, much further effort is needed to render all of the extant cost-utility analyses of various intervention types comparable to each other. Although there is a strong trend toward methodological standardization, it has not yet been sufficiently achieved. Additionally, research must be done on "bundles" or "mixtures" of interventions to determine the optimal way to align interventions within a comprehensive program.

Still, the economic evaluation of HIV prevention interventions is a rapidly emerging field and excellent beginnings have been made. Further challenges in methodological standardization, conceptual work, and application to more intervention types appear surmountable. Perhaps more daunting are challenges in assisting policy makers in actually using these studies in their decision making. That is the topic of the next section of this book.

ACKNOWLEDGMENT. Preparation of this chapter was supported by grants R01-MH55440, R01-MH56830, and P30-MH52776 from the National Institute of Mental Health.

REFERENCES

1. Centers for Disease Control and Prevention. Cooperative agreements for human immunodeficiency virus (HIV) prevention projects, program announcement and availability of funds for fiscal year 1993. *Federal Register* 57:40675–40683.
2. Holtgrave DR, Valdiserri RO, West GA. Quantitative economic evaluations of HIV-related prevention and treatment services: A review. *Risk: Health, Safety and Environment* 1994; 5:29–47.
3. Farnham PG. Economic evaluation of HIV counseling and testing programs: The influence of program goals on evaluation. In Holtgrave DR, ed. *Handbook of Economic Evaluation of HIV Programs.* New York: Plenum; 1998.
4. Owens DK. Economic evaluation of HIV screening interventions. In Holtgrave DR, ed. *Handbook of Economic Evaluation of HIV Programs.* New York: Plenum; 1998.
5. Holtgrave DR, Vaidiserri RO, Gerber AR, Hinman AR. Human immunodeficiency virus counseling, testing, referral, and partner notification services: A cost-benefit analysis. *Arch Intern Med* 1993; 153:1225–1230.
6. Holtgrave DR, Qualls NL, Graham JD. Economic evaluation of HIV prevention programs. *Annu Rev Public Health* 1996; 17:467–488.
7. Kamb ML, Douglas JM, Rhodes F, et al. A multi-center, randomized, controlled trial evaluating HIV prevention counseling (Project RESPECT): Preliminary results. Poster presented at the *11th International Conference on AIDS*, Vancouver, British Columbia (abstract ThC4380), July 1996.
8. Holtgrave DR, Pinkerton SD. The cost-effectiveness of small group and community-level interventions. In Holtgrave DR, ed. *Handbook of Economic Evaluation of HIV Programs.* New York: Plenum; 1998.
9. Holtgrave DR. Public health communication strategies for HIV prevention: Past and emerging roles. *AIDS* 1997; 11(Suppl. A):S183–S190.

10. Gentry EM, Jorgensen CM. Monitoring the exposure of 'American Responds to AIDS' PSA campaign. *Public Health Rep* 1991;106:651–655.

11. Woods DR, Davis D, Westover BJ. 'American Responds to AIDS': Its content, development process, and outcome. *Public Health Rep* 1991; 106:616–622.

12. Soderlund N, Lavis J, Broomberg J, Mills A. Costs of HIV prevention strategies in developing countries. *Bull WHO* 1993; 71:595–604.

13. Pinkerton SD, Abramson PR. The Bernoulli-process model of HIV transmission: Applications and implications. In Holtgrave DR, ed. *Handbook of Economic Evaluation of HIV Programs.* New York: Plenum; 1998.

14. Pinkerton SD, Holtgrave DR. Assessing the cost-effectiveness of HIV prevention interventions: A primer. In Holtgrave DR, ed. *Handbook of Economic Evaluation of HIV Programs.* New York: Plenum; 1998.

15. Kahn JG. Economic evaluation of HIV prevention interventions for persons who inject drugs. In Holtgrave DR, ed. *Handbook of Economic Evaluation of HIV Programs.* New York: Plenum; 1998.

16. Institute of Medicine Committee on Prevention and Control of Sexually Transmitted Disease. Executive summary. In Eng TR, Butler WT, eds. *The Hidden Epidemic: Confronting Sexually Transmitted Disease.* Washington, DC: National Academy Press; 1997; pp. 1–18.

17. Gilson L, Mkanje R, Grosskurth H, et al. Cost-effectiveness of improved STD treatment services as a preventive intervention against HIV in Mwanza region, Tanzania. Paper presented at the *11th International Conference on AIDS*, Vancouver, BC (abstract MoC444), July 1996.

18. Moore RD, Bartlett JG. Combination antiretroviral therapy in HIV infection. *PharmacoEconomics* 1996; 10:109–113.

19. Pinkerton SD, Holtgrave DR, Pinkerton HJ. Cost-effectiveness of chemoprophylaxis after occupational exposure to HIV. *Arch Intern Med*, in press.

20. Pinkerton SD, Holtgrave DR, Bloom FR. Is post-exposure prophylaxis for sexual or injection-associated exposure to HIV cost-effective? *N Engl J Med* (letter), in press.

21. Centers for Disease Control and Prevention. Case-control study of HIV seroconversion in health-care workers after percutaneous exposure to HIV-infected blood—France, United Kingdom, and United States, January 1988–August 1994. *MMWR Morb Mortal Wkly Rep* 1995; 44:929–933.

22. Sweat MD, Denison J. Changing public policy to prevent HIV transmission: The role of structural and environmental intervention. In Holtgrave DR, ed. *Handbook of Economic Evaluation of HIV Prevention Programs.* New York: Plenum; 1998.

10

Resource Allocation and the Funding of HIV Prevention

A. DAVID PALTIEL and AARON A. STINNETT

INTRODUCTION

Issues of priority setting in the health sector force decision makers to confront a tangled web of competing obligations. Confronted with limited resources and a seemingly infinite array of attractive programs, decision makers face a constant struggle to balance their ethical duty to do what is best for the individual against their responsibility to use society's resources to promote the collective safety and well-being efficiently and fairly. In HIV prevention, these painful trade-offs are further complicated by the fact that they must be made against the backdrop of a tragic epidemic, contentious political and social debate, aggressive community activism, and limited information regarding the costs and consequences of intervention.

Economic evaluation has been promoted as one means of stimulating a reasoned approach to this difficult challenge. As described elsewhere in this volume, cost-effectiveness analysis (CEA) assists decision makers in organizing and understanding information about complex choices with uncertain outcomes. By making explicit the economic costs and health benefits of health-related investments, CEA is a powerful tool for assessing program performance. Moreover, because it sheds light on comparative cost consequences and the benefits forgone when funds are devoted to one activity rather than another, CEA provides valuable information for resource allocation decisions. It might even, in principle, be used for purposes of priority setting between health-related initiatives and other social investment alternatives. For these reasons, cost-effectiveness analyses are becoming increasingly common, in evaluations of HIV prevention programs[1] and more generally in the health and social policy literature.[2,3]

Despite the increased use and acceptance of economic evaluative methods, however, there is evidence that real-world spending decisions continue to deviate substantially from what so-called "rational" economic models would suggest. Economists have long recognized the inefficiency of society's investment choices. Relatively cost-effective programs are often passed by whereas more costly, less effective alternatives are implemented.[4–7] Even when credible cost-effectiveness information is made available to decision makers, the evidence shows that it is often ignored. It seems that the economic principles of efficient

A. DAVID PALTIEL • School of Medicine, Yale University, New Haven, Connecticut 06520. *AARON A. STINNETT* • Department of Health Care Organization and Policy, University of Alabama, Birmingham, Alabama 35294.

Handbook of Economic Evaluation of HIV Prevention Programs, edited by Holtgrave. Plenum Press, New York, 1998.

resource allocation fail to capture qualitative criteria that play an important role in individual and social priority setting in the health sector. Research in the theory of risk perception and social choice aims to step beyond the simple observation of economic inefficiency and to explore what some of these "softer" preference criteria might be. Investigators have learned that people do not value all lives and deaths equally, that some hazards and perilous situations elicit greater degrees of social sympathy than others, and that what people are prepared to give up to prevent a loss of life or health is very much a question of context.[8,9]

These findings have a special significance for HIV prevention policy. Many of the "gut feel" considerations that influence societal attitudes toward health programs, such as the controllability of the risk in question, the degree to which blame can be assigned, the age, wealth, productivity, and visibility of the individuals in peril, and whether the hazard is a naturally occurring (as opposed to a man-made) phenomenon, have a particular salience in the context of the AIDS epidemic and the communities at greatest risk of HIV infection. Moreover, it is not clear that education or outreach efforts appreciably change the visceral human responses that these issues provoke. Whatever one's view on these matters might be, it has become clear that the perceptual obstacles to "rational" decision making in AIDS policy can be anticipated and must be addressed. An appreciation for these issues and their role in the decision making process is necessary if the role of economic evaluation and formal analysis in priority setting is to be appropriately defined.

This chapter explores the tension between the theory of resource allocation and the reality of priority setting in the public arena. It is divided into three distinct parts. The first section "The Theory of Resource Allocation" provides a formal presentation of the intellectual foundations of cost-effectiveness analysis for priority setting. We define the concept of a threshold cost-effectiveness ratio, discuss how this threshold can serve as a guide to choosing among competing alternatives under constrained budgets, and examine alternative approaches for determining where the threshold lies (or "where to draw the line"). In the next section "Risk Perception and the Policy Process," we shift our focus away from the theory of resource allocation and toward the realities of decision making in the public setting. We examine evidence of discrepancies between the guidance offered by economic theory and the actual choices revealed by real-world policy decisions, and we suggest that many of the societal decisions that seem puzzling from a purely economic perspective are rooted in strongly held beliefs about personal responsibility and compassion. Some issues in the perception of risk that may explain society's unwillingness to adhere to a single-minded, efficiency-driven recipe for decision making are discussed. The final section "Blending Theory and the Policy Process: The Role of Formal Analysis" seeks to identify ways in which formal analysis may be employed to reconcile the divergence between human nature and the pursuit of so-called "rational" HIV prevention policy. We propose what we believe is an appropriate role for quantitative program evaluation in the HIV prevention policy process—one that recognizes the importance of efficiency while simultaneously affording human values their rightful place.

THE THEORY OF RESOURCE ALLOCATION

The Constrained Optimization Problem

Broadly stated, the challenge of health resource allocation is to confer the greatest possible good, subject to financial and other limitations. In the context of HIV prevention, the problem can be framed as choosing how to allocate the limited resources available to achieve the greatest possible reduction in HIV-related morbidity and mortality. Problems such as this, in which an explicit objective function is maximized or minimized subject to specified limitations, are referred to as "constrained optimization" problems. These problems can be formally expressed using the language of mathematical programming:

$$\text{maximize: } \Sigma \; x_j \, e_j \tag{1}$$

$$\text{subject to: } \Sigma \; x_j \, c_j \leq B \tag{2}$$

$$0 \leq x_j \leq 1 \text{ (for all } j) \tag{3}$$

Here, e_j and c_j denote the effectiveness and cost of activity j if fully implemented, B is the total budget available, and x_j represents the percent implementation of activity j. Note that the x_j's are the decision variables in this problem, whereas all other terms represent input data. The objective function (1) measures the total health effectiveness conferred by a given allocation of funds. The first constraint (2) requires that the total resources consumed not exceed the available budget, and the second constraint (3) restricts each activity's implementation level to between 0% and 100%.

The following simple algorithm offers a general solution to the optimization problem[10–13] and serves as the theoretical foundation for cost-effectiveness analysis:

0. Immediately eliminate from consideration any activities with positive costs and negative health effects. At the same time, fully implement any programs that produce net savings and confer positive health gains.
1. Rank order all remaining activities according to their ratio of c_j to e_j.
2. Select activities for funding in order of increasing c_j/e_j ratio.
3. Repeat step 2 until the budget is exhausted.

Activity j's cost-effectiveness ratio c_j/e_j is a measure of value for money. It can be interpreted as the additional resources that would be consumed in producing one extra unit of health benefit via activity j. By ranking programs in ascending order of cost per unit benefit conferred and by selecting programs for implementation from the top of the list downward until the budget is depleted, the solution algorithm ensures that each dollar is devoted to the most productive option available and that, consequently, the total benefits conferred are maximized.

This simple solution algorithm applies only to a hypersimplified and restrictive decision environment. Yet, the basic structure is flexible enough to accommodate a range of complicating factors, including diminishing marginal returns to scale, application of a single intervention to multiple population subgroups (at different costs and benefit levels), and issues of program "lumpiness" and indivisibility.[11,14,15] It can also be adapted to situations where subsets of the activities under consideration are mutually exclusive. In such instances, an algorithm based on *incremental cost-effectiveness analysis*[13,16] must be employed. Even in these more realistic instances, however, the general approach and spirit of the solution algorithm are unchanged. Funds are apportioned to activities in ascending order of cost per additional unit of benefit conferred.

The Critical Ratio

The solution method presented can be interpreted as a search for a value-for-money threshold. Viewed from this perspective, the purpose of the analysis is to ascertain what managers might call the "hurdle rate" and what we will refer to as the "critical" or "threshold" cost-effectiveness ratio. Full finding is assigned to activities that deliver a unit of benefit for less than this threshold dollar amount. Activities whose cost per unit of benefit conferred exceeds the cutoff go unfunded.

A critical cost-effectiveness ratio serves many useful purposes. First, it offers the decision maker guidance in distinguishing those health investments that produce sufficient value for money, in light of the available alternatives, from those that do not. Secondly, it provides a framework for evaluating all subsequent claims against the budget. The critical ratio establishes a standard against which any new investment option can be judged, without requiring that the entire constrained optimization problem be solved over again.[11,17] Perhaps most useful of all, the critical ratio is a shorthand way of conveying the value of the health benefit foregone by diverting resources from their most productive alternative use. This is what economists call the *opportunity cost*, a useful measure in understanding the potential impact of funding increases or cutbacks.

Of course, it is one thing to appreciate the potential utility in the abstract of a cost-effectiveness threshold and quite another to estimate one credibly for decision making. There is perhaps no question more frequently asked of cost-effectiveness analysts than what the value of the critical ratio *ought* to be. Sometimes, the answer is straightforward and follows directly from the theory. In the formal statement of the problem given previously, for example, the threshold can be assigned an explicit value in units of dollars spent per unit of health gained. In the language of mathematical programming, the critical cost-effectiveness ratio is computed as the reciprocal of the shadow price of the budget constraint. This represents the opportunity cost of decreasing the budget by a single dollar. The solution algorithm produces this hurdle rate as the ratio of cost to benefit for the final program to receive funding before the budget is exhausted.

The direct approach to drawing the line is possible only because of the special circumstances we have created in our formal specification of the problem: first, our adoption of a known, finite budget constraint; secondly, our assumption that there exists an individual decision maker (or, at least, a single decision making entity) charged with the task of allocating the budget; and thirdly, our use of an explicit objective function to be optimized. Real-world circumstances where such a situation arises are rare but not unheard of. Managed-care organizations aim to maximize profits by making fixed-budget coverage and reimbursement choices from among sets of competing alternatives. The State of Oregon confronted more or less this situation in 1989 when it sought to broaden Medicaid eligibility by rationing the set of medical services that would be provided under its plan on the basis of cost-effectiveness.[18] On a still larger scale, some nations with universal health insurance programs (notably Australia and Canada) operate under global budget constraints and have begun to consider cost-effectiveness as a criterion for choosing among drugs eligible for reimbursement.[19-21]

Obstacles to Estimating the Threshold Cost-Effectiveness Ratio

In many practical situations, there simply is no unequivocal answer to what the threshold cost-effectiveness ratio ought to be. More often than not, the assumptions that lead to the direct, endogenous evaluation of the threshold (as described previously) do not hold. It is rarely possible, for example, to identify a single decision maker with the authority to make a budget allocation across the universe of competing alternatives.[14,22] In most health policy settings, moreover, there is neither an explicit budget nor a clear understanding of which public spending opportunities will be precluded by a decision to fund a particular intervention. For example, when the FDA approves a new drug, it does so knowing that such a decision is likely to crowd out some other medical expenditures, but it is unlikely to know exactly which programs will be affected or how they are likely to evolve with changes in the overall size of the budget. Thus, even though choices may be made with increasing regard to their economic consequences, cost-consciousness rarely translates into an explicit understanding of the true opportunity costs of a decision.

Perhaps the most daunting obstacle to the direct assessment of a threshold cost-effectiveness ratio is the assumption that a well-specified and generally accepted objective function exists to be optimized. In the realm of HIV and AIDS, for instance, it is easy to identify situations where explicitly constrained resources must be allocated across competing alternative uses, but it is hard to imagine a unique statement of objective that would satisfy all parties to the decision. Stakeholders may assign varying degrees of weight to a diversity of performance attributes, including changes in infection incidence, reductions in infection prevalence, and increases in life expectancy, all of which may be further confounded by differing views regarding the importance of individual preferences and quality-of-life considerations.[23]

These issues get even thornier when the discussion is extended beyond HIV to embrace the wider menu of health-related investment alternatives. In such instances, a standard measure of health benefit is required that can be applied to widely varying diseases, treatments, and conditions. The fix, in principle, is a preference-based measure of outcome, such as the quality-adjusted life year (QALY).[24-26] The QALY merges considerations of survival and quality of life into a single measure of "health" or "well-being." Each year of survival is assigned a weight according to one's preferences regarding the health state in which that year is spent. A year spent in perfect health is equal to one QALY, and a year spent in less than perfect health is assigned a value less than one QALY. Thus, the QALY establishes a common metric in which a variety of health outcomes can be reported and compared. The practical difficulties of collecting, standardizing, and understanding preference-based measures of quality of life are, of course, enormous. Nevertheless, efforts have been made to apply them to HIV- and AIDS-related decisions.[27-33]

Some theorists advocate valuing health benefits in monetary terms by assessing people's willingness to pay for reductions in risks to their lives and health. Following this approach, a program is selected for implementation if and only if the willingness to pay for its benefits exceeds the program's costs.[34,35] Here again, however, the methodological challenges are daunting, and the ethical implications of basing resource allocation on people's willingness (and, hence, ability) to pay are open to debate.

League Tables

When direct estimates of the critical cost-effectiveness ratio cannot easily be obtained, one may still make inferences about opportunity costs by performing comparisons. By way of illustration, consider the following argument. It has been estimated that home dialysis for patients with renal failure, widely considered a justifiable, noncontroversial use of public funds, extends lives at a cost to society of about $20,000 to $50,000 per year of life gained.[36–38] By comparison, the cost of hypertension screening in men age 45–54 is estimated at roughly $5,000 to $10,000 per year of life gained.[39] These results clearly compare favorably with those for home dialysis. Based on this comparison, it would be inconsistent for a society that considers home dialysis an acceptable use of public funds not to support hypertension screening for 45–54-year-old men.

A tool that facilitates this type of analysis is the *league table*, a rank ordering of investment alternatives by cost-effectiveness ratio.[40] League tables help decision makers get a relative feel for what is expensive, what is cheap, and, most important, what is "worth it" in some comparative sense. A league table recently constructed by researchers at the Harvard Center for Risk Analysis offers a valuable resource for exploring comparative program performance.[3] The "Lifesaving Database" contains cost-effectiveness information on 587 health programs, drawn from a range of domains, including medicine (preventive and curative), transportation safety, environmental health, consumer product safety, and occupational health. The interventions compiled in this league table range from mandatory seat belt use regulations and smoking cessation campaigns to pesticide control and home dialysis for end-stage renal disease. HIV- and AIDS-related interventions in the database include screening interventions (mandatory and voluntary, in various populations); antiretroviral therapy at various stages of disease progression; prophylaxis against opportunistic infections; and prophylaxis following needle-stick injury in health-care workers. Costs per year of life gained for programs compiled in the Lifesaving Database range across 11 orders of magnitude, from programs that actually save money (e.g., immunizing children against rubella, mumps, and measles; requiring stricter flammability standards for some children's sleepwear; and targeted, voluntary screening for HIV in high-risk populations) to those that cost as much as $100 billion per life-year saved (e.g., chloroform emission standards at paper mills). Most of the programs in the database deliver life years at a cost of $10,000 to $1 million, with a median cost of $42,000 per year of life gained. The median medical program costs $19,000 per year of life gained.

Although these observations offer some useful insight into the comparative cost-effectiveness of health programs, Drummond and others[41,42] caution against the indiscriminate and unthinking use of league tables for estimating societal cost-effectiveness cutoffs. First among the many pitfalls they have identified is the questionable assumption of comparability across studies. The usefulness of the league table hinges on the assumption of comparability, that the methods employed to produce the various entries are consistent enough to justify a meaningful comparative assessment of worth. In most instances, however, league tables represent little more than compilations of disparate analyses. It is difficult to ascertain what effort was devoted to standardizing the methods of study design (e.g., choice of discount rate; year of study origin; methods of estimating outcome and utility values; the range of costs and consequences considered; and the choice of comparator programs). Secondly, league tables say nothing about a program's level of implementation. Inclusion of a program in a table does not mean that anyone considers it a justifiable use of funds, nor does it imply that any money has actually been devoted to that purpose. Finally, the availability of programs for inclusion in a league table is not random. Not all health-related interventions are the subject of economic evaluations. Publication and other biases may favor the analysis and reporting of counterintuitive or nonrepresentative instances where researchers have obtained either surprisingly favorable or surprisingly unfavorable cost-effectiveness results.

Practical Approaches to Drawing the Line

Where does all this leave decision makers? Practical people looking for an explicit, ready-to-use threshold value will no doubt be disappointed by our reluctance to provide one. Our bottom line is that there is no general answer that applies uniformly across contexts of time, place, and circumstance. Indeed, the pursuit of a "one-size-fits-all" cutoff value seems to us a counterproductive exercise. Quantitative analysis should be motivated by a search for qualitative insight into how assumptions affect choices. What really matters is not so much the precise, numerical value of the cutoff but rather an exploration of how robust the analysis is to small changes in whatever value is employed. The crucial question with regard to the threshold value, therefore, is the range over which it can fluctuate and the impact that such fluctuations have on a given resource allocation decision.

Nevertheless, we recognize that choices are inevitable and that on occasion, a bright line must be drawn. The best we can offer the practical reader facing such a situation are some rules of thumb that have proved useful in the realm of HIV prevention and in the health sector more generally. Owens and colleagues,[43] for example, employed a $45,000/QALY hurdle rate in evaluating the cost-effectiveness of HIV screening. Holtgrave and Qualls[44] used this same figure to compute a societal threshold cost per HIV infection averted. Kaplan and Bush[45] reviewed existing health economic evaluations and found that medical interventions with cost-effectiveness ratios of $20,000/QALY were usually deemed "cost-effective," whereas programs with ratios in excess of $100,000/QALY were judged "questionable." According to their review of the literature, the threshold cost-effectiveness ratio lies somewhere in the range of $20,000 to $100,000 per QALY gained. Laupacis and colleagues[46] produced an identical estimate of the range for the critical ratio. Although the consistency of these results must be viewed with caution—it has been noted, for example, that Kaplan and Bush reported costs in 1982 U.S. dollars whereas Laupacis measured them in 1992 Canadian dollars[47]—this loosely defined triage of the cost-effectiveness range provides reasonable guidance for HIV prevention effectiveness planners. Programs that deliver QALYs for less than about US$20,000 compare favorably with a host of other noncontroversial, HIV-related uses of public funds and may comfortably be labeled "cost-effective" whereas programs costing in excess of US$100,000 per QALY are difficult to justify on comparative economic grounds. Moreover, as the body of HIV-related evaluations continues to grow, the HIV-specific league table will become more credible, and it may soon be possible to narrow these dollar ranges considerably.

RISK PERCEPTION AND THE POLICY PROCESS

The discussion to this point has focused on the theory of efficient resource allocation. We have suggested, in general terms, how the cost-effectiveness criterion might be used to inform decisions regarding the allocation of scarce health resources. Now we turn to the realities of priority setting in the public arena. Here, we find abundant evidence that the rules of cost-effective resource allocation have little influence on society's health investment choices. Americans frequently support expensive programs that promise little health benefit, while, at the same time, forgoing opportunities to invest in much more cost-effective strategies for health improvement.[48,49] To cite just one example, the United States spends approximately $115 million per year on benzene emission control to save an estimated five years of life.[50] If this same amount were instead spent on collapsible automobile steering columns, the nation could save an additional 1684 life years.[51]

Inconsistencies of this kind have devastating consequences for both the public health and the public purse. Tengs[52] performed an analysis of 287 lifesaving interventions for which information on both cost-effectiveness and current levels of implementation were available. She determined that a simple redistribution of resources among those programs could prevent 60,000 premature deaths (resulting in a long-run gain of over 600,000 life years) each year in the United States without a net increase in resource consumption. Viewed another way, these findings suggest that a reallocation of lifesaving resources to the most cost-effective activities would free up $31 billion per year in the United States without a net loss of life. How do we explain this apparent inefficiency in the public prioritization of health risks?

Part of the answer lies in the diffusion of authority. Lifesaving resources are not easily transferred from one domain of intervention (such as occupational safety, environmental health, or infectious disease control) to another. One would be hard-pressed to identify a single policy maker who has the authority to shift funds from pollution abatement to childhood immunization or from mammography for premenopausal women to automobile airbag installation. Indeed, entirely different funding mechanisms operate from one domain to the next. The compliance costs of many environmental interventions, for example, are borne by private businesses and their customers, whereas other health programs, such as epidemiological outbreak investigations, are funded directly with tax dollars. In addition, although some public health measures are implemented at the behest of individual decision makers, many others (such as screening women for cervical cancer) rely on the participation of millions of independent decision makers with widely varying priorities, information, and resources.

Issues of fungibility and the concentration of decision making authority notwithstanding, it is clear that society could be making better use of its lifesaving resources. Even in instances where a single decision making entity is identified, programs with the potential to save both lives and dollars are often passed over in favor of interventions that consume vast amounts of money with little promise of improved health. In the realm of HIV prevention, for example, one need only look at the State of Illinois' 1988 decision to institute a mandatory prenuptial screening program. This program, adopted against the advice of public health experts, was abandoned 11 months after its inception, when it was found that of 150,000 persons tested, only 23 HIV-positive individuals were identified, with a cost per case identified of $228,000. According to one public health official, the cost of screening the first 12,000 persons (to identify four HIV-positive individuals) would have been sufficient to quadruple the state's expenditure on AIDS education or to pay for zidovudine for one year for all persons with AIDS in Illinois.[53–55]

Perhaps even more troubling than these inefficiencies and inconsistencies is the fact that policy makers are generally not upset to learn that their preferences deviate from what might be suggested by a more "rational" model of decision making. In the State of Oregon, for example, policy makers undertook—and then more or less ignored—an ambitious, formal evaluation in 1989 to guide them in rationing the state's Medicaid services. A draft priority list, derived on the basis of the cost-effectiveness criterion, was revealed in May 1990. In the face of overwhelming criticism and ridicule, it was almost immediately withdrawn. Commissioners went back to the drawing board and began work on a revised ranking scheme. By the time the dust had settled in March 1993, the commission members had virtually abandoned the priorities suggested by the formal analysis in favor of a softer, intuitive apportionment process.[56–59]

Clearly, the economic principles of cost-effective resource allocation fail to capture elements of choice that—although perhaps irrational to the dispassionate observer—are essential to achieving a socially acceptable outcome. In this section, we explore some of the qualitative criteria that play an important role in both individual and social priority setting.[60]

Blame and Controllability

The attribution of death to a voluntary, controllable cause appears to play an important role in determining the degree of social sympathy it is likely to provoke.[61] Consider, for example, the recent comments of Senator Jesse Helms (R-N.C.) who argues for a reduction in federal funds for AIDS medical care because it is the "deliberate, disgusting, and revolting conduct" of AIDS patients that is responsible for their infection.[62] Or the suggestion that baseball legend Mickey Mantle's history of drinking ought to have disqualified him as a candidate for a precious liver transplant.[63]

Where issues of blame are concerned, perception is more important than reality. For example, much of the public believes (incorrectly!) that most people with mental health problems somehow brought their difficulties upon themselves. Owing in part to this belief, public support for the funding of mental health care programs is low compared to other illness categories. Similarly, because HIV infection is perceived as a voluntary, controllable risk, public funding for HIV prevention generally meets a great deal of opposition, despite evidence that many such programs actually save society money and lives over the long run.[3] By contrast, even the specter of cancers from involuntary, uncontrollable sources (such as air pollution, second-hand tobacco smoke, and electromagnetic fields) provokes widespread calls for greater research and funding.

The human propensity to feel less charitable toward those perceived to be taking on voluntary or controllable risks is particularly pertinent in the light of findings by psychological researchers that people almost universally underestimate the importance of situational (or environmental) factors, as opposed to personal qualities, in determining the behavior of individuals. Indeed, this tendency appears to be so deep-rooted and so widespread that psychologists have termed it the *fundamental attribution error*.[64] Studies also show that the proclivity to overassign blame to the individual when considering other peoples' behavior does not extend to the evaluation of one's own behavior. We usually give ourselves credit for our successes while blaming our failures on the surrounding environment. With these findings in mind, it is perhaps not too surprising that people feel less sympathy for cigarette smokers (a distinct minority of the population) who contract lung cancer than for inactive people with poor dietary habits (a group with which all too many of us can identify) who fall victim to coronary heart disease. For similar reasons, it is not surprising that people favor increasing taxes on tobacco but not on beer or wine, despite the conclusions of numerous economic studies that alcohol is significantly undertaxed (based on a comparison of alcohol tax revenues and alcohol-related costs to society, such as those resulting from drinking and driving accidents) whereas the tax revenues from cigarettes more than outweigh the tobacco-related health-care costs imposed on society by smokers.[65,66]

A clear, if inconsistent, sense of fairness seems to be at work here. We are less sympathetic to lives in peril when the individuals at risk are judged to have "brought it on themselves." Although it is often easy to sympathize with these views, it is also important to note that what is perceived as fair from the viewpoint of causation may be inefficient with regard to final outcomes. An allocation of resources guided by considerations of blame and controllability will generally diverge significantly from the economically efficient allocation prescribed by the cost-effectiveness criterion.

Identifiable Lives and the "Rule of Rescue"

A second consideration that plays an important role in shaping people's attitudes toward various health programs is the so-called "Rule of Rescue"—the ethical sense of duty to a particular life in peril. Economists have long known that when identifiable individuals are at risk of death, the demand for intervention is high.[67] The case of the trapped mine worker or the child who will die of acute lymphocytic leukemia unless he or she receives a bone marrow transplant are two good illustrations.

The Rule of Rescue exerts a powerful force on human intuition.[68] People find it comforting to know that everything possible is being done to save a particular life at risk. We all bask in the joy of rallying together to rescue a toddler from the bottom of a well. A dispassionate analysis might reveal that an equal expenditure could have prevented the deaths of many more children if it were devoted either to building fences around wells or to vaccination programs and improved automobile safety, but these opportunity costs are measured in faceless statistics and rarely appear on the nightly newscast. They are invisible and, hence, they are easier to ignore.[69]

This propensity to tune out the anonymous victim has particular relevance for funding HIV prevention. Epidemic control activities, by their very nature, are aimed at saving "statistical lives." Nobody can point with certainty to the particular individual whose life was unequivocally "saved" by a preventive intervention. By contrast, it is possible to identify the double-transplant recipient who would absolutely, positively have died without the heroic measures taken by surgeons on his behalf. In this sense, the Rule of Rescue gives a comparative advantage to aggressive treatment activities in competing for public sympathy and resources.

Errors of Commission and the Natural Occurrence of Risk

Another fundamental discrepancy between human choice and the principles of cost-effective resource allocation lies in people's tendency to distinguish between deaths due to errors of omission and those that are traceable to a particular deed.[70] To illustrate this point, consider the following hypothetical example: A particular birth defect is present in one out of every thousand children born. A child who has the defect and does not receive early treatment faces a 50% chance of dying from the condition. Fortunately, a perfectly accurate diagnostic test is available, and all newborns in whom the birth defect is identified before the onset of symptoms can be completely cured. However, the procedure used to test for the defect can be lethal; four out of every ten thousand infants tested will die as a direct and observable result of the test itself. A decision must be made of whether or not newborns should be routinely tested.

A simple analysis which sought to minimize the total number of expected deaths would favor the testing strategy. To see why this is so, consider a population of 100,000 newborns. Testing results in the expected death of $(0.0004 \times 100,000) = 40$ children, while not testing produces $(0.001 \times 0.5 \times 100,000) = 50$ expected deaths. Closer inspection, however, reveals that the specific lives lost under the two strategies are quite different. In the absence of the testing program, all 50 expected deaths occur within the group of children afflicted with the birth defect and may be attributed to "natural causes." By contrast, virtually all 40 of the children expected to be killed through the testing program are infants not possessing the birth defect. For many people, this distinction makes a crucial difference. The children who die from testing are "innocent victims" who actually had nothing to gain from the testing program.

The problem, of course, is that we have no way, before the fact, of identifying those newborns who do not carry the fatal defect and who stand to gain nothing from the testing program. But therein lies the rub. Our errors of commission are more immediately tangible and, hence, more emotionally distressing to us than our errors of omission. If we choose not to proceed with the testing program, we seem to be able to ignore the fact that it was our inaction that led to the "natural" death of the infants possessing the birth defect. Although their loss is tragic, there is solace in reasoning that these children were somehow destined to die. We would have a harder time accepting the loss of "innocent lives" directly attributable to our intervention. Intuition instructs us to err on the side of making the less discernible, less disruptive mistake. The result, however, is that we treat one child's death as more tolerable than that of some other newborn—even though we have no way, before the fact, of distinguishing one infant from the other.[71]

The relevance of these issues to questions of HIV policy is perhaps best illustrated by the drug approval processes of the U.S. Food and Drug Administration (FDA). Since the passage of the landmark 1962 Amendments to the Federal Food, Drug, and Cosmetic Act, the FDA has pursued a single-minded strategy of protecting consumers from unsafe or ineffective drugs. It has steadfastly chosen to err on the side of caution, even at the cost of delaying the approval of potentially useful drugs. Celebrated instances where prudence has averted disaster, such as the FDA's role in insulating the United States from the thalidomide catastrophe, have reinforced the benefits of restraint. Only recently have AIDS activists begun to sensitize the public to the less visible costs that delayed access and higher prices have imposed on society.

BLENDING THEORY AND THE POLICY PROCESS: THE ROLE OF FORMAL ANALYSIS

Powerful economic forces exerted over the last two decades have compelled the United States to reconsider its priorities with regard to the nation's health and to examine whether it can afford to continue allocating its lifesaving resources inefficiently. Dramatic technological innovation, explosive growth in costs, and intense pressure to restrain budgets have forced Americans to acknowledge that resources devoted to prolonging lives in one area are not available for investment in other domains. There is growing acceptance of the claim that the nation can no longer afford all the health care and prevention it would like to consume and that painful trade-offs are inevitable. In the first section of this chapter we presented a formal justification of cost-effectiveness analysis as a tool for allocating a constrained budget across competing alternatives. In the second section we examined evidence suggesting that these formal rules have little or no influence on real-world priority setting in the health sector. This final section seeks to identify ways in which formal analysis can be employed to bridge the gap between rational efficiency and other human values.

At the heart of the dilemma is a persistent tension between two deeply rooted convictions.[72] Pulling us in one direction is the utilitarian conviction that society ought to allocate its scarce resources to confer the greatest possible benefit, subject to resource constraints. A more informed, more sophisticated, and more distrustful public detects some unfairness in the Rule of Rescue and other qualitative risk attributes when applied at the population level. Simply stated, we cannot continue to make choices without regard to severity, equity, or the alternatives forgone. From this perspective, formal analysis based on the cost-effectiveness criterion offers much-needed guidance for improving the efficiency of our health investment decisions.

Pulling us in the other direction are the perceptions of risk, responsibility, and blame enumerated previously. As guides to global resource allocation, these perceptual forces may be both inequitable and financially disastrous. Nevertheless, they reside deep in the human psyche, and it would be futile and naïve to suggest that we simply abandon them as rules of conduct and decision making. For physicians who have a Hippocratic obligation to "do no harm" and a duty to place the interests of the patient ahead of the collective well-being, issues of responsibility will almost invariably trump the more "rational" economic arguments. For the public official seeking reelection, the seductive power of the Rule of Rescue and the assignability of blame may also be impervious to logical argument and considerations of statistical lives and opportunity costs. One need only look at the recent debate over the rationing of Medicaid resources in Oregon to appreciate how painful the tension between these two mutually incompatible imperatives can be.[73]

The finding that our gut instincts are rarely aligned with the results of formal analysis takes on added significance in the context of AIDS. HIV illness is distinguished from most other diseases by the characteristics of the patient population and by the scope of the social crisis occasioned by the AIDS epidemic. The uniqueness of the situation and the emergence of influential patient advocacy groups have contributed to the evolution of a view that traditional conceptions of ethical duty, personal responsibility, and societal concern may be inadequate for guiding societal resource allocation decisions in matters affecting people with HIV illness and AIDS. The unique set of circumstances—a young, marginalized population suffering from a chronic illness for which only a few, expensive, life-prolonging therapies exist—conspire to create a heightened sense of urgency and a need to expedite and tailor-fit the process by which new medical technologies are developed, evaluated, approved, and brought to market. The often conflicting considerations of the Rule of Rescue, the controllability of risk, the drive to avoid errors of commission, and the desire to achieve the greatest overall good for society come to loggerheads in the AIDS policy arena perhaps more saliently than in any other health policy domain.

This calls for new thinking about the role of formal analysis in the policy process. Is the absence of such concerns as identifiability and attribution of blame a weakness or a strength of standard decision analytic models? What do we consider to be "rational" and is rationality an ideal we wish to pursue? What role do we wish human values to play in our decision making and in the policy process? These are difficult questions, and they have no (or perhaps many) "correct" answers.[74] Reflecting the range of views expressed on these matters, a variety of approaches to policy analysis and decision modeling have emerged. Although the individual models advanced vary widely in theoretical foundations and structure, it is informative to consider them in three classes: descriptive, normative, and prescriptive models.[75]

Descriptive Models

Descriptive models attempt to answer the question, How do we make decisions? The goal is to reproduce and to predict human choice processes. Issues such as the Rule of Rescue and other psychological phenomena feature prominently in these models. By investigating the ways in which people process, interpret, and respond to information, analysts in this line of research aim to capture and portray the key elements of human choice, however rational or irrational those elements may be. It is this type of research that has identified and explored the phenomena discussed in the preceding section of this chapter.

Within the policy process, this framework offers assistance by helping to predict people's responses to various policy changes. For example, descriptive models of decision making are useful for anticipating the public's response to health promotion programs. These models also explicitly identify pitfalls in human decision making (such as a tendency to assign disproportionate weight to low-probability risks) that we may wish to avoid. Because they are not designed for such purposes, however, descriptive models generally offer little assistance in developing new policies. They do not offer guidelines for "improved" decision making.

Normative Models

Normative models, in contrast, seek to answer the question, What *should* we do? The analyst begins by stating the objectives to be pursued. Then formal decision rules designed to attain those goals are specified. In the field of welfare economics, for example, criteria for decision making have been elaborated to achieve the objective of allocating society's scarce resources as efficiently as possible—conditional, of course, on a particular definition of efficiency. Any values not considered germane to the goal pursued are simply disregarded in the decision process. Doing otherwise would be considered "irrational."

Because normative models are managerial in their very design, it is not surprising that they offer the advantage of providing clear guidance in developing and assessing policies. It must be borne in mind, however, that the directions given by these models may—once again, by design—exclude from consideration issues and values (such as personal responsibility and the Rule of Rescue) that are important to many people. Thus, for example, a normative approach to decision modeling may dictate that it would be better to spend $6,000 on dental caps to alleviate the pain of pulp exposure for 150 patients than to spend that money on a single operation to save the life of a woman with an ectopic pregnancy.[57-59] By treating the human "gut feel" as irrelevant, strict adherence to a normative decision model carries with it an emotional price tag that many find unacceptable. Indeed, people's discomfort with the economic evaluation of health interventions arises, quite understandably, from a fear that research results will be interpreted as blueprints for social choice and that such a dispassionate process would fail to reflect human values.

Prescriptive Models

Lying midway on the spectrum bounded by descriptive models at one end and normative models at the other, *prescriptive* (or *suggestive*) models for evaluation seek to provide decision makers with information that can help them to make better choices but stop short of telling them what to do. The prescriptive approach does not provide a policy maker with rigid marching orders, nor does it take sides on the question of what role the Rule of Rescue and related concepts should play in the policy process. The goal of the approach is merely to structure choices to force decision makers to acknowledge their subjective assessments of value and to confront their implications. Unlike the descriptive approach, the decision maker is given some assistance in the choice process. At the same time, unlike the normative approach, the decision maker is not bound by the results of the formal analysis. Rather, he or she is invited to weigh the analytic results against other values and concerns, such as the assignability of blame and the Rule of Rescue, and authority and responsibility ultimately lie in the hands of the human decision maker.

Prescriptive Models in Action

To illustrate the potential of a prescriptive approach to program evaluation for contributing to the development of sound health policy decisions, it is helpful to consider those situations in which the results of formal economic analyses are likely to be considered most (or least) valuable. First, consider the case where formal evaluation suggests that a particular program is highly attractive from the perspective of economic efficiency. If this program also appeals to people's values and gut feelings, then the additional, quantitative support may prove a useful spur to action and may also help to sway others to support the program. For example, findings that many prenatal and well-baby care programs save lives and money (by averting downstream medical care costs) have proven valuable in helping to secure support for programs in maternal and children's health.

On the other hand, if the program in question has encountered strong political or community opposition, favorable results from a formal evaluation may prompt policy makers to state and explain their reasons for not supporting the program more explicitly. The result may be a more open discussion of values, principles, and objectives in the public policy process. In some cases, a formal analysis may prompt decision makers to reevaluate previously held positions. To illustrate, let us return to our earlier hypothetical example of a risky diagnostic test for a birth defect. The general unwillingness of physicians and parents alike to accept the risks of the test suggests that people place a higher value on avoiding the 40 iatrogenic deaths (the "errors of commission") than on preventing 50 natural deaths from the birth defect (the "errors of omission"). Faced with this data, however, some people may revise their choices. It is not uncommon for decision makers to discover that their fears of regret—left unexamined—had been magnified out of proportion.[76] After reflection, others may remain firm in their positions. Even these people, however, may benefit from the process. For example, in considering this decision, most people would agree that some level of test-related mortality risk is low enough that a policy of routine testing of newborns would be justified. One decision maker might opt for the testing strategy if the risks of iatrogenic death were reduced to 20 in every 100,000 infants tested. Another might be willing to accept only 5 such test-related deaths for every 50 "natural" deaths averted. By being forced to address these trade-offs explicitly, people may—whatever their final decision—benefit from scrutinizing and coming to grips with values to which they had previously given little thought.

Finally, consider the situation in which formal analysis finds that a particular program is relatively cost-ineffective. If the program in question was relatively unpopular to begin with, this information may confirm people's convictions and help them to feel more secure and justified in their positions. On the other hand, after being confronted with this data, people who had supported the program might reevaluate their positions and either modify their choices or more carefully delineate the other reasons why they consider the program worthwhile. For example, the plight of AIDS patients without access to potentially valuable, experimental treatments has forced the FDA to reconsider some of the costs associated with their bias towards preventing errors of commission (approving potentially harmful treatments) at the expense of errors of omission (leaving people without access to treatments that might be their best hope for prolonged survival). Although changes at the FDA have been incremental and have been the exception rather than the rule, they help to illustrate the benefits gained when formal study results are used to inform a reevaluation of existing policies and the reasoning on which they have been based.

Phillips and Rosenblatt have argued that the success of health services research hinges on the degree to which investigators can span disciplinary boundaries.[77] With specific regard to understanding choice in the health sector, they maintain that successful scholarship must integrate the perspectives and methods of both economics and psychology. We submit that the prescriptive approach to formal analysis (including, but not limited to, medical cost-effectiveness analysis) is one means of effecting Phillips and Rosenblatt's assertion. Viewed in this light, the purpose of policy evaluation is emphatically not to supplant the human decision maker, nor is it to question the legitimate role played by the Rule of Rescue and other "gut feelings" or value judgments in the resource allocation process. Rather, it is to provide information in the service of a subjective but reasoned decision making process that still affords compassion and humanity their rightful place. Such an approach is essential for developing ethically defensible and carefully reasoned HIV prevention policies.

REFERENCES

1. Holtgrave DR, Qualls NL, and Graham JD. Economic evaluation of HIV prevention programs. *Annu Rev Public Health* 1996; 17:467–488.
2. Elixhauser A, Luce BR, Taylor R, Reblando J. Health care CBA/CEA: An update on the growth and composition of the literature. *Medical Care* 1989; 27:S190–S204.
3. Tengs TO, Adams ME, Pliskin JS, Safran DG, Siegel JE, Weinstein MC, Graham JD. Five hundred life-saving interventions and their cost-effectiveness. *Risk Analysis* 1995; 15:369–390.
4. Zeckhauser R. Procedures for valuing lives. *Public Policy* 1975; 23:419–464.
5. Zeckhauser R, Shepard D. Where now for saving lives? *Law and Contemporary Problems* 1976; 40:5–45.
6. Bailey MJ. *Reducing Risks to Life: Measurement of the Benefits.* Washington, DC: American Enterprise Institute; 1980.
7. Lave LB. *The Strategy of Social Regulation.* Washington, DC: Brookings Institution; 1981.
8. Slovic P. Perception of risk. *Science* 1987; 36:280–285.
9. Fischhoff B, Slovic P, Lichtenstein S, Read S, Combs B. How safe is safe enough? A psychometric study of attitudes towards risks and benefits. *Policy Sci* 1978; 9:127–152.
10. Torrance GW, Thomas WH, Sackett DL. A utility maximization model for evaluation of health care programs. *Health Serv Res* 1972; 7:118–133.
11. Weinstein MC, Zeckhauser R. Critical ratios and efficient allocation. *J Public Econ* 1973; 2:147–157.
12. Weinstein MC. Principles of cost-effective resource allocation in health care organizations. *Int J Technol Assessment Health Care* 1990; 6:93–103.
13. Johannesson M, Weinstein MC. On the decision rules of cost-effectiveness analysis. *J. Health Econ* 1993; 12:459–467.
14. Birch S, Gafni A. Cost effectiveness analyses: Do current decision rules lead us where we want to be? *J Health Econ* 1992; 11:279–296.

15. Stinnett AA, Paltiel AD. Mathematical programming for the efficient allocation of health care resources. *J Health Econ* 1996; 15:641–653.
16. U.S. Department of Health and Human Services and the Foundation for Health Services Research. *The Comparative Benefits Modeling Project. A Framework for Cost-Utility Analysis of Government Health Care Programs*. A report to the Office of Disease Prevention and Health Promotion, Public Health Service; 1992; pp. 15–17.
17. Weinstein MC. Tutorial: Economic assessments of medical practices and technologies. *Medical Decision Making* 1981; 1:309–330.
18. Klevit HD, Bates AC, Castanares T, et al. Prioritization of health care services: A progress report by the Oregon Health Services Commission. *Arch Intern Med* 1991; 151:912–916.
19. Drummond MF. Basing prescription drug payment on economic analysis: The case of Australia. *Health Aff* Winter, 1992; 191–196.
20. Bloom BS. Issues in mandatory economic assessment of pharmaceuticals. *Health Aff* Winter, 1992; 197–201.
21. Freund DA, Evans D, Henry D, Dittus R. Implications of the Australian guidelines for the United States. *Health Aff* Winter 1992; 202–206.
22. Birch S, Gafni A. Changing the problem to fit the solution: Johannesson and Weinstein's (mis) application of economics to real world problems. *J Health Econ* 1993; 12:469–476.
23. Keeney RL, Raiffa H. *Decisions with Multiple Objectives: Preferences and Value Trade-Offs*. New York: Wiley; 1976.
24. Garber AM, Phelps CE. *Economic foundations of cost-effectiveness analysis*. Working paper #4164, Cambridge, MA: National Bureau of Economic Research; 1992.
25. Torrance GW. Utility approach to measuring health related quality of life. *J Health Econ* 1986; 5:1–30.
26. Kaplan RM. Utility assessment for estimating quality-adjusted life-years. In FA Sloan, ed. *Valuing Health Care: Costs, Benefits, and the Effectiveness of Pharmaceuticals and Other Medical Technologies*. New York: Cambridge University Press; 1995.
27. Patrick DL, Erickson P. *Health Status and Health Policy: Quality of Life in Health Care Evaluation and Resource Allocation*. New York: Oxford University Press; 1993.
28. Paltiel AD, Stinnett AA. AIDS. In B Spilker, ed. *Quality of Life and Pharmacoeconomics in Clinical Trials*, 2nd ed. New York: Raven Press; 1996.
29. Wu AW, Rubin HR. Measuring health status and quality of life in HIV and AIDS. *Psychol Health* 1992; 6: 251–264.
30. Owens DK, Sox HC. Medical decision making: Probabilistic medical reasoning. In Shortliffe EH, Perreault LE, Fagan LM, Wiederhold G, eds. *Medical Informatics: Computer Applications in Medicine*. Reading, MA: Addison-Wesley; 1990; 70–116.
31. Tsevat J. Methods for assessing health-related quality of life in HIV-infected patients. *Psychol Health* 1994; 9:19–30.
32. Gelber RD, Lenderking WR, Cotton DJ, et al. Quality-of-life evaluation in a clinical trial of zidovudine therapy in patients with mildly symptomatic HIV infection. *Ann Intern Med* 1992; 116:961–966.
33. Wu AW, Lamping DL. Assessment of quality of life in HIV disease. *AIDS* 1994; 8:S349–S359.
34. Phelps CE, Mushlin AI. On the near equivalence of cost-effectiveness and cost-benefit analysis. *Int J Technol Assessment Health Care* 1991; 7:12–21.
35. Pauly MV. Valuing health care benefits in money terms, in FA Sloan, ed. *Valuing Health Care: Costs, Benefits, and the Effectiveness of Pharmaceuticals and Other Medical Technologies*. New York: Cambridge University Press; 1995.
36. Bulgin RH. Comparative costs of various dialysis treatments. *Peritoneal Dialysis Bull* 1981; 1:88–91.
37. Ludbrook A. A cost-effectiveness analysis of the treatment of chronic renal failure. *Appl Econ* 1981; 13: 337–350.
38. Churchill DN, Lemon BC,Torrance GW. A cost-effectiveness analysis of continuous ambulatory peritoneal dialysis and hospital hemodialysis. *Medical Decision Making* 1984; 4:489–500.
39. Bryers E, Hawthorne J. Screening for mild hypertension: Costs and benefits. *J Epidemiol Community Health* 1978; 32:171–174.
40. Torrance GW. Measurement of health state utilities for economic appraisal: A review. *J Health Econ* 1986; 5:1–30.
41. Drummond MF, Torrance GW, Mason J. Cost-effectiveness league tables: More harm than good? *Soc Sci Med* 1993; 37:33–40.

42. Mason J, Drummond MF, Torrance GW. Some guidelines on the use of cost-effectiveness league tables. *Br Med J* 1993; 306:570–572.

43. Owens DK, Nease RF, Harris RA. Use of cost-effectiveness and value of information analyses to customize guidelines for specific clinical practice settings. *Medical Decision Making* 1993; 13:395 (Abstract).

44. Holtgrave DR, Qualls NL. Threshold analysis and programs for HIV prevention. *Medical Decision Making* 1995; 15:311–317.

45. Kaplan RM, Bush JW. Health-related quality of life measurement for evaluation research and policy analysis. *Health Psychol* 1981; 1:61–80.

46. Laupacis A, Feeny D, Deetsky A, Tugwell PX. How attractive does a new technology have to be to warrant adoption and utilization? Tentative guidelines for using clinical and economic evaluations. *J Can Medical Assoc* 1992; 146:473–481.

47. Weinstein MC. From cost-effectiveness ratios to resource allocation: Where to draw the line? In FA Sloan, ed. *Valuing Health Care: Costs, Benefits, and the Effectiveness of Pharmaceuticals and Other Medical Technologies.* New York: Cambridge University Press; 1995.

48. Schwing R. Longevity benefits and costs of reducing various risks. *Technol Forecasting Soc Change* 1979; 13:333–345.

49. Graham JD, Vaupel J. Value of a life: What difference does it make? *Risk Anal* 1981; 1:89–95.

50. Van Houtven G, Cropper ML. *When is a life too costly to save: Evidence from US environmental regulations.* World Bank Policy Research Paper No. 1260; 1994.

51. Graham JD. How to save 60,000 lives. *Electric Perspect* 1995; 20:14–21.

52. Tengs TO. The opportunity costs of haphazard societal investments in life-saving. Optimizing societal investments in the prevention of premature death. Unpublished doctoral dissertation, Harvard University; 1994.

53. Wilkerson I. Prenuptial AIDS screening a strain in Illinois. *New York Times* January 26, 1988; p 1.

54. Illinois may end premarital AIDS testing. *New York Times* January 23, 1989; p 10.

55. Belongia EA, Vergeront JM, Davis JP. Border hopping as a consequence of premarital HIV screening: The Kenosha diamond (letter). *JAMA* 1988; 260:1883–1884.

56. Tengs TO, Meyer G, Siegel JE, Pliskin JS, Graham JD, Weinstein MC. Oregon's Medicaid ranking and cost-effectiveness: Is there any relationship? *Medical Decision Making* 1996; 16:99–107.

57. Hadorn DC. Setting health care priorities in Oregon: Cost-effectiveness meets the rule of rescue. *JAMA* 1991; 265:2218–2225.

58. Eddy DM. Oregon's methods: Did cost-effectiveness analysis fail? *JAMA* 1991; 266:2135–2141.

59. Hadorn D. The Oregon priority-setting exercise: Cost-effectiveness and the rule of rescue, revisited. *Medical Decision Making* 1996; 17:117–119.

60. Slovik P, Fischhoff B, Lichtenstein S. Characterizing perceived risk. In Kates RW, Hohenemser C, Kasperson JX, eds. *Perilous Progress: Managing the Hazards of Technology.* Boulder, CO: Westview Press; 1985.

61. Douglas M. *Risk Acceptability According to the Social Sciences.* New York: Russell Sage Foundation; 1985.

62. Freedland J. Life could be in good Carolina. *The Observer.* May 5, 1996; p 21.

63. Goodstein L. Crying foul over Mantle; liver transplant sparks ethics, alcoholism debate. *The Washington Post.* June 10, 1995; p. B01.

64. Plous S. *The Psychology of Judgment and Decision Making.* New York: McGraw-Hill; 1993.

65. Manning WG, Keeler EB, Newhouse JP, et al. *The Cost of Poor Health Habits.* Harvard University Press: Cambridge, MA; 1991.

66. Viscusi WK. *Cigarette taxation and the social consequences of smoking.* NBER Working Paper No. 4891. Cambridge, MA: National Bureau of Economic Research; 1994.

67. Schelling TC. The Life You Save May Be Your Own. In Chase SC, ed. *Problems in Public Expenditure Analysis.* Washington DC: Brookings Institution; 1968.

68. Jonsen A. Bentham in a box: Technology assessment and health care allocation. *Law Med Health Care* 1986; 14:172–174.

69. Raiffa H, Schwartz WB, Weinstein MC. Evaluating health effects of societal decisions and programs. In *Decision Making in the Environmental Protection Agency.* Selected Working Papers, Washington, DC: National Academy of Science; 1977.

70. Ames B, Gold LS. Chemical Carcinogenesis: Too many rodent carcinogens. *Proc Nat Acad Sci USA* 1990; 87:7782–7786.

71. Brett AS. Hidden ethical issues in clinical decision analysis. *N Engl J Med* 1981; 305:1150–1152.

72. Paltiel AD, Stinnett AA. Making health policy decisions: Is human instinct rational? Is rational choice human? *Chance* 1996; 9:34–39.
73. Eddy DM. The individual vs. society: Resolving the conflict. *JAMA* 1991; 265:2399–2406.
74. Etzioni A. Normative-affective factors: Toward a new decision making model. *J Econ Psychol* 1988; 9: 125–150.
75. Bell DE, Raiffa H, Tversky A, eds. *Decision Making: Descriptive, Normative, and Prescriptive Interactions.* Cambridge: Cambridge University Press; 1988.
76. Kasperson RE, Kasperson JX. The social amplification and attenuation of risk. *Ann Am Acad Political Soc Sci* 1996; 545:95–105.
77. Phillips KA, Rosenblatt A. Speaking in tongues: Integrating economics and psychology into health and mental health services outcomes research. *Medical Care Rev* Summer, 1992; 49:191–231.

11

Economic Evaluation and HIV Prevention Decision Making

The State Perspective

BETH WEINSTEIN and RICHARD L. MELCHREIT

HISTORY OF HIV PREVENTION PROGRAMS

The first cases of AIDS were recognized in the early 1980s. Federal funds for HIV prevention were first allocated in 1985, when Congress appropriated $9,773,263. Eleven years later, in fiscal year 1996, Congress appropriated $222,807,596 to state and local health departments for HIV prevention,[1] an increase of 2,179% over the 1985 appropriation.

According to a survey by the Intergovernmental Health Policy Project of George Washington University, states appropriated $7,891,967 in state funds for HIV prevention in fiscal year 1986.[2] By fiscal year 1992, the last year in which the survey was conducted, that amount had risen to $401,894,973.[3]

This rapid growth in funding for HIV prevention indicates the great concern of U.S. and state policy makers about the spread of AIDS. Such a substantial increase also implies confidence that the programs being carried out with these funds are effective and that wise decisions are being made how best to spend the funds to maximize prevention benefits. Alas, such is not the case. Fifteen years after the first cases of AIDS were recognized and hundreds of millions of dollars of public funds have been spent, surprisingly little has been scientifically demonstrated about the effectiveness and the cost-effectiveness of many HIV prevention programs carried out with state and federal funds, and there is no substantial and useful body of knowledge for state health departments to consult in deciding how to allocate funds to best prevent new cases of the disease.

This chapter reviews the history of federal and state roles in allocating HIV prevention funds and describes barriers to the use of cost, effectiveness and cost-effectiveness data. It also describes the experiences of Connecticut and other states in developing and using such information.

BETH WEINSTEIN and RICHARD L. MELCHREIT • Connecticut Department of Public Health, Hartford, Connecticut 06134-0308.

Handbook of Economic Evaluation of HIV Prevention Programs, edited by Holtgrave. Plenum Press, New York, 1998.

Early Funding for HIV Prevention Programs in State Health Agencies: Federal Leadership and Direction

State health agencies (SHAs) in the United States have been carrying out HIV prevention programs since the early 1980s. Most states began such work with community education programs aimed at teaching the public and communities at risk how the disease is spread and reassuring them that it is not spread by "casual contact." With the discovery of a test for antibodies against HIV in 1985, blood collection agencies began testing blood donations for HIV, leading to concerns that some people might donate blood to learn whether they were infected. Therefore, in 1985, the U.S. Centers for Disease Control (CDC) began funding HIV counseling and testing programs through SHAs to protect the blood supply by providing other testing sites for people who wanted to know their HIV status.

Later in the 1980s and continuing into the 1990s, HIV prevention programs in state health agencies continued to grow and diversify. All SHAs received funds from the CDC for prevention activities, and through 1994 CDC guidelines spelled out the types of programs which could be carried out with federal funds. There was no indication at the time that the choice of these programs was based on studies of costs, effectiveness, or cost-effectiveness.

Congress also mandated that a certain portion of the total funding available to states be allocated to HIV counseling, testing, referral, and partner notification (CTRPN). Conversely, federal funds also came with prohibitions. Beginning in 1988, Congress mandated that no federal funding could be used for syringe exchange programs.[4] Many states also allocated their own funds for AIDS prevention. In some cases, these state funds were designated for specific kinds of HIV prevention programs by the legislatures which appropriated the funds.

In September 1993, the Public Health Service of the U.S. Department of Health and Human Services issued a document entitled, "Planning and Evaluating HIV/AIDS Prevention Programs In State and Local Health Departments: A Companion to Program Announcement #300."[5] This document was issued in response to the need for technical assistance on planning and evaluation, identified by state and local health departments in meetings in 1992, and was intended for use by states in preparing their applications to CDC for HIV prevention funding. It described methods for assessing outcomes, designing studies, and collecting data. The document included a chapter on cost analysis, which cited the requirement of the CDC guidance for SHA HIV prevention applications that "detailed consideration should be given to cost per service unit delivered."

States Take Control: Community Planning for HIV Prevention

In December 1993, CDC issued guidance to SHAs requiring that they develop a new process for deciding how to spend federal HIV prevention funds[6] and that this new process be used for the first time for funds to be spent in 1995. This guidance required each state to convene at least one HIV prevention community planning group (CPG) to direct the state in its expenditure of CDC HIV prevention funds. The CDC required that these groups be composed of people at risk for HIV infection; representatives of government, academia, and public health; and other interested parties. The guidance mandated "experts in epidemiology, behavioral and social sciences, evaluation research, and health planning" but did not require that economists be included, nor did it mention them specifically in any way. These groups were charged with assessing prevention needs, designating priority populations for prevention interventions, and deciding which interventions should receive CDC prevention funds from the SHAs. The steps of the decision making process were spelled out clearly in the guidance, and they encouraged examining different interventions to determine their effectiveness. Although SHAs may have made implicit assumptions about effectiveness and cost-effectiveness under previous federal guidance, the new process of HIV prevention community planning suggested that there would be increased rigor in examining costs and effectiveness of HIV prevention interventions.

Moving control of allocations of prevention funding from the federal government (Congress and the CDC) to the states also left states on their own to a more substantial degree. Thrown quickly into a new process for HIV prevention planning which required organization of and cooperation with interested participants, SHAs and CPGs spent much of the first two years of HIV prevention community planning creating workable processes and in many cases were unable to focus on program effectiveness as much as many had hoped.

In February 1994, the National Alliance of State and Territorial AIDS Directors and the Association of State and Territorial Health Officers issued a report commissioned by the CDC entitled, "A Resource Guide to Selected Outcome, Impact and Economic Evaluations of State and Local HIV Prevention Programs."[7] The document reviewed outcome and impact evaluations of HIV prevention programs. It also contained a chapter on economic evaluations of HIV prevention programs, which noted that 15 states had conducted 20 economic analyses, the majority of which were evaluations of CTRPN programs. The remainder evaluated safe needle devices, education and training programs, and primary/early intervention programs.

As a result of more control over the use of federal funds, the community planning guidance, and the more rigorous examination of program effectiveness needed to carry out the intent of the guidance, states have become more conscious of the need to determine the effectiveness of HIV prevention programs. This has led to increased concern about the costs per "prevention unit" for the variety of programs that could be funded, in some cases because of the recognition that some funded programs may not be a "good buy" in the supermarket of potential HIV prevention programs.

EXISTING ECONOMIC EVALUATIONS OF HIV PREVENTION PROGRAMS

A review of the literature of economic evaluations of HIV prevention interventions by Holtgrave et al. shows that three kinds of interventions have been the most frequent subjects of analysis: (1) large-scale HIV screening programs (e.g., premarital HIV testing and HIV testing of hospital patients); (2) medical treatments to decrease the occurrence of specific illness related to HIV; and (3) partner notification.[8] In the first two kinds, the impacts and costs of the programs can be identified relatively easily. For example, studies of screening interventions have estimated the costs of screening for a particular population and the number of cases which would be identified. Thus, the cost per case identified can be calculated. More difficult is identifying the costs that can be averted by such screening programs, presumably resulting from the cessation of behavior that transmit the virus (e.g., unprotected sex or sharing of contaminated syringes) from an infected partner to an uninfected partner. Similarly, both the cost of a medical treatment to prevent an opportunistic infection (OI) in a population of infected individuals and the number of cases of the OIs prevented can be calculated. For partner notification programs, estimates can be made of the number of partners who can be warned of potential infection and tested for HIV, but assumptions as to the number of infections averted by those who cease risky behavior are more speculative.

The HIV prevention programs that have received the most funding, HIV counseling and testing targeted at individuals at risk and HIV education/outreach, have been poorly evaluated for effectiveness or cost-effectiveness. Although publicly funded HIV counseling and testing sites can identify the number of clients served and the number who tested positive during a specific time period, there have been few studies of the impact that counseling has had on reducing behavior that transmits the virus to partners. Education and outreach programs are also very difficult to evaluate for a number of reasons. Although interventions established for research purposes are well defined, community interventions are more flexible, and therefore more difficult to study. For example, it is often difficult to identify even the population that has received the message, as is often the case in street outreach efforts. Although the target audience may be injection drug users, others, such as commercial sex workers and homeless people, may be reached as well. Messages may also differ significantly depending on the risk behavior identified. Therefore, defining the intervention may be difficult. In addition, very intensive and expensive education interventions may be necessary to show significant changes in behavior.

BARRIERS TO USE OF COST, EFFECTIVENESS, AND COST-EFFECTIVENESS INFORMATION BY STATES

A number of barriers limit the extent to which SHAs and their community planning groups use cost, effectiveness, and cost-effectiveness data to determine funding for HIV prevention programs. They are as follows:

Lack of Useful Studies

As described previously, studies of cost, effectiveness, and cost-effectiveness are often difficult to carry out or are limited in their usefulness to program planning. Cost studies can describe the resources needed to provide a unit of service of a particular type. This may be of some benefit for CPGs, SHAs and other decision makers as it allows comparing costs of units of service for different interventions, e.g., the cost of HIV counseling and testing, syringe exchange, or outreach education per client. However, it does not provide a basis for determining the cost of a unit of changed behavior or of averting one new infection.

Effectiveness studies require study samples of sufficient size to determine significant changes. Studies of such size are difficult for many states to conduct, especially if the number of people involved in the intervention studied is small. Multisite studies beyond the ability of many individual SHAs may be needed. However, applying the results of studies carried out in other jurisdictions may be difficult if the intervention evaluated is not carried out in the same way, especially if the effect of the intervention is relatively small. For example, studies of the cost-effectiveness of HIV counseling and testing in one state may be of limited usefulness in estimating the cost-effectiveness in another state because of differences in the interventions or the target populations.

On the other hand, if there are sufficient numbers of studies of similar interventions in different jurisdictions yielding similar results, then applying those results to other locales may be more valid. For example, studies of syringe exchange in diverse locations have yielded substantially similar effectiveness results,[4] making it reasonable to assume similar results in new programs carried out in the same general manner.

HIV prevention and care are rapidly evolving fields, so that new studies must be conducted and older studies regularly updated if they are to be relevant. For instance, a current analysis of costs avoided by averting a case of HIV infection must include the cost of the newest treatments. Similarly, an analysis of the anticipated costs of an HIV prevention activity, such as HIV testing, should recognize recent changes in prevention technology, such as rapid assessment tests for HIV and home collection kits for HIV testing.

Lack of In-House Scientific Expertise in Cost and Effectiveness Evaluation

Few states have staff allocated specifically to program evaluation. Therefore, other program staff with less familiarity and experience in using such information are looked to for expertise by community planning groups and program administrators. In some cases, however, community planning groups have members with such expertise. Thus, the ability of states to gather and use cost and effectiveness data with existing staff or community planning group expertise may vary widely. This may necessitate that some states hire outside experts to evaluate effectiveness and costs.

Conflicts of Interest

There are often members of community planning groups or people in important positions in the community who have interests in a particular program intervention. These participants may resist changes in the way that programs are carried out or in the amount of funding the programs receive, despite evidence that the programs may not be effective or cost-effective. Conversely, they may promote changes in funding for a program without adequate justification.

Community planning groups are required by CDC guidance to include individuals who represent certain populations, including people with HIV infection, racial/ethnic minorities, or men who have sex with men. In addition, CPGs also often include former inmates, former injection drug users, and former commercial sex workers. Each of these individuals brings to the table personal expertise based on experience and the desire to assure that programs target people at risk. Their support for a certain intervention or for services to the population they represent may not match the relative importance of that population in the epidemic or the effectiveness of the intervention in reducing HIV risk.

Perceived Differences among States

Community planning groups and SHAs may feel that evaluations of programs carried out in other states do not apply in their own states. Likewise, they may perceive that the demographics, infrastructure, and epidemiology of HIV in their own states are very different from the places where interventions have been analyzed for economic costs. They may decide that these differences are great enough to render the studies irrelevant. Whether the perceived differences are important or not, these perceptions may mean that published economic analyses are not used by HIV prevention planners from some states, greatly limiting the scientific information base with which to work. The onus is on health economists to explain to an HIV prevention planner from a rural, low-incidence state whether and why studies done in Manhattan are applicable to other states. Although perceptions of differences and lack of applicability in other places may be correct in some cases, in other cases they may reflect an isolationist belief that a state's programs are different and perhaps better than those evaluated elsewhere in the country.

Studies' Views of Interventions in Isolation

To evaluate the cost and/or effectiveness of HIV prevention programs, studies generally focus on narrow, definable programs or program components. In the real world, these programs exist side by side with other intervention messages that promote or detract from prevention messages. Thus, it is sometimes difficult to determine how much of the effectiveness or lack of effectiveness is due to the actual program itself and how much may be contributed by outside forces.

Resistance to Controversial Interventions

Interventions, such as syringe exchange, legal access to syringes in pharmacies without prescriptions, and laws that allow possession of syringes, have been shown to be effective in reducing HIV risk behaviors. However, federal law still prohibits use of HIV prevention funds for syringe exchange.[4] Many states also continue to limit sale of syringes in pharmacies and to prohibit possession of syringes despite evidence showing the effectiveness of such changes in reducing risk behavior.[4,9]

Possible Unintended Consequences of Use of Economic Evaluations

It is reasonable to ask what would happen if economic analysis were to become widespread and routine in states' HIV prevention planning. Because no states have used economic analysis systematically, there are no studies of the effect of economic analysis in implementing states' HIV prevention programs. Therefore, we are left to speculate. One possible consequence is a skewing of planning decisions not based on real benefits, but on the ease of documenting benefits. For example, programs with hard-to-measure but potentially great benefits might lose out to other equally costly programs with lesser but easy-to-measure benefits. This factor may have a conservative tendency. If economic analysis is the norm, decision makers are at some risk in deciding to try a program that has not been evaluated but has great theoretical promise, rather than a heavily evaluated program that is only moderately cost-effective.

Economic analysis might have other unintended consequences. It might be anticipated that the media and state legislatures interpret and use the data to support their own political agendas, though according to our survey of states, this has not happened very often. However, prevention planners are concerned that economic analyses could become politicized, especially if interventions are not shown to be cost-effective. Thus, some states may resist such analyses.

CONNECTICUT'S EXPERIENCE IN COST AND EFFECTIVENESS EVALUATIONS AND IN USE OF COST AND EFFECTIVENESS DATA

In 1992, CDC funded an economic evaluation of HIV counseling and testing of injection drug users in treatment in methadone clinics in Connecticut and Massachusetts[10] to complement an effectiveness evaluation which was already underway.[11] The study estimated the costs of the counseling and testing services and concluded that if more than one in 260 participants changed his or her behavior to the extent that one HIV infection is averted, the medical care savings from that averted infection would exceed the costs of the services. The effectiveness evaluation itself showed little in the way of significant behavioral impacts of HIV counseling and testing in the methadone clinics, because any potential impacts were overwhelmed by the dramatic reduction in the use of heroin and thus of needle sharing because clients were being treated with methadone. In fact, there was no significant reduction in sexual risk in those who tested HIV-negative. Therefore, although an economic evaluation was performed and provided theoretical information on cost effectiveness of HIV counseling and testing in methadone clinics, the prevention intervention was not sufficiently robust to allow the conclusion that the program is cost-effective. However, the study did establish a methodology for estimating costs of counseling and testing which could be used in other states.

In another case, Connecticut implemented significant changes in its laws which had a dramatic impact on risk behavior among injection drug users at no cost. Prescription and paraphernalia laws for syringes were partially repealed by the state legislature in 1992, allowing injection drug users to legally purchase and possess up to 10 sterile syringes. A CDC-sponsored evaluation of this legal change was performed. The evaluation showed that syringe sharing among injection drug users in the community decreased from 52 percent to 31 percent in the one-year period following the statutory changes.[9] Because the intervention of making these legal changes cost no money but instead relied on drug users' desire to purchase clean, sharp, and less expensive syringes and pharmacists' willingness to sell them, an economic evaluation was unnecessary to demonstrate the cost-effectiveness of this no-cost intervention.

EXPERIENCE OF OTHER STATES IN COST AND EFFECTIVENESS EVALUATIONS AND IN USE OF COST AND EFFECTIVENESS INFORMATION

The 1994 study by the National Alliance of State and Territorial AIDS Directors and the Association of State and Territorial Health Officers[7] reported on cost benefit studies and cost effectiveness studies done by or for the states, as reported by the states in 1993. However, the report did not examine studies of program costs alone. Of the 53 respondents to their survey, 15 (28%) had completed a total of 20 cost benefit or cost-effectiveness studies.

We conducted a brief survey to update the findings (Table 1). Unlike the previous study, this survey was hampered by a lack of response from some of the larger and high AIDS-incidence states. Of the 57 states and large cities with CDC HIV prevention cooperative agreements that we surveyed, only 26 (46%) responded. Fourteen of the 26 respondents

Table 1.   State Studies on Cost and Effectiveness

Type of Analysis	Number of Studies	Target Populations	Type of Intervention	Staff
Cost	25	Various, partners, counseling and testing site (CTS) clients, injection drug users (IDUs), high-risk persons, women of childbearing age, sexually tranmitted disease (STD) patients	Counseling, testing, referral and partner notification (CTRPN), CTS in methadone programs, health education/risk reduction (HERR) programs, public information (PI) campaigns, prevention case management (PCM), condom social marketing, street outreach	Program staff[a]
Cost-effectiveness	9	Various, partners, CTS clients, high-risk persons, STD patients	CTS, partner notification (PN), educational outreach, prevention case management, testing and follow-up	Program staff[a]
Cost-utility	0			
Cost-benefit	5	Various, partners, childbearing age women, STD patients	PN, counseling and testing, prenatal testing, testing and followup	Program staff
Total	39			

[a]One study in each of these categories involved a collaboration between state health department staff and academic institutions.

(54%) had completed at least one economic analysis since 1993. The 14 respondents had done 39 studies. However, one respondent had performed thirteen, one-third of the total.

Twenty-five of the studies were carried out to determine the costs of conducting specific HIV prevention interventions. Only 14 (36%) had examined effectiveness or benefit. Nearly all reported relying on existing staff not specifically trained in economics or in cost or effectiveness analysis to conduct this work. Several reported that the state community planning group was interested in cost-effectiveness information to have a factual basis for decisions on allocations of funds.

We followed up with structured interviews of several of the states which were more active in doing economic analyses. In general, they found that economic analysis was very labor intensive and that the results were not comprehensive or clear enough to help in setting direction for program planning.

Though conclusions about all states cannot be drawn from this survey because of the response rate, it is clear from those states that responded that many of the evaluations they are doing are solely to estimate the costs of interventions and are being done by existing staff without training in economic analysis. Thus, relatively simple analyses are the rule for many SHAs.

CONCLUSIONS

Funding for HIV prevention continues to grow as the epidemic continues. State and federal governments and local governments and private funders invest hundreds of millions of dollars each year to prevent the further spread of the disease. The federal government has now vested authority for decisions on expenditure of federal HIV prevention funds with state health agencies and their community planning groups.

Many barriers exist to economic and effectiveness evaluation of HIV prevention programs. Evaluation of the programs is often expensive and time consuming, and the interventions must be carried out with a population large enough to allow detection of anticipated behavioral changes. Defining the intervention and the population it targets can be more complicated than may appear to be the case. Expertise in evaluation is needed to construct and conduct valid studies which have results that can be applied in the real world of HIV prevention.

A number of nontechnical issues can make evaluation of programs challenging. Communities, target populations, and staffs of programs may oppose evaluations from fear that they aim to prove that the programs are ineffective. Alternatively, they may feel that the target population of a program is not receiving sufficient prevention services and that an analysis showing that an intervention targeting that population is not effective could result in the population not receiving any intervention.

States may also feel, rightly or wrongly, that an evaluation conducted elsewhere does not apply to their own intervention. Indeed, the level of risk in different communities may lead to different results, and differences in program implementation may also mean that an evaluation of one program cannot be applied directly to another.

The fact remains, however, that states and community planning groups desperately need information regarding the costs and effectiveness of prevention interventions if they are to make wise choices in investing prevention funds. Joint efforts by states to define a research agenda and to carry out studies, perhaps multistate in nature, are needed to develop the information for decisions about funding. Cooperation among the states in defining the agenda, purchasing expertise to carry out studies, and determining how to apply the results can only increase the effectiveness of HIV prevention activities in the country and maximize the impact of every dollar spent on HIV prevention.

National leadership is still needed to work with states in defining an agenda for cost and effectiveness research, identifying expertise for carrying out studies, and for funding. Studies which have already assessed the effectiveness of particular interventions can be made more useful by adding economic evaluations. A national agenda for producing information needed for HIV prevention planning can be constructed with the cooperation of the National Institutes of Health, the National Centers for Disease Control and Prevention, state health agencies, community planning groups, and prevention planners. It is an effort which is long overdue, but it is not too late to undertake it.

REFERENCES

1. West G. Personal communication, National Centers for Disease Control and Prevention. Sept. 1996.
2. Intergovernmental Health Policy Project of The George Washington University. National Survey of State Funding for AIDS. *Intergovernmental AIDS Reports* Sept.-Oct. 1989; Vol. 2 No. 3A.
3. Intergovernmental Health Policy Project of The George Washington University. National Survey of State HIV/AIDS Funds-FY 1992; Apr. 1993.
4. Normand J, Vlahov D, Moses L, eds. *Preventing HIV Transmission: The Role of Sterile Needles and Bleach.* Washington, DC: National Academy Press; 1995.

5. U.S. Department of Health and Human Services, Public Health Service, Centers for Disease Control and Prevention. *Planning and Evaluating HIV/AIDS Prevention Programs in State and Local Health Departments: A Companion to Program Announcement 300.* Washington, DC; Sept. 1993.
6. U.S.Department of Health and Human Services, Public Health Service, Centers for Disease Control and Prevention. *Supplemental Guidance on HIV Prevention Community Planning for Noncompeting Continuation of Cooperative Agreements for HIV Prevention Projects.* Washington, DC; Dec. 1993.
7. National Alliance of State and Territorial AIDS Directors, Association of State and Territorial Health Officers. *A Resource Guide to Selected Outcome, Impact and Economic Evaluation of State and Local HIV Prevention Programs.* Feb. 1994, Washington, DC.
8. Holtgrave DR, Qualls NL, Graham JD. Economic evaluations of HIV prevention programs. *Annu Rev Public Health* 1996; 17:467–488.
9. Groseclose SL, Weinstein B, Jones TS, et al. Impact of increased legal access to needles and syringes on practices of injecting drug users and police officers—Connecticut 1992–1993. *J Acquir Immune Defic Syndr Human Retrovirol* 1995; 10:73–81.
10. Gorsky RD, MacGowan RJ, Swanson NM, et al. Prevention of HIV infection in drug abusers: A cost analysis. *Prev Med* 1995 Jan; 24(1):3–8.
11. MacGowan RJ, Brackbill RM, Rugg DL, et al. Sex, drugs and HIV counseling and testing: A prospective study of behavior among methadone maintenance clients in New England. *AIDS* 1997; 11:229–235.

12

Adapting Cost Analytic Techniques to Local HIV Prevention Programs

ANNA FAY WILLIAMS, CHARLES BEGLEY,
ANDREW FOURNEY, PAUL MASOTTI,
and ANA JOHNSON MASOTTI

INTRODUCTION: WHY BOTHER WITH ASSESSING THE COST OF LOCAL HIV PREVENTION EFFORTS?

Community planning groups and program managers have the difficult task of managing limited resources when they fund HIV prevention. They attempt to identify and reach target audiences within a geographic area with a variety of prevention programs, including counseling, testing, and community education. Their task involves allocating scarce resources among the interventions and the target populations. Those resources are not adequate to fund all interventions to all the target populations that could benefit, so the problem is one of selecting the most effective methods of preventing HIV infections at the least cost.

Community planning groups require information to make these allocation decisions and to evaluate the relative performance of agencies implementing the interventions.[1] The Centers for Disease Control (CDC) and the state health agencies that fund local planning groups have recommended that the planning groups prioritize their choices using unit cost analysis and cost-effectiveness analysis (CEA). Unit cost analysis is often used as a measure of program efficiency among similar programs with the same goal. CEA is a reasonable tool for allocational decisions when the goal is to compare the relative costs and benefits of different interventions that are pursuing the same underlying goal, such as averting future cases of HIV infection.

Although CEA promises considerable assistance in prioritizing programs, many methodological questions arise about how to gather the necessary data and how to conduct the analysis. The opportunity to explore the use of CEA in HIV prevention community planning was presented in Houston when the Department of Health and Human Services HIV/STD Prevention Bureau funded a University of Texas School of Public Health (UTSPH) study to assess the feasibility of using CEA assessments in the HIV prevention community planning

ANNA FAY WILLIAMS • Consultant, Houston, Texas 77005.   *CHARLES BEGLEY, ANDREW FOURNEY, and PAUL MASOTTI* • Center for Health Policy Studies, School of Public Health, The University of Texas at Houston, Houston, Texas 77030.   *ANA JOHNSON MASOTTI* • Center for AIDS Intervention Research (CAIR), Medical College of Wisconsin, Milwaukee, Wisconsin 53202.

Handbook of Economic Evaluation of HIV Prevention Programs, edited by Holtgrave. Plenum Press, New York, 1998.

process. The goals of this study were (1) to determine the steps that must be taken to measure behavioral change in the programs and locate the instruments that are appropriate for measuring behavioral change; (2) to determine the requirements for reporting costs and service performance on a consistent basis across prevention programs; and (3) to develop a framework for relating costs and benefits that can be used by planners with community-based projects.

The purpose of this chapter is to describe the UTSPH experience in Houston in carrying out these tasks. Although the Houston study has many unique characteristics, we believe that it should provide some insight and general guidance for those in other communities considering CEA analysis and other cost methodologies. The following sections review the role of CEA in the Houston community planning process, provide an overview of the general guidelines and data requirements for CEA, and describe the steps in developing the data for applying cost and CEA methodologies.

CEA AND THE HOUSTON COMMUNITY PLANNING PROCESS

Community planning groups are challenged with choosing among many different interventions. CDC has recognized the importance of several priority interventions including individual level interventions, group level interventions, community level interventions, and outreach interventions, but the planning group must develop a prioritization process among the possible interventions.[2]

In its decision processes, the Houston HIV Prevention Community Planning Group (CPG) regularly solicits input from other groups in the community and conducts its business through consensus building. The membership of the CPG, which was established in 1994 to provide the city's comprehensive HIV prevention plan, was chosen to closely reflect the characteristics of the populations in the HIV epidemic in Houston. It is an ethnically diverse group with African-American, Hispanic, and white members, representatives of sexual orientation diversity, and those with HIV/AIDS. Two co-chairs were named, one designated by the city and another by CPG members.

A number of factors are considered in prioritizing prevention programs for funding among target populations, including prevalence of risky behavior, HIV seroprevalence in the population, and the size of the high-risk population. Although the CPG considers evidence of cost effectiveness when considering possible interventions, it is only one of several determinants for prioritizing interventions. In its process, the CPG assigns different weights to many other factors, which are presented in some detail in the *Handbook for HIV Prevention Community Planning*.[3] Because CEA data have not been available on Houston projects, the CPG has considered evidence from similar interventions in the literature.

GENERAL GUIDELINES AND DATA REQUIREMENTS

The Panel on Cost Effectiveness in Health and Medicine, formed by the U.S. Public Health Service, has recommended methods and procedures to assist analysts in conducting CEA studies that will be comparable.[4] The PHS panel defines CEA as a method for evaluating the outcomes and costs of interventions designed to improve health. The outcomes are the benefits of the program, which may include a number of different outcomes, such as additional years of life gained.

The PHS panel recommends that a societal perspective be taken in conducting CEA to require that the costs of illness prevention or treatment include the direct costs of the intervention and all other costs to society including patient time in accessing the intervention, any care by family members, travel, and child care. Costs of treatment should also include those for treating any adverse effects resulting from the intervention and costs of the disease associated with the program because of prolonged life spans, but should exclude treatment costs not associated with the program and non-health-care costs incurred because of extended life years.

Several approaches are recommended for measuring improvements in health or morbidity resulting from a program, including a recommendation for quality-adjusted life years (QALYs). QALYs are obtained by having individuals in the community, not investigators or patients, value various health states by assigning a value between and including "1" for perfect health and "0" for death and then applying these values to life years gained in a particular health state. If community assessments are not available, patients may provide the valuation of health states.

Recommendations were made for studies extending over several years, such as adjusting monetary terms for any inflationary effects and discounting costs and outcomes to present values at the same rate. The effect of a program can be calculated with data from randomized clinical trials and descriptive or observational data from uncontrolled experiments. When adequate data do not exist, expert opinion or simulation modeling may be considered.

Although the Panel's recommendations provide useful guidelines, they do not deal with the practicalities of implementing CEA for a given illness, nor applying it to local governmental and community-based projects. Modifications are needed to adapt these guidelines within the context of community HIV prevention. Although QALYs have been identified for HIV, their application is not necessary within the HIV prevention planning process.

Holtgrave has identified several CEA information needs for HIV prevention programs, including the need to identify the types of interventions available that are effective, how much they cost, and whether they can be custom-tailored to local circumstances.[6] Yet, searches of the literature find few CEA studies, and many of those few cases use different methodologies and approaches with are not comparable.[6]

However, methodological literature is emerging now which points to some requirements for conducting CEA with prevention programs. CEA requires behavioral change measurements (effects) and information on the costs and services performed for each intervention. The benefits measured are changes in behavior that reduce the risk of transmission, such as increased condom use before and after an intervention. These measurements become the basis for estimating averted cases of HIV infection. Estimates can be developed when the expected behavior is related to the frequency of sexual activities (condom use per sex act) and the probabilities of transmission and seroprevalence within the target populations. Survey instruments for reporting behavior are required for pretest and posttest evaluation of behavioral change.

The cost methodologies and service measurements for CEA require detailed reporting. All resource costs must be identified and related to program services. Staff members and facilities devoted to more than one intervention must be allocated to each intervention.

Funded resources must be combined with volunteers and other donated resources that are used in the delivery of services. Accounting systems must be developed to allocate costs for all resources used for different programs and to document the services delivered to various target populations.

CEA may be confused with unit cost analysis, which requires similar cost data and resource units. CDC's Order 300 specifically requires that detailed consideration be given to the cost per service unit delivered, which may be accomplished by detailed allocations of budget costs to service units and careful tracking of service units delivered over a short time.[7] Unit cost analysis provides a measure of program efficiency for projects with the same effectiveness, the same results in terms of clients served. However, unit cost analysis is not adequate when comparisons are made between different types of interventions, such as media advertisements versus counseling and testing, which are likely to differ in their relative effectiveness. For example, interventions that appear costly because they have a higher unit cost per client contact may be cost-effective if they reach high risk populations where small behavioral changes lead to significant reductions in HIV transmission.

Methods for Assessing Effectiveness

Although HIV prevention planning groups may already consider a number of process measures of program effectiveness, such as numbers of clients served, CEA requires a common measure of program impact that can be used across several interventions.[8] Because changes in risk of transmission are related to sex and drug use behavior, planners need measures of such behavioral change that can be implemented within their own community prevention interventions.

Kelly et al.[9] developed an instrument to measure knowledge, locus of control, peer norms, and sexual and drug use behavior that provided the basis for a Houston survey. The Kelly instrument used several questions to form three scales: a measure of knowledge of HIV and AIDS; locus of control (LOC), and peer norms. There were 23 HIV/AIDS knowledge questions, e.g., "pre-ejaculatory fluids carry the AIDS virus" with true/false responses. Nine questions concerned locus of control, e.g., "more than anything else, chance determines whether I get the AIDS virus." Peer norms were measured with five items, e.g., "my friends always use condoms during oral, anal, and vaginal sex." The choice of responses for the peer norms and locus of control scales ranged from 1 ("strongly disagree") to 5 ("strongly agree").

The questions from the Kelly instrument were modified to make them appropriate for programs and populations in Houston. The wording of some of the behavioral questions were changed to simplify them. For example, the term "intercourse" was changed to "sex." The behavioral questions on the original surveys, which were developed for a homosexual population, were rephrased so they would be more appropriate for a heterosexual population. Some questions were added to measure drug use behavior.

The modified version was tested in a focus group that included outreach workers, education program directors, and other staff at a community-based organization. Based on this feedback, changes were made in the formats, skip patterns were added, and some response categories were collapsed from a 10-point scale to a 4-point scale. These changes resulted in an instrument with a score of 6.3 on a Fleish–Kinkaid test, indicating that it was appropriate for someone with a sixth grade reading level. The final modified version was referred to as the HIV Intervention Outcome Survey (HIOS).

The HIOS survey was administered in a pilot test to 125 individuals from three HIV/ AIDS agencies in Houston. These individuals represented diverse populations including college students, incarcerated youth, and homeless individuals. The purpose of the pilot test was to identify problems unanticipated by the focus group and to determine if the changes made resulted in a reliable survey instrument. The reliability of the instrument was assessed in three ways. A factor analysis was conducted to confirm that the groups of questions on each scale measured the same factor, i.e., knowledge, locus of control, and peer norms. Two assessments were made: internal consistency to see how well the items measured these factors and test–retest reliability, to determine if the survey instrument is reliable over time. The results of these analysis indicated that the instrument is reliable.

The pilot test revealed that there were difficulties with the behaviorally related questions, and they were reformatted accordingly. After reformatting, the pilot test indicated that the HIOS could be used to measure changes in behavior for the Houston high-risk population and that the three scales could be used to measure factors associated with risk-related behavior.

Because the pilot survey was administered before an intervention was conducted, it did not measure the impact of the intervention, which requires follow-up data from a post-test implementation. However, it does provide some data on knowledge levels, LOC, and peer norms, which may be used for future CEA analysis and program design. For the pilot samples, the mean number of correct knowledge answers was 8.6 (standard deviation, 2.1) out of 23. On the internal LOC questions, there was a mean score of 4.2 out of a possible score of 5 (standard deviation, 0.79), indicating that the subjects believe that they largely control behavior that determine whether or not they get AIDS. Peer norm results indicated that subjects feel their peers are neutral on practicing unsafe sex (mean 2.7 out of a 5; standard deviation, 0.90) and on practicing safe sex (mean 3.0 out of 5; standard deviation 0.87). Table 1 is a summary of the responses to the behavioral questions, showing the means, standard deviations, and maximum values for the number of times that respondents reported each sexual behavior and the average number of male and female partners.

Table 1. Mean, Standard Deviation, and Maximum Values
for Number of Times by Type of Activity[a]

	Mean	Standard Deviation	Maximum Value
Receptive anal intercourse without a condom	1.32	2.77	10
Insertive anal intercourse without a condom	0.59	1.67	10
Receptive anal intercourse with a condom	0.68	2.33	12
Insertive anal intercourse with a condom	0.98	5.03	43
Receptive oral intercourse without a condom	3.06	6.61	43
Insertive oral intercourse without a condom	3.14	11.74	102
Receptive oral intercourse with a condom	1.42	10.68	102
Insertive oral intercourse with a condom	0.19	1.11	10
Vaginal intercourse without a condom	5.30	14.93	102
Vaginal intercourse with a condom	3.68	11.91	102
Number of male partners	2.44	5.64	50
Number of female partners	1.83	6.03	50

[a]n = 125.

The pilot testing demonstrated that the HIOS is an appropriate and reliable instrument for measuring knowledge, loci of control, peer norms and provides information about high-risk behavior in the Houston populations tested. The process discussed here covers the important first steps for any planning group in developing a survey instrument.

Methods for Assessing the Unit Costs of Interventions

The cost methodology requires developing consistent cost reporting across projects, units of service specific to the differing types of interventions, and an allocation of costs that reflects the resources required for each intervention. The cost team determined that the development of a plan for obtaining cost data and implementing cost methods involved four tasks: (1) to investigate community-based organization (CBO) accounting data to determine whether it is appropriate and complete enough to provide an accurate determination of unit cost; (2) to determine data requirements for deriving unit costs; (3) to determine measures of service delivery and the availability of such information from the CBOs; and (4) to gather reactions from the CBOs on additional reporting requirements and their ability to obtain the required data. Several references are helpful for those implementing cost methodologies.[10–13]

Investigating CBO Accounting Data

A resource inventory was initially developed for each of 17 funded projects to understand the resources and costs for delivering services within the existing projects. An inventory provides a complete list of all resources used for the project, the dollar cost of those resources, and the volume of resources consumed in each project. The list of resources used in delivering a service in a project was based on the standard accounting classifications used in the Houston CBO contracts, including both fixed costs supporting the provision of a service and variable costs, such as staffing, supplies, and travel that vary with the services offered.

The next major step was to review reports and interview staff to determine whether existing expense reports captured the costs of each resource. Typically, projects captured their direct costs (personnel and supplies) but differed in accounting for indirect costs, rent-mortgage, and depreciation. For example, the initial survey of project expenses from HDHHS reports indicated various practices in reimbursing rent, space, and equipment. The percentages of the projects reporting expense reimbursements in the different cost categories are shown in Table 2.

Determining Common Service Measurements

Existing reports and CBO interviews were used to determine measures of services that are similar in terms of their resource requirements and descriptions. Several differences were found with the program descriptions and the manner in which services were provided. For instance, it was determined that both counseling and testing and intensive counseling and testing, now administered under two separate contracts, may be grouped together for cost analysis. CBOs providing these services generally treat all their clients on an "as needed" basis, and the intensity level is dictated by the client situation. A CBO which has a Counseling, Testing, Referral and Partner Notification (CTRPN) contract for "nonclinic

Table 2. CBO Expense Reimbursement Reporting

Cost Category	% of CBOs Reporting	Cost Category	% of CBOs Reporting
1. Personnel	78	7. Indirect	17
2. Fringe benefits	78	8. Brochures	6
3. Travel	72	9. Advertising	6
4. Supplies	89	10. Auto insurance	6
5. Rent/space	33	11. Equipment	22
6. Other[a]	67	12. Computing	6

[a]Other categories included a wide variety of cost items, such as telephone, utilities, postage, liability insurance, some supplies, and sometimes, rent.

testing" may actually be delivering services similar to a CBO that has separate contracts to deliver both Health Education and Risk Reduction (HE/RR) "outreach" and "nonclinic testing" interventions targeted to the same population. Those CBOs doing nonclinic testing had to provide some education before high-risk individuals volunteered to be tested. In another CBO, the outreach program also fed the nonclinic testing program. In some cases, the same employees were involved in more than one program.

Several large groupings are frequently used for grouping the intervention services: Health Education and Risk Reduction (HE/RR): Counseling, Testing, Referral, and Partner Notification (CTRPN); and Early Intervention Prevention (EIP). The cost team recommended more narrowly defined categories within these broad groups, such as clinic-based counseling, community-based counseling and testing, and combined counseling and testing. New service categories were defined that would be useful in the cost methodologies for comparing the relative performance of agencies providing similar services. The services are listed in Table 3, and definitions are provided in Table 4.

Table 3. Service Categories and Service Units

	Service Units
Counseling, Testing, Referral, and Partner Notification (CTRPN)	
1. Clinic-based counseling and testing	# clients tested
2. Community-based counseling and testing	# clients tested
	# client contacts
3. Combined counseling and testing	# clients tested
	# client contacts
Health Education and Risk Reduction (HE/RR)	
1. Outreach (no testing, nonclinic-based)	# client contacts
2. Large group	# client contacts
	# clients
	# client contact hours
3. Small group	# client contacts
	# clients
	# client contact hours
4. Mass media	# events
Early Intervention Prevention (EIP)	
1. Early intervention	# clients
	# client contact hours

Table 4. Definitions of the Service Categories and Service Units

Client Test. A test consists of three completed items: a) pretest counseling, b) laboratory testing, and c) posttest discussion of the laboratory results and additional counseling.

Clinic Counseling and Testing (Clinic C&T). Clinic C&T consists of CTRPN activities that usually or always take place at a central location, such as a clinic, office, or hospital.

Community Counseling and Testing (Community C&T). Community C&T consists of all CTRPN activities that usually take place at locations other than a central location, such as a clinic, office, or hospital. Another name for this could be "Field Counseling and Testing" (Field C&T).

Combined C&T. This is appropriate for CBOs that perform both community and clinic counseling and testing as part of one program.

Outreach. Outreach differs from other HIV prevention and health care programs by providing services outside the clinic setting. Service providers go to the client's community rather than clients coming to the service providers. Outreach is a way to (1) reach populations that have not been part of the traditional health care delivery system, (2) refer these "hard-to-reach" clients to health and social services and/or, (3) deliver health information, risk reduction materials, and prevention services at the point of contact.

Small Group. Small group consists of delivering a structured education session to 3 to 15 participants. Education, instruction, and counseling activities may consist of any combination or all of safe sex activities; skills training, such as condom use; training to improve negotiation and communication skills; risk reduction strategies; and the emotional impact of sexual activities. The small-group program is more structured than outreach programs and may take place at locations such as clinics, schools, places of employment, apartment complexes, or community centers.

Large Group. The large group category consists of structured educational sessions for groups which are larger than 15 participants and usually exceed 20 or more participants. Education, instruction, and counseling activities may consist of any combination or all of safe sex activities; skills training, such as condom use; training to improve negotiation and communication skills; risk reduction strategies; and the emotional impact of sexual activities. Large group programs are more structured than outreach programs and may take place at locations, such as clinics, schools, places of employment, apartment complexes, or community centers.

Mass Media. Mass Media uses mass media methods (radio, TV, brochures, posters, bill boards, and hotlines) that address topics such as counseling, testing, reporting, partner notification, and sexual barriers.

Clients. "# clients" or the "# clients tested" refers to separate individuals. Each person served is counted once even if they receive multiple contacts or visits as part of the service.

Client Contacts. "# client contacts" consists of each contact with a client regardless of whether that client has previously been seen, tested, counseled, or educated. A minimum time period should be determined as part of the definition of a client contact.

Client Contact Hours. "# client contact hours" is the amount of time a certain number of clients have had interaction with an HIV intervention program. "# client contact hours" is calculated by multiplying the "# clients" and the "# hours" (or fractions of hours) for each contact, i.e., education or counseling session.

Example # 1: Number of clients = 40
Intervention: One-hour large group presentation
Client contact hours = 40 × 1 = 40 client contact hours
Example # 2: Number of clients = 40
Intervention: Two-hour large group presentation
client contact hours = 40 × 2 = 80 client contact hours

Calculating Unit Costs

Using existing performance reports and cost information, preliminary calculations of unit costs showed a wide variance. For example, CTRPN reimbursement rates per client ranged from $15 to $156, a range which likely reflects the variation in cost reporting and cross-subsidization.

To gain a better understanding of the true unit cost of delivering a program, a method must be developed that (1) allocates resources required for different interventions when an agency is conducting multiple programs with the same resources and (2) accounts for any cross subsidization. For example, an HE/RR contract might include both a large group program and an outreach program and both programs share CBO resources, such as employee time and room space. The cost of each intervention must be separated and related to service units to accurately estimate the unit costs. When programs share overhead, an allocation formula must be employed. The distribution of personnel time may serve as a basis for this allocation. For instance, if employees spend 30% of their time delivering outreach services and 70% delivering large group services, then a portion of the total overhead cost may be allocated to each of these interventions based on these percentages.

The CBOs were asked about the methods that they were using to define units of services, their cost categories in their accounting systems, how they distinguish one intervention from another, their unreimbursable cost categories, and the cost team recommendation for collecting additional cost data. CBO staff reactions varied when informed of the purpose of the measures and the possibilities of additional reporting requirements to obtain data. Although some were not enthusiastic, others saw it as a means to prove the quality and value of their programs. CBOs seemed to like the idea of providing their unreimbursed costs and seemed willing to undertake additional reporting requirements. Most did not see any problem in adding the recommended service units in the quarterly performance reports. Some CBOs indicated that they were giving the city a "good deal" and that the amount of unreimbursed costs would support this belief. The allocation method was acceptable to the CBOs as a method for determining the shared costs. The administration of the HIOS tool was of interest to the CBOs and was viewed as an acceptable method for measuring effects.

The steps, which are described previously in evaluating the existing cost data, are important for implementing the cost methodologies. In this part of the Houston study, the cost team accomplished its goals in providing a method for calculating unit costs, methods for identifying the categories of costs and service units for measurement, and the allocation formulas. Among its recommendations were an unreimbursable cost report that would include those cost items that may be cross-subsidized by other CBO programs or financially absorbed by the CBO. Consequently, all direct and indirect costs, whether reimbursed or not, could be included because an unreimbursable cost report would allocate these costs to the interventions.

The Planning Group supported the study team's efforts throughout the study. Reports were made at Planning Group meetings and subcommittee meetings. An extension on the study provided an opportunity for further field tests to determine the steps that must be established to gather the cost and behavioral data and to develop guides for administering the cost methodologies.

Practical Methods for CEA: A Spreadsheet Approach

A spreadsheet approach was developed for the HIV Prevention Community Planning Group to apply CEA formulas and methodologies. The spreadsheet conveys the basic data requirements, rather than centering on the details of the calculations that were explained more informally. For instance, condom usage and other factors affecting transmission of disease, such as the numbers of partners, the numbers of sexual acts, and the types of sexual acts, can be related to the probabilities of disease transmission from other studies. An illustration of a spreadsheet approach was based on a previous study by Holtgrave and

Kelly[14] because behavioral or cost data were not available for Houston interventions. The illustration deals with counseling sessions for a group of women at an urban, primary health clinic and consisted of four, weekly, 90-minute group sessions and a one-month group follow-up. The counseling sessions, an example of small group counseling, included skills training in condom use, problem solving, assertiveness in sexual situations, peer support, and self management. The top section of the spreadsheet (Table 5) lists the required behavioral data for estimating the numbers of cases averted, such as prevalence rates within the target group, probability of being infected, and efficacy of condoms for those participating in small-group counseling sessions. Data which will be collected from the clients includes the numbers of partners, the numbers of sex acts, and the percentage of times that condoms are used before the intervention and after the intervention. Other interventions, such as needle exchange, would also include other risk variables.[15]

The formula for estimating the cases averted, as cited in the Holtgrave and Kelly article,[14] is given as follows:

$$A = G\{[1 - (p(1 - r_a(1 - ef_{ca}))^n + (1 - p))^m] - [1 - (p(1 - r_a(1 - ef_{ia}))^n + (1 - p))^m]\}$$

where p is the sex partners' HIV seroprevalence; r_a the single sex act transmission probability; e condom effectiveness; f_{ca} condom use, control condition, per act; f_{ia} condom use with intervention, per act; n number of contacts with one partner; and m number of partners per client. In addition to the Holtgrave and Kelly article,[14] further information on

Table 5.   Spreadsheet Analysis for Cost-Effectiveness

Intervention:	Small group counseling sessions	
Target population:	Women (87% African-American) with multiple partners	
Number of women served:	100	
Behavior:	Proportion of sex encounters protected by a condom (vaginal sex)	
	Number of sex encounters with same partner	
	Number of partners	
DATA BEFORE INTERVENTION	DATA AFTER INTERVENTION	
0.03	0.03	Prevalence of HIV infection in partners
0.0155	0.0155	Probablility of being infected per sex act with infected partner
0.32	0.56	Proportion of sex encounters protected by a condom
0.95	0.95	Efficacy of condoms in preventing transmission of HIV virus
31.25	31.25	Number of sex encounters with same partner
1.5	1.5	Number of partners
3	3	Number of months for recall period in survey data
Risk of becoming infected before intervention	Risk of becoming infected after intervention over 3 months	
0.0129	0.0091	
Cases averted over three months	0.3766	
Costs of program (1992 dollars)		
Total societal costs of intervention	$26,914	
Cost per client	$269	
Cost-effectiveness ratio (Cost per case averted)	$71,466	

the formula and discussions may be obtained from Fineberg,[16] Gold,[4] Pinkerton,[17] and Weinstein.[18]

The behavioral data for estimating the cases averted in Houston may be obtained from the HIOS survey questionnaire, which covers the use of condoms, the numbers of sexual partners, and the number and type of sexual acts. Epidemiological data for the spreadsheet may be obtained from the local health department. The literature provides estimates of condom effectiveness and HIV transmission rates.[17] Additional worksheets, not shown here, may be required to adjust calculations for multiple sexual partners (both heterosexual and homosexual) and multiple engagements (both anal and vaginal sex).

The program costs are provided on the lower part of the spreadsheet, along with an average cost per client served and a cost-effectiveness ratio. The cost-effectiveness ratio divides changes in the effects of the program (cases averted) into total program costs. The total program costs are accumulated for each program separately, as discussed in the previous section. Additionally, unit costs may be calculated separately for each program based on the service units, such as average cost per client served. Other adjustments may be made to annualize the effects of a program across a one-year period. For instance, the study may cover three months, providing a fraction of the numbers of cases that would be averted, which can be adjusted to an annual basis and presented in terms of larger population groups.

This phase of the project demonstrated an approach to presenting study results in a spreadsheet analysis. Further field tests in Houston will provide the opportunity for demonstrating program impacts.

CONCLUSION AND FUTURE RESEARCH

The Houston project accomplished its goals (1) in identifying, adapting, and testing an instrument for gathering behavioral data; (2) in providing a general method of cost accounting combining existing expense reports and a new unreimbursable expense report; and (3) in demonstrating the CEA methodology with a spreadsheet approach.

In developing tools for applying cost effectiveness analysis within Houston's community based projects, we learned the following:

- *The importance of planning.* The success in implementing cost-effectiveness methodology depends on having time to address a number of major steps in gathering data and making decisions regarding the appropriate methodologies. Funding and expertise must be available for collecting the cost and behavioral information. Sufficient time must be provided for selecting survey instruments and modifying them so that they are appropriate for implementation within the community. The process requires training and cooperation from the CBOs. Alternative routes should be explored for gathering the required information and integrating the cost data collection as much as possible into existing report formats. Possibilities may exist for cooperative arrangements in gathering the cost data within city health departments or accounting departments.
- *Agreements on the methodologies.* Consistent measures of cost that may not currently exist in accounting systems must be adopted for defining service units and unit costs. Acceptance of these measures requires educational programs and discussions within the planning groups, the CBOs and with other city officials involved

in the accounting process. Changes in the manner of contracting with CBOs could also affect the development of the methodology. For instance, if contracts are undertaken on a per unit basis, i.e., so much paid for each client, then CBOs may well want to consider these cost methodologies for calculating their units costs.

- *Taking the first steps in implementation.* Planning groups may first want to apply CEA within one or two different interventions to have adequate time to address any problems in data collection.
- *A realistic assessment of the difficulties.* The tasks of gathering behavioral data will continue to challenge the creativity of CBO evaluators and those who administer the behavior and other surveys. First, those receiving services from CBOs may not want to participate to maintain their confidentiality or anonymity which will result in low response rates. Second, the validity of such evaluations may be threatened by self-reporting methods, which still appear to be the only route for obtaining the estimates. Finally, even though individuals with a sixth-grade reading level can complete the survey, some may need to have it read to them or translated into another language. Some clients may not want to participate, especially if such participation incurs additional time and travel for them. In such cases, incentives should be considered to encourage participation. Special care must be taken to provide privacy for those participating in the surveys. Since follow-up may be time-consuming in contacting those who participated initially in the surveys, it may be necessary to consider other means of follow-up.
- *The importance of CBO involvement.* The responses from the CBOs proved crucial in developing the overall cost methodology and in adapting and implementing the pretest surveys. Ultimately, their involvement will be very important to the successful implementation of any cost methodologies.

Despite these concerns over implementing these methodologies, unit cost analysis and CEA hold promise for prioritizing projects and for resource decisions. Importantly, they can assist planning groups and CBOs in establishing some measures of their program effectiveness, which should assist them in designing more effective interventions in the future. The process may have other benefits for the planning groups and the CBOs in providing technical assistance to CBOs on how to define their service units and cost categories and in terms of understanding what is significant and why. The ongoing program will provide a template and continuing education to the program and accounting staff. Successful implementation is likely to require an interactive process over time, so that adjustments can be made after field tests to improve the survey instruments and cost reporting formats and improve responsiveness to them.

The next steps being considered in Houston are applications of the recommended methodologies in selected interventions. In this manner, it will be possible to test the formats for collecting cost data, to refine the processes for administering the surveys and analyzing the data, and to provide the templates for implementing CEA across future prevention programs.

ACKNOWLEDGMENTS. This project was supported by a grant from the City of Houston Department of Health and Human Services (HDHHS). The authors would like to thank those at HDHHS and the Houston HIV Prevention Community Planning Group for their assistance in the project: Glenda Gardner, HDHHS Bureau Chief, Bureau of HIV/STD

Prevention; Bill Comeaux, HDHHS Senior Community Liaison; Peggy Rogers, Ph.D., MPH, Chief of Health Planning for HDHHS and the designated Co-Chair for the Houston HIV Prevention Community Planning Group; Mike Mizwa, Community Co-Chair of the Houston Prevention Community Planning Group Data Management and Needs Assessment Committee, HIV Prevention Community Planning Group, and Education Director, AIDS Foundation of Houston. We have also benefited from consultations with David Holtgrave, Ph.D., Director, Division of HIV/AIDS Prevention: Intervention Research and Support, Centers for Disease Control and Prevention, in the early design and implementation of this study. The paper reflects the experience of the research team, not necessarily that of the HDHHS program officers.

REFERENCES

1. Centers for Disease Control. *Overview of HIV/AIDS Prevention Interventions: An Approach to Examining Their Effectiveness*, May 1995, The Academy for Educational Development funded by CDC.
2. U.S. Department of Health and Human Services, Centers for Disease Control and Prevention, *Announcement No. 704*, Washington, DC; 1997.
3. Academy for Educational Development. *Handbook for HIV Prevention Community Planning*, Washington, DC; 1994.
4. Gold MR, Siegel JE, Russell LB, et al. *Cost-Effectiveness in Health and Medicine*. Oxford University Press; 1996; Chap. 6.
5. Holtgrave DR, Qualls NL. HIV Prevention programs. *Science* 1994; 266:16.
6. Holtgrave DR, Qualls NL, Graham JD. Economic evaluation of HIV prevention programs. *Annu Rev Public Health* 1996; 17:467–488.
7. Centers for Disease Control, Department of Health and Human Services. *Cooperative Agreements for Human Immunodeficiency Virus (HIV) Prevention Projects Program Announcement, Order 300*. Washington, DC, 1993; pp. 28–29.
8. Conference of Mayors, *Technical Assistance Reports*, Washington, DC, November 1990.
9. Kelly JA, St. Lawrence JS, Hood HV, et al. An objective test of AIDS risk behavior knowledge: Scale development, validation and norms. *J Behavior Therapy Exp Psychiatry* 1989; 20(3):227–234.
10. Mandelblatt JS, et al. Assessing the effectiveness of health interventions. In Gold MR, et al. *Cost Effectiveness in Health and Medicine*. New York: Oxford University Press; 1996.
11. Drummond MF, Stoddart GL, Torrance GW. *Methods for Economic Evaluation of Health Care Programs*. New York: Oxford University Press; 1987; Chaps 4 and 5.
12. Haddix AC, Teutsch SM, Shafer PA, et al. *Prevention Effectiveness*. New York: Oxford University Press; 1996; Chaps 2, 5, and 8.
13. U.S. Department of Health and Human Services, Public Health Survey. *Determining the Unit Cost of Services—A Guide for Estimating the Cost of Service*. Funded by the White Care Act of 1990. Health Resources and Services Administrator, Washington, DC; 1992.
14. Holtgrave DR, Kelly JA. Preventing HIV/AIDS among high-risk urban women: The cost-effectiveness of a behavioral group intervention. *Am J Public Health* 1996; 86:1442–1445.
15. Kahn JG, Washington AE, Showstack JA, et al. *Updated Estimates of the Impact and the Costs of HIV Prevention in Injection Users, Final Report*. San Francisco: Institute of Health Policy Studies, School of Medicine, University of California. Prepared for the Division of STD/HIV Prevention, Center for Prevention Services, Centers for Disease Control, Department of Health and Human Services; September, 1992.
16. Fineberg H. Education to prevent AIDS: Prospects and obstacles. *Science* 1988; 239:592–596.
17. Pinkerton SD, Abramson PR. Effectiveness of condoms in preventing HIV transmission. *Soc Sci Med* 1997; 44(9):1301–1312; Implications of increased infectivity in early-stage HIV infection—application of Bernoulli-process model of HIV transmission, Pinkerton SD, Abramson PR, *Evaluation Rev* 1996; 20(5): 516–540.
18. Weinstein MC, et al. Recommendations of the panel on cost-effectiveness in health and medicine. *JAMA* 1996; 276(15):1253–1258.

Economic Evaluation and HIV Prevention Community Planning
A Policy Analyst's Perspective

EDWARD H. KAPLAN

INTRODUCTION

In 1994, a new approach to implementing publicly funded HIV prevention programs was introduced. Roughly $190 million in federal funds in fiscal year 1994 allocated to the Centers for Disease Control were in turn reallocated to 65 different planning areas (the 50 states, eight territories, and seven of the U.S. cities hardest hit by AIDS).[1] Each of these jurisdictions undertook a *community planning process* to establish priorities for HIV prevention. The planning groups formed were intended to reflect the local communities affected by the HIV/AIDS epidemic, providers of HIV prevention programs and services, and local health officials (and in some cases local AIDS experts). Thus the role of the community planning group was envisioned as one of providing guidance to local health departments with respect to HIV prevention activities. The actual allocation of HIV prevention funds to specific programs and tasks remained within the jurisdiction of the local health department.[1–3] The overriding goal of this process is stated clearly: "The purpose of the HIV Prevention Cooperative Agreement Program is to assist State and local health departments in preventing the transmission of HIV . . ."[4] The 1997 budget further underlines this focus: "At the historic White House Conference on HIV and AIDS, the President made his commitment to HIV prevention clear: "We have to reduce the number of new infections each and every year until there are no more infections.' "[5]

How should federal HIV prevention funds be allocated? To be consistent with the goals of the community planning process and the intentions of the President, the money should be spent in a manner that *arguably* induces a large (if not maximal) reduction in new HIV infections. To create such an argument requires a framework that recognizes the relationships between existing HIV infection rates, the preventive capabilities of public programs at different funding levels, and prevented infections.

This chapter is about developing and illustrating such a policy analytic framework. The community planning process can be couched in the general economic language of resource allocation problems as shown in the next section. Viewing community planning as an

EDWARD H. KAPLAN • School of Management, Yale University, New Haven, Connecticut 06520-8200.

Handbook of Economic Evaluation of HIV Prevention Programs, edited by Holtgrave. Plenum Press, New York, 1998.

instrument for resource allocation naturally leads to the consideration of HIV prevention production functions in the third section. Such functions reflect the expected number of infections that can be prevented at different funding levels for various families of HIV interventions. The fourth section tackles the problem of allocating HIV prevention resources. The key is a standard for evaluating any proposed allocation of the prevention budget in terms of the number of prevented infections that such an allocation could be expected to produce. Given such a standard, it is possible to determine allocations that, consistent with previously assessed HIV prevention production functions, maximize the number of prevented infections for any given budget. It is also possible to value social constraints, such as equity and fairness by this approach.

Though the methods suggested here represent a departure from HIV community planning practice, they are by no means incompatible with the work of existing community planning groups. Much of the data collection, arguments, and discussion in which planning groups currently engage would also surface as described in the third section. The analysis to be described is not intended to replace community planning groups with mathematical formulas. Rather, the intent is to provide new tools for HIV prevention community planning that will lead to arguably better outcomes.

COMMUNITY PLANNING AS RESOURCE ALLOCATION

The community planning process recommends prioritization of HIV prevention activities to maximize the impact of publicly funded HIV interventions. To have any force, such recommendations must ultimately translate into actual budget allocations across existing and/or proposed prevention programs. Indeed, a stated core objective by CDC is to foster "... strong, logical linkages between the community planning process, plans, application for funding and *allocation of CDC HIV prevention resources.*"[4] (emphasis added)

Given the importance of community planning for funding decisions, it is not surprising that many planning groups saw fit to issue funding recommendations. For example, in Arizona, a formula was developed for allocating HIV prevention funds to the three different planning regions in that state. "The formula took into account population size, AIDS cases, land area, border issues, and the number of Native American reservations in each region."[3] Similarly, the community planning group in Massachusetts proposed changes in the formula used by that state to allocate both state and federal HIV prevention dollars.[3] In Vermont, community planners created a "risk times need" index based on factors such as seroprevalence, prevalence of risky behavior, population size, and degree of access to services, and applied this index to potential target populations. Then available funds for prevention activities were allocated in proportion to group scores on this index.[6] As another example, Wisconsin community planning group members initially voted budget allocations by risk groups. Individual votes were reviewed and revised by the entire group.[6] Bibus et al.[7] provide a detailed description of an allocation formula used by the Seattle-King County Department of Public Health to help distribute HIV prevention funds across risk groups, and the Academy for Educational Development has proposed a general approach to priority setting in community planning.[8] These approaches have been adapted for use by specific planning groups, including some of the states mentioned.[6]

Thus HIV prevention community planning can be viewed as an instance of a familiar problem in economics: How should one divide a fixed budget among different activities?

There is a key difference, however, between the examples cited previously and the approach taken by economists. The economist asks how budgets can be divided to achieve some objective.[9] Budget allocations derived via economic reasoning are linked to an associated performance model that quantifies the "goodness" of an allocation in terms of this objective. Although the examples previously cited offer proposals for allocating budgets, there are no associated performance models linking resource allocations to progress toward a clearly stated goal.

In the community planning context, the overriding goal is to prevent new HIV infections. Therefore one can offer the following interpretation of the community planning exercise: How should available public HIV prevention money be allocated to prevent a substantial (and perhaps the maximum) number of HIV infections? Viewed from this perspective, community planning requires a different set of working assumptions. The critical ingredients are a set of shared beliefs regarding how many HIV infections are prevented via incremental expenditures on a given set of HIV prevention activities. Viewing prevention dollars as an input and prevented infections as an output, these shared beliefs are tantamount to what economists refer to as *production functions* that transform inputs into outputs.[10] Such production functions, combined with a fixed HIV prevention budget and a goal to maximize the number of prevented infections, define a well-posed economic resource allocation problem, the solution to which is a recommended expenditure for each of the prevention activity classes under consideration. The resulting *optimal resource allocation* will have the important property that no alternative division of the prevention budget could better achieve the overriding HIV prevention goal, given the shared beliefs relating expenditures on HIV prevention activities to the number of infections prevented.

To think about community planning in this framework forces one to think about the effectiveness of HIV prevention as a function of investment. Such thinking is largely absent in existing approaches to community planning. Even those planning groups that have attempted to quantify budget allocations have not done so with any explicit reference to the relationship between dollars spent and infections prevented. Given that the goal of HIV prevention is in fact to prevent HIV infections, however, one would like some assurances that the recommended division of HIV prevention money reasonably achieves this goal. To begin addressing these important issues, we must take a closer look at the details of production functions and resource allocation for HIV community planning.

PRODUCTION FUNCTIONS FOR HIV PREVENTION

Preliminaries

There are different ways to approach the construction of production functions for HIV prevention. Usually economists seek empirical data relating outputs to inputs that enable the statistical estimation of production functions. Given the paucity of data describing the costs of alternative HIV prevention activities and their preventive impact in terms of infections prevented, statistically estimating production functions is not currently possible. The approach advocated here is to *subjectively construct* HIV production functions based on planning group beliefs informed by whatever data are in fact available.

To proceed, first consider a single group targeted for HIV prevention. The methods that follow would be applied to all groups of interest. Let $I(x)$ denote the number of new HIV infections that would occur in this group over some agreed upon planning horizon (e.g., one year) if x *incremental* dollars are spent on HIV prevention activities. The proper duration of this planning horizon is itself an interesting question, but we will not address it here. If *no* money is allocated to the group then $I(0)$ infections will result. We assume that $I(x)$ is nonincreasing in x, which is equivalent to saying that HIV prevention activities cannot cause more infections than would have resulted otherwise.

Then the number of infections prevented as a result of spending x dollars is given by

$$\Delta I(x) = I(0) - I(x). \tag{1}$$

The relative reduction in new infections if x dollars are spent on HIV prevention in this group, denoted by $\alpha(x)$, is given by

$$\alpha(x) = \frac{\Delta I(x)}{I(0)} \tag{2}$$

and thus we can rewrite Eq. (1) in the more revealing form

$$\Delta I(x) = I(0)\alpha(x). \tag{3}$$

Note that $\alpha(x)$ is a nondecreasing function of x, which again reflects our assumption that HIV prevention cannot hurt and can only help. Also, $\alpha(0) = 0$, so spending nothing on prevention yields no incremental benefits, whereas $\alpha(\infty) \leq 1$, which states that irrespective of how much money is allocated to HIV prevention in the group, it is impossible to prevent more infections than would have occurred in the absence of any intervention.

Equation (3) shows that the number of prevented infections depends on two factors, the baseline rate of new infections $I(0)$ and the effectiveness of prevention programs *as a function of investment* $\alpha(x)$. Estimating the term $I(0)$ is a problem in HIV epidemiology, and determining $\alpha(x)$ is fundamentally a problem of program evaluation. Decomposing the production function into these two components enables community planners first to agree on baseline incidence and then argue about program effectiveness in *relative* terms conditional upon an already agreed upon baseline rate of new infections. Now we consider each of these problems.

Estimating Baseline HIV Incidence

As previously mentioned, determining the baseline rate of new infections (the $I(0)$s) is a common problem in HIV epidemiology. This is an area where community planning groups can turn naturally to epidemiologists for advice. What follows is a very brief listing of various methods that have been proposed for estimating the rate of new HIV infections.

Cohort studies, where a representative sample of initially uninfected persons are tested over time to detect new infections, yield empirical estimates of HIV incidence that enable estimating the overall number of new HIV infections one might expect in the population.[11] In the small number of settings where cohort studies have been undertaken (such as among gay men in San Francisco[12] or drug injectors in Baltimore[13]), such studies do provide a guide. Most community planning groups, however, will not be able to refer to incident cohort studies conducted locally.

Absent the ability to make direct measurements, epidemiologists and statisticians have proposed various techniques for estimating HIV incidence. Back-calculation, for example, enables reconstructing HIV infection rates from AIDS data by exploiting the statistical distribution of the time from HIV infection through AIDS, a distribution that is assumed known on the basis of AIDS natural history studies.[11] Recent incidence estimates produced via back-calculation, however, are not precise because the likelihood of progressing to AIDS within one or two years after infection is tiny. Still, back-calculation provides very helpful information regarding trends of historical incidence that can lead to better informed guesses regarding current incidence.

Newer methods based on immunological markers of infection offer hope for rapidly estimating recent HIV incidence from a single representative sample of the population of interest. For example, Brookmeyer and Quinn have developed a model based on the time delay of roughly three weeks between the detection of HIV p24 antigen and HIV antibody in infected persons,[14] and Kaplan and Brookmeyer have developed a more general approach for application to any immunologic marker that varies as a function of time since infection.[15] However, these studies are also not widespread at present.

Finally, Holmberg has proposed a "components model" of HIV incidence and prevalence for men who have sex with men (MSM), drug injectors (IDUs), and high risk heterosexuals (HET) for all metropolitan statistical areas with populations over 500,000.[16] These estimates were prepared with the idea that they could contribute to the targeting of HIV interventions. Although statistically unorthodox, the figures presented in this study could form a starting point for local planning groups to begin a discussion.

At this point the reader will note that it is essentially impossible for a planning group to know just what the baseline rate of new HIV infections is among the local populations of interest. Such uncertainty, however, does not excuse one from thinking hard about the rate of new HIV infections. The key is that the planning group needs to arrive at an agreement regarding a plausible value (or range of values) for these infection rates. The input of health department experts and local researchers is especially crucial in helping the planning group reach this consensus.

Assessing the Relative Impact of HIV Prevention

Though much has been written regarding the effectiveness of HIV prevention programs, the majority of intervention programs remain unevaluated. Most of the published studies suggest how such interventions help to mediate risky sexual and drug injecting behaviors.[17] Very few studies have attempted to estimate the actual number of infections averted by prevention programs, and fewer still have reported the price tag associated with preventing a given number of infections (though there are some important studies addressing the cost-effectiveness of individual programs[18–24]). Then how can planning groups even begin to consider the relative reduction in new HIV infections that results from prevention programs funded at different levels?

Although empirically linking infections prevented to money spent is a serious challenge for researchers, *subjectively* creating such a link is possible. Doing so results in the $\alpha(x)$ functions discussed earlier. Consider the following hypothetical example: in an area where an additional 350 infections among IDUs are expected, absent any interventions in the next year, a planning group is free to recommend any amount up to $3,000,000 for prevention activities in this population. As a benchmark question, planning group members first argue about the likely impact of spending all $3,000,000. Taking into consideration the types of interventions available, the number of injectors served by these interventions in the past, the costs of the programs and the quality of the services delivered, an argument ensues. Some members contend that recent reports show that cheap outreach programs are quite effective at preventing infections among program participants, but that the main issue is getting injectors to participate in such programs. A $3,000,000 commitment could expand existing programs to the point of reaching perhaps one quarter of all injectors, and assuming that infections emanating from those reached could also be reduced by half, the conclusion is that 12.5% of those infections that would have occurred can be prevented. Other members disagree, arguing that, in their view, the outreach programs have prevented "easy" infections. More expensive and intensive counseling and treatment options are the appropriate route in their view. In their view, the maximum allotment of $3,000,000 could only be expected to avert 5% of all infections. Intermediate positions are also stated, and finally a consensus emerges: the group *agrees to believe* that spending $3,000,000 would avert 10% of the 350 infections that would otherwise occur.

A different benchmark question that the planning group considers is this: How much money would have to be spent on prevention activities to prevent *any* infections? Here a different argument develops, for the issue has to do with the smallest program that could be established that would have some sort of an impact. Some argue that small yet effective programs have been launched with shoestring budgets as low as $50,000 per year relying largely on volunteer or low-cost, peer-group efforts. Others question whether these costs have been underestimated. The group settles on $100,000 as the minimum expenditure needed to have any preventive effect at all.

Now the group tackles intermediate assessment issues. Having earlier agreed that 10% of infections could be averted from funding $3,000,000 in prevention activities, how much money would be required to avert 5% of the infections? How much money would be needed to prevent 2.5% or 7.5%? As a consistency check, the group struggles with questions like, What percentage of infections could be prevented for $1,000,000, $1,500,000, or $2,000,000?? At the end of the exercise, the group has converged on a graph which represents their shared beliefs regarding the relative effectiveness of prevention activities as a function of spending for IDUs. This graph is shown in Figure 1.

Figure 1 reflects the following beliefs about the effectiveness of interventions targeting

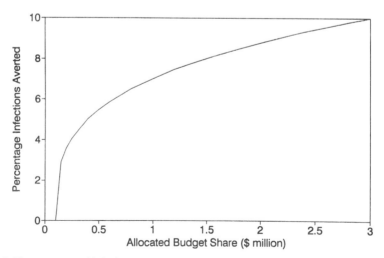

Figure 1. The percentage of infections averted among injection drug users as a function of budget share.

IDUs. A minimum of $100,000 is required to achieve any benefit at all. Once available funds exceed $100,000, the impact of prevention grows rapidly. Spending $500,000 on prevention activities for IDUs is expected to prevent almost 5.5% of avertable infections in this group (or about 19 infections) during one year. However, the impact of such prevention activities increases at a decreasing rate as the available budget increases. Such *diminishing returns to scale* are to be expected for various reasons. For example, if the prevention activities involve some form of outreach and the outreach programs access IDUs from the easier to the more difficult to reach, then the cost of contacting each additional injector increases (because of the increased time and effort required to make such contacts), resulting in a reduction in preventive impact per dollar spent. The simple fact that there is a finite number of preventable infections in any given year is itself sufficient to force diminishing returns to scale, as available funds become very large. As an empirical example of these properties, see the production function for the prevention effectiveness of needle exchange that was derived using data from New Haven.[23]

Returning to the community planning example, the assessment exercise described for IDUs is repeated for each of the key target populations. In each case, the exercise is geared toward producing a graph relating the percentage of infections averted to money spent. Figures 2 and 3 report hypothetical curves for relative prevention effectiveness among MSM (where 100 infections are expected next year in the absence of intervention) and among HET (with a base rate of 50 infections), respectively. Figure 2 has a different shape than Figure 1. Though there is little preventive impact on new infections among MSM for expenditures less than $200,000, prevention effectiveness in this group actually grows at a *marginally increasing* rate for expenditures up to $1,000,000. This situation could be attained by interventions where the likelihood of someone not contacted becoming involved is a function of the number of people already participating. Contact tracing plausibly possesses this property, because the number of referrals increases geometrically at the beginnings of such programs. Interventions in social settings, such as bars, where the attractiveness of the intervention to nonparticipants depends on the number of people already participating, could also yield initial increasing returns to scale. Beyond the first million

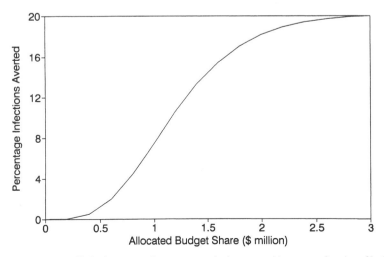

Figure 2. The percentage of infections averted among men who have sex with men as a function of budget share.

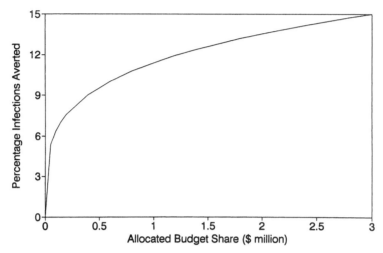

Figure 3. The percentage of infections averted among high risk heterosexuals as a function of budget share.

dollars allocated, however, the curve in Figure 2 bends to exhibit decreasing returns. An expenditure of $3,000,000 on MSM would avert 20% of infections in this group.

Figure 3, reflecting prevention effectiveness among HET, looks more like Figure 1. Here, however, there are essentially no fixed costs, the jump in prevention effectiveness is rapid (9.5% of infections are prevented after spending only $500,000), but subsequent improvements grow slowly as a function of available money. One possible reason for such a curve is that a sizeable number of these women can be located inexpensively (in STD clinics for example), thus prevention activities, such as counseling and condom distribution, can begin almost immediately. Diminishing returns could result from the difficulties of locating the rest of the women, and also if these same women are in situations that themselves render behavior modification more challenging.

The approach described is certainly not the only approach available for subjectively assessing prevention effectiveness as a function of spending. A different approach would be for individual group members or smaller subgroups to create their own graphs independently, and then arrive at a consensus by comparing these individual results. Or the planning group might appoint working groups for each of the target populations or geographic subareas under consideration. Whichever approach is taken, the task proposed is not easy, and would certainly occupy much of the time available in a planning cycle. Although while time-consuming, however, the assessment of production functions does serve the purpose of structuring the already difficult discussion of HIV prevention needs and priorities.

ALLOCATING HIV PREVENTION RESOURCES

Evaluating Alternative Resource Allocations

Combining the results of the previous sections enables a simple formula for evaluating the *implied* preventive impact of any particular budget allocation. Framing the problem in terms of allocating funds across target populations is consistent with the existing practice of many planning groups as described earlier in the second section. Thus, suppose that there are n subgroups being targeted and that a particular proposal calls for allocating x_i dollars to the ith subgroup. Letting $I_i(0)$, and $\alpha_i(x_i)$ denote the base rate of new infections in group i and the relative reduction in this rate if x_i dollars are spent on prevention programs in group i, the implied *number* of infections prevented in group i, $\Delta I_i(x_i)$, equals $I_i(0)\alpha_i(x_i)$ as in Eq. (3). Then the total number of infections prevented, $\Delta I(x_1, x_2, \ldots, x_n)$, is given by

$$\Delta I(x_1, x_2, \ldots, x_n) = \sum_{i=1}^{n} \Delta I_i(x_i) = \sum_{i=1}^{n} I_i(0)\alpha_i(x_i) \tag{4}$$

Thus Eq. (4) enables a community planning group to compute the number of prevented infections implied by a particular allocation of resources, given the production functions already assessed.

The additive representation in Eq. (4) is a pragmatic choice, as it enables community planning groups to think about subpopulations individually. In stating Eq. (4), however, an additional assumption has been made: money directed towards prevention activities in a particular subgroup translates into infections prevented *in that subgroup*. Programs for IDUs, for example, are recognized as preventing infections in IDUs, but not among noninjecting women who have unprotected sex with IDUs. If such overlap is believed to be substantial, one approach would be to estimate the baseline infection rates $I_i(0)$ as the number of infections that would be *transmitted by* members of the ith risk group (as opposed to the number of infections that would *occur* in members of this group). Of course, this approach would make the estimation of $I_i(0)$ more difficult. In theory, one could imagine more complicated functions than Eq. (4) to represent the total number of infections prevented from any particular allocation across the subpopulations, but such analysis is beyond the scope of this paper.[25]

Before continuing, it is important to reiterate that there is no guarantee that the numbers of infections *actually* prevented by any given resource allocation follow from Eq. (4). Equation (4) reports the number of infections prevented that are both *implied by and consistent with* planning group beliefs, beliefs that are themselves represented by production functions *as assessed by the planning group*. In what follows, then, when we speak of the number of infections prevented by alternative resource allocations, what we mean is an implied number consistent with planning group beliefs.

With the above caveat in mind, suppose that a community planning group is faced with allocating $3,000,000 across the three target populations discussed in the previous section. Recall that the three target groups are IDUs, MSM, and HET. The baseline numbers of infections that would occur in the absence of intervention have been estimated as 350, 100 and 50 in these groups, and Figures 1 through 3 report relative program effectiveness (the functions $\alpha_i(x)$ for $i = 1, 2, 3$).

Table 1 presents several examples of infections averted via different divisions of the $3,000,000 budget. The first three rows of Table 1 report all-or-nothing strategies. Spending all $3,000,000 on IDUs would prevent 35 infections, and dedicating the entire budget to MSM or HET would prevent 20 and 7.5 infections, respectively. It is unreasonable to expect that an all-or-nothing strategy would be perceived as fair in any situation, nor would such a strategy be terribly effective (unless only one subpopulation was alone in experiencing new HIV infections). Still, it is important to note the near factor of 5 difference in prevented infections that results across these strategies.

Table 1. Alternative Allocations of $3 Million
HIV Prevention Budget and Infections Prevented

Budget Allocation ($ Million)			Infections Prevented			
IDU	MSM	HET	IDU	MSM	HET	Total
3	0	0	35	0	0	35
0	3	0	0	20	0	20
0	0	3	0	0	7.5	7.5
1	1	1	24.5	7.5	5.7	37.7
2.1	0.6	0.3	31.2	1.9	4.2	37.4
1.15	1.74	0.11	25.7	16.6	3.3	45.5
0.88	1.62	0.5	23.4	15.6	4.8	43.8
0.75	1.5	0.75	22.2	14.4	5.3	41.9

The fourth row in Table 1 proposes assigning $1,000,000 to each of the three groups. Doing so would prevent 24.5 infections among IDUs, 7.5 among MSM, and 5.7 among HET, a total of 37.7 prevented infections. This equal splitting of the budget ensures that equal money is allocated to each group, and the total number of infections prevented is higher than what could be achieved by giving all of the money to any single group.

Of course, there is no particular reason why each group should receive the same amount. Perhaps a more reasonable proposal is to allocate the budget in proportion to the baseline infection rates. Doing so would assign $2.1 million to IDUs, $600,000 to MSM, and only $300,000 to HET. The result would be that 31.2, 1.9, and 4.3 infections would be prevented among IDUs, MSM, and HET, respectively, a total of 37.4 prevented infections. Oddly enough, slightly fewer infections are prevented by allocating money in proportion to the baseline HIV infection rates than by giving each group the same amount. Indeed, to the extent that "targeting" means allocating money to either the highest incidence group or in proportion to incidence,[26] targeting is outperformed in this example by a more "broad-based" HIV prevention plan (which gives $1 million to each group). This paradox quickly disappears if "targeting" is defined instead to mean "allocate resources to prevent the maximum number of infections."

Optimal Resource Allocation

Now it should be apparent that even for the example under discussion with only three groups, there is any number of alternative allocations that could be evaluated using Eq. (4). Although such "if then" analysis is useful in arriving at a final decision, it would also be of interest to know the *maximum* number of infections that could be prevented as a function of the prevention budget and the corresponding *optimal resource allocations* to each of the groups. Mathematically, we face the following optimization problem: given n target populations [the ith of which is represented by a production function $\Delta I_i(x_i) = I_i(0)\alpha_i(x)$] and a total HIV prevention budget of B dollars to allocate, find those amounts $x_1, x_2, \ldots, x_n$ to allocate to each of the respective groups that solve

$$\max_{\{x_1, x_2, \ldots, x_n\}} \sum_{i=1}^{n} I_i(0)\alpha_i(x_i) \qquad (5)$$

subject to

$$\sum_{i=1}^{n} x_i \leq B \tag{6}$$

and

$$x_i \geq 0 \text{ for } i = 1, 2, \ldots, n. \tag{7}$$

The problem posed in Eqs. (5–7) is known as a *knapsack problem*, and well-known techniques are available for obtaining its solution.[27] In particular, as a function of the budget B, we are interested in the optimal resource allocations denoted $x_i(B)$ for the ith target population and the corresponding maximum number of prevented infections denoted by $\Delta I^*(B)$.

Figure 4 reports $\Delta I^*(B)$ for our three group example where the budget B runs from $0 through $3 million. That the total infections averted increases with the budget is unsurprising, but the scalloping nature of Figure 4 requires some explanation. For very low total budgets (less than $100,000), all money is allocated to interventions among HET. The reason for this is clear. Figures 1 and 2 imply that no infections would be prevented by giving only $100,000 to programs targeting either IDUs or MSM, whereas Figure 3 suggests that even such small amounts of money could have an effect if targeted toward HET. For budgets between $100,000 and $1.73 million, the prevention budget is split between activities targeting HET and IDUs. Only when the budget reaches $1.73 million is money allocated to programs for MSM.

The specific allocations to each of the three targeted groups, the $x_i^*(B)$, are shown in Figure 5. As already stated, no money is allocated to programs for MSM until the overall prevention budget reaches $1.73 million, at which point programs for MSM receive $1.2 million. From this point, the commitment to MSM increases to $1.74 million when the total budget is $3 million. Activities targeting IDUs are supported increasingly as the overall budget grows from $100,000 to $1.73 million. The dollars allocated to IDUs reach $1.57

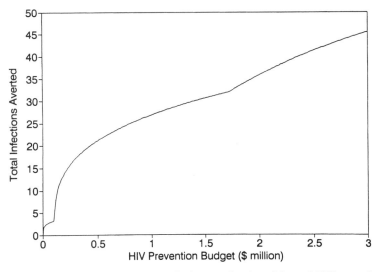

Figure 4. Total infections averted by optimal budgeting as a function of the total HIV prevention budget.

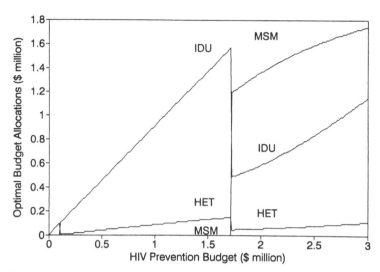

Figure 5. Optimal budget allocations by risk group as a function of the total HIV prevention budget.

million when the total budget is just below $1.73 million. However, the allocation to IDUs drops sharply to $490,000, once funding for MSM enters the picture. Funding grows for IDU activities from this point, reaching an allocation of $1.15 million when the total budget is $3 million. The optimal allocations to HET bounce the most in this example. They grow from zero to $100,000 as the total budget does the same, drop to nearly zero and then grow to $150,000 as the total budget increases to $1.73 million, and drop to $40,000 and then grow to $111,000, when the total budget reaches $3 million.

The optimal allocations shown in Figure 5 appear odd, but it must be remembered that these allocations maximize the number of prevented infections at any given total budget level. Returning to Table 1 where various allocations of a $3 million budget have been evaluated, the *optimal* allocation of $1.15 million to IDUs, $1.74 million to MSM, and $110,000 to HET averts 45.5 infections. *No alternative division of the $3 million budget could prevent more infections.* Still, the dramatic switching in optimal allocation exhibited in Figure 5 raises serious concerns. Suppose that in our three group example, the initial budget is originally $1.75 million and the optimal allocation is determined. Now suppose that the total budget is cut by $30,000 to $1.72 million. Could one really imagine using the optimal budget allocations of Figure 5, which would entail reducing the allocation to activities targeting MSM from roughly $1.2 million to zero? Of course not.

Valuation of Social Constraints

The problem is that the optimal budgeting problem expressed in Eqs. (5–7) does not recognize social constraints, such as fairness or equity. Although preventing HIV infections is surely the major goal of HIV prevention community planning, it is not the only goal. The resource allocation framework developed thus far, however, allows one to value social constraints in terms of the loss in efficiency in preventing infections. Having computed the maximum number of infections that can be prevented, one can explore alternative allocations that are attractive by other political or social criteria and ask whether the political or social gains from the alternatives justify the reduction (from the optimal allocation) in the number of prevented infections.

As an example of such an analysis, consider the discomfort caused by the switching budget allocations of Figure 5. Such switching would not be considered fair by some. Given a total budget increase, the amount of money available to any set of activities should not be *allowed* to decrease. One way around this is to consider only *monotonic* budget allocations. The principle of monotonic allocations is that the amount of money allocated to prevention activities in a particular group cannot decrease as the total budget increases. To obtain monotonic allocations as a function of the budget, one first solves the optimal budgeting problem in Eqs. (5–7) to obtain the optimal allocations $x_i^*(B)$ where B now represents the largest total budget the group is willing to consider. Having obtained these allocations, one then re-solves the optimal allocation problem for a *smaller* total budget, say $(B - b)$, with the constraints

$$0 \leqslant x_i \leqslant x_i^*(B) \text{ for } i = 1, 2, \ldots, n \qquad (8)$$

substituted for Eq. (7). Iterating this process leads to monotonic budget allocations.

Returning to our numerical example, Figure 6 shows the monotonic budget allocations that result from the procedure described above. Unlike Figure 5, now the allocations to each group increase only as the total prevention budget increases. However, there is a small price to be paid in infections averted. Figure 7 reports the total infections averted by the optimal and the monotonic allocations. For budgets of at least $1.73 million, the monotonic and optimal allocations are identical. However, for intermediate total budgets from $500,000 through $1.73 million, the monotonic allocations prevent slightly fewer infections. The same is true for very small budgets.

As a second example, again a planning group seeks to optimally allocate a $3 million prevention budget but now decides to guarantee at least $c for activities targeting each of these groups. Mathematically this corresponds to substituting

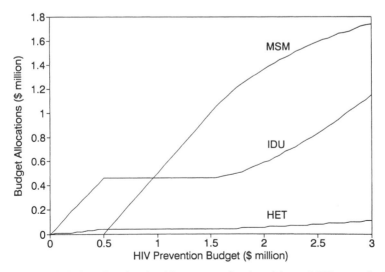

Figure 6. Monotonic budget allocations by risk group as a function of the total HIV prevention budget.

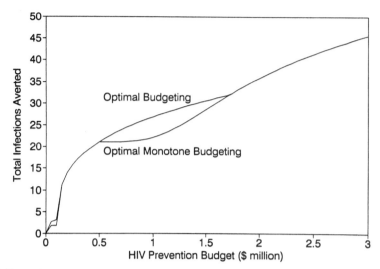

Figure 7. Total infections averted by monotonic budgeting as a function of the total HIV prevention budget.

$$x_i \geq c \text{ for } i = 1, 2, \ldots, n \tag{9}$$

for the nonnegativity constraints of Eq. (7) in the knapsack problem. Figure 8 reports the total number of infections averted as a function of c. For any value of c below \$110,000, these minimum allocation guarantees have no effect, and the total infections averted remains equal to 45.5, for as already shown, the solution to the original knapsack problem awards at least c dollars to each group. Once c increases beyond \$110,000, however, the situation changes, and the total number of infections averted declines. The extent of the decline depends on the magnitude of c. At the extreme where each groups receives \$1 million,

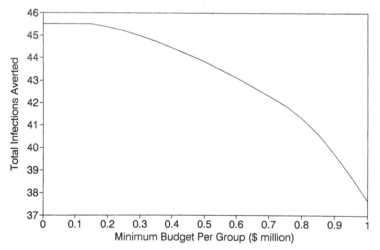

Figure 8. Total infections averted by constrained optimal allocation of a \$3 million HIV prevention budget as a function of the minimum budget allocation guaranteed per risk group.

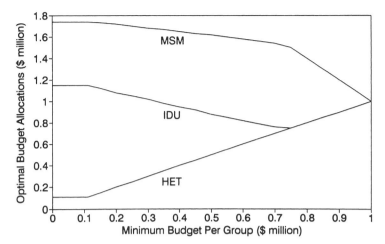

Figure 9. Constrained optimal budget allocations by risk group as a function of the minimum budget allocation guaranteed per group.

only 37.7 infections are prevented, a loss in efficiency of 7.8 infections or 17%. Figure 9 reports the constrained optimal allocations for the three groups. The amount of money allocated to HET equals the guarantee c, once c exceeds $110,000. As a result, the money assigned to both MSM and IDUs is reduced. For guarantees as high as $750,000, IDUs and HET receive the guaranteed amount, and the remaining funds are allocated to MSM.

In principle, any number of social constraints can be imposed on the resource allocation process. The contribution of the framework proposed here is its ability to value such constraints. By comparing the total number of prevented infections from a socially constrained resource allocation to the optimal allocation, we arrive at a measure of the penalty imposed by these social constraints. Computing such efficiency losses can help planning groups decide whether imposing such social constraints is justified. For example, Figure 9 shows that guaranteeing $500,000 at a minimum for each of the three groups in our example results in an allocation that prevents 43.8 infections, a loss in efficiency of 1.7 infections or 3.7%. Is it worth sacrificing 1.7 prevented infections to ensure that all groups receive at least $500,000 in prevention money? There is no right or wrong answer to this question. Different planning groups could decide to take different actions. However, our framework offers the opportunity to assess the consequences of these different actions.

Finally, it is worth mentioning that although social constraints will impose efficiency losses for any fixed budget, the magnitude of such efficiency losses will typically decline as the total budget to be allocated becomes very large. In the absence of a budget constraint, maximal prevention can be achieved in various ways. Unfortunately, HIV prevention budgets are not likely to expand, so budget-constrained resource allocation is the reality that planning groups must face.

CONCLUSION: DECISIONS MUST BE MADE

The HIV prevention community planning process is designed to allow making decisions regarding how best to prevent the further spread of HIV at the local level. Regardless of the particular approach taken by a community planning group, at the end of the process, decisions must be made. I have argued that, ultimately, such decisions translate into budget allocations for alternative HIV prevention activities that are supposed to prevent infections. Therefore it stands to reason that thinking through the linkage between public HIV prevention expenditures and prevented infections should play an important role in allocating HIV prevention resources.

Many will oppose the use of such formalism. They would protest that it is not realistic to expect community planning groups (or panels of HIV intervention researchers for that matter) to be able to construct production functions for HIV prevention, given the lack of epidemiological and evaluation data. This same state of uncertainty, however, pervades any approach to decision making in HIV prevention community planning. Existing approaches to community planning appear immune to criticisms regarding the relationship between allocated resources and infections prevented only because such approaches fail to raise the question!

How to spend public HIV prevention money is one of the most important public health decisions facing the nation. The HIV prevention community planning process launched 65 natural experiments in response to this challenge. Decisions must be made. The framework suggested here represents an alternative approach to reaching such decisions. By recognizing the linkage between resource expenditures and the prevention of HIV infection, planning groups can produce a measure of the effectiveness of any resource allocation, and thus compare and contrast alternative proposals. This capability can help planning groups focus on the implications of their decisions, enabling arguably better decisions to be reached.

ACKNOWLEDGMENTS.   Supported in part by the Societal Institute of the Mathematical Sciences, via Grant DA09531 from the National Institute on Drug Abuse, and the Center for Interdisciplinary Research on AIDS at Yale University, via Grant PO1-MH/DA-56826 from the National Institutes on Mental Health and Drug Abuse.

REFERENCES

1. Valdiserri RO, Aultman TV, Curran JW. Community planning: A national strategy to improve HIV prevention programs. *J Community Health* 1995; 20:87–100.
2. Renaud M. *HIV Prevention Community Planning Profiles: Assessing Year One*. Washington, DC: United States Conference of Mayors; 1995.
3. Renaud M. *HIV Prevention Community Planning Profiles: Assessing the Impact*. Washington, DC: United States Conference of Mayors; 1996.
4. *Guidance and Supplemental Information, Non-Competing Continuation of Cooperative Agreements for Human Immunodeficiency Virus (HIV) Prevention Projects*. Announcement No. 300. Atlanta: Centers for Disease Control and Prevention; 1995.
5. *Budget of the United States Government, Fiscal Year 1997*. Washington, DC: Government Printing Office; 1996.
6. Hoffman C, de Palomo FB, Greabell L. *HIV Prevention Priorities: How Community Planning Groups Decide*. Washington, DC: Academy for Educational Development and National Alliance of State and Territorial AIDS Directors, 1996 (Draft).
7. Bibus DP, Wood RW, Hartfield K, et al. A model for distributing HIV-Prevention Resources. *AIDS Public Policy J* 1994; 9:197–207.
8. *Priority Setting in HIV Prevention Community Planning*. Washington, DC: Academy for Educational Development; 1994.

9. Pollack H, Zeckhauser R. Budgets as Dynamic Gatekeepers. *Manage Sci* 1996; 42:642–658.

10. Nicholson W. *Microeconomic Theory*, 2nd ed. Hinsdale, Illinois: The Dryden Press; 1978.

11. Brookmeyer R, Gail MH. *AIDS Epidemiology: A Quantitative Approach*. Oxford: Oxford University Press; 1994.

12. Bacchetti P. Estimating the incubation period of AIDS by comparing population infection and diagnosis patterns. *J Am Stat Assoc* 1990; 85:1002–1008.

13. Nelson KE, Vlahov D, Solomon L, et al. Temporal trends of incident human immunodeficiency virus infection in a cohort of injecting drug users in Baltimore, MD. *Arch Int Med* 1995; 155:1305–1311.

14. Brookmeyer R, Quinn TC. Estimation of current human immunodeficiency virus incidence rates from a cross-sectional survey using early diagnostic tests. *Am J Epidemiol* 1995; 141:166–172.

15. Kaplan EH, Brookmeyer R. Snapshot estimators of recent HIV incidence rates. *Operations Research* (in press).

16. Holmberg SD. The estimated prevalence and incidence of HIV in 96 large US metropolitan areas. *Am J Public Health* 1996; 86:642–654.

17. Choi K-H, Coates TJ. Prevention of HIV infection. *AIDS* 1994; 8:1371–1389.

18. Holtgrave DR, Valdiserri RO, West GA. Quantitative economic evaluations of HIV-related prevention and treatment services: A review. *Risk* 1994; 5:29–47.

19. Holtgrave DR, Qualls NL. Threshold analysis and programs for prevention of HIV infection. *Medical Decision Making* 1995; 15:311–317.

20. Holtgrave DR, Qualls NL, Curran JW, et al. Effectiveness and efficiency of HIV prevention services: An overview. *Public Health Rep* 1995; 110:134–146.

21. Holtgrave DR, Kelly JA. HIV infection among high-risk women: The cost-effectiveness of a behavioral intervention. *Am J Public Health*, in press.

22. Kahn JG. Are NEPs cost-effective in preventing HIV infection? In Lurie PG, Reingold AL, eds. *The Public Health Impact of Needle Exchange Programs in the United States and Abroad*. San Francisco: Institute for Health Policy Studies, University of California, San Francisco; 1993.

23. Kaplan EH. Economic analysis of needle exchange. *AIDS* 1995; 9:1113–1119.

24. Kaplan EH, Brandeau ML. *Modeling the AIDS Epidemic: Planning, Policy, and Prediction*. New York: Raven Press; 1994.

25. Keeney RL, Raiffa H. *Decisions with Multiple Objectives: Preferences and Value Tradeoffs*. New York: John Wiley and Sons; 1976.

26. Kahn JG. The cost-effectiveness of HIV prevention targeting: how much more bang for the buck? *Am J Public Health*, in press.

27. Hillier FS, Lieberman GJ. *Introduction to Operations Research*, 6th ed. New York: McGraw-Hill; 1995.

14

Threshold Analysis of AIDS Outreach and Intervention

EDWARD C. NORTON, ROBERT F. MARTIN, and WENDEE M. WECHSBERG

INTRODUCTION

One of the most important public health policy issues is how best to prevent the further spread of the human immunodeficiency virus (HIV). The federal government spends hundreds of millions of dollars each year on prevention programs and more than $1.5 billion on medical care and on research. In 1993 the Centers for Disease Control and Prevention spent $358.6 million on extramural HIV prevention activities and an additional $139.5 million on intramural HIV prevention activities.[1] In addition, state and local governments also fund prevention programs.

Although the government spends an enormous amount to control HIV transmission, the money may not be well spent. The effectiveness and cost-effectiveness of the majority of HIV education and intervention programs have not been evaluated because the need was to get programs into communities.[2] Given that government resources are limited, it is important to spend wisely on those programs that yield the most benefits. Now economic methods are being used to evaluate whether programs are effective at producing benefits that exceed their cost.

This study estimates the costs of one exemplary HIV prevention program and applies threshold analysis to estimate the level of benefits needed to exceed the costs. We believe that it is the first study to estimate the costs of an AIDS outreach and intervention program. This prevention program is especially interesting because it is part of a larger national efficacy study, and this program is specifically measuring the process and quantity of outreach and intervention services. Furthermore, it targets the high-risk populations of most interest to the National Institute on Drug Abuse (NIDA), injecting drug users and crack users, and subpopulations, such as African-American women, younger drug users, and drug users outside urban areas.

Beginning in the late 1980s, NIDA sponsored two national research studies of HIV intervention efficacy among injecting drug users who are not in treatment. These two studies,

EDWARD C. NORTON • Department of Health Policy and Administration, University of North Carolina at Chapel Hill, Chapel Hill, North Carolina 27599-7400.   ROBERT F. MARTIN • Department of Economics, University of Chicago, Chicago, Illinois 60637.   WENDEE M. WECHSBERG • Research Triangle Institute, Research Triangle Park, North Carolina 27709.

Handbook of Economic Evaluation of HIV Prevention Programs, edited by Holtgrave. Plenum Press, New York, 1998.

the National AIDS Demonstration Research (NADR) Project and the current Cooperative Agreement for AIDS Research (CoOp), include intake and follow-up data on HIV risk patterns for large samples of substance abusers not in treatment. The primary goal of these prevention programs is to prevent the spread of HIV by targeting those considered most at risk and changing their behavior. Although these programs vary, most consist of an outreach and an intervention component. Outreach workers identify and contact the target populations and provide brief prevention messages. Intervention workers attempt to alter high-risk behavior through further education and HIV antibody testing.

Although these two national research studies have improved our understanding of efficacy, until recently they did not study whether prevention programs provide net positive benefits. Prevention programs must justify their existence by showing health benefits to their target population and also by showing economic benefits to society.[3] The prevailing mood in Congress is to reduce spending and social programs. In addition, taxpayers want public health programs to produce quantifiable benefits. Therefore, limited government resources place the onus on prevention programs to show that they are cost-beneficial. This can be done through economic analysis that compares the costs to the benefits. However, disentangling research costs from program costs can be problematic.

Although a large body of economic evaluation literature exists, most studies of HIV prevention programs do not compare costs to benefits in a way that shows directly whether a program is cost-beneficial. A review by Holtgrave, Qualls, and Graham[4] found 93 published papers that compared quantitative estimates of the program costs and outcomes for either a domestic or international prevention or care and treatment program. Of these studies, only five were cost-benefit analyses of domestic interventions aimed at changing behavior. None were done on the NADR or CoOp projects or for outreach programs. Given the recent emphasis of NIDA in these areas, there is a considerable gap in the literature.

If it is too early in the evaluation to estimate actual benefits, as is the case in this study, then one can use threshold analysis to estimate the level of benefits that just balance costs. Threshold analysis estimates two things, the program cost, and the monetary benefit per outcome. (Unlike cost-benefit analysis it does not estimate the actual number of outcomes, like cases of HIV infection avoided, because the data are not available yet.) Then threshold analysis compares the program cost to the monetary benefit per outcome to estimate the number of outcomes needed to be achieved to just balance the costs. Threshold analysis is useful because it gives a sense of how effective the program must be to achieve benefits greater than the cost.

Several recent studies have used threshold analysis. Holtgrave and colleagues[5] used threshold analysis to compare the total costs and benefits of the CDC's extramural HIV prevention activities. They concluded that if 758 cases of HIV were avoided per year, then the program would be cost-effective. Gorsky and colleagues[6] used threshold analysis to determine the likely cost-savings of HIV counseling and testing at three methadone treatment centers. They performed their analysis using as benefits only the avoided medical costs of HIV infection, which they estimated to be $56,000 in 1991 dollars. With this conservative estimate, they concluded that if more than one person in 260 changes behavior as a result of counseling and testing, then the program would be a cost-saving prevention strategy. In another study of HIV counseling and testing, Holtgrave and colleagues[7] used data from Wisconsin to estimate whether estimated benefits exceeded costs. Under a variety of assumptions they found that the answer is yes, although the exact amount depends critically on whether avoided productivity losses are included and on other assumptions. Clark and Corbett[8] used threshold analysis to evaluate whether needle exchange programs are cost-effective based on results from studies in London and Connecticut. Although their estimates of benefits included both medical and lost productivity, their cost estimates were rough. They concluded that given the effectiveness of avoiding two HIV infections per 100 attendees found in both studies, the expected benefits far outweigh the costs. To our knowledge, no study to date has applied threshold analysis to a community-based outreach and intervention program aimed at avoiding the spread of HIV infection.

METHODOLOGICAL FRAMEWORK

This study estimates the annual costs of the North Carolina CoOperative Agreement Program (NC CoOp), a part of the NIDA Cooperative Consortium. We estimated the monthly and annual cost of the program through extensive on-site interviews and budget reviews. We included all economic costs, accounted for depreciation, and excluded all research costs. We calculated costs separately for outreach and intervention and for five different cost categories. All costs are reported in 1995 dollars. The details of the cost calculations are explained here.

We did not estimate rigorously how the program affected risk behavior, the chance of getting HIV, or other long-term outcomes because the NC CoOp has not yet produced the long-term data necessary for a definitive benefit analysis. Instead, we used threshold analysis to answer a simple question: What level of benefits must be achieved for the NC CoOp to be cost-beneficial? We also used preliminary data on outcomes to indicate whether the NC CoOp is likely to be effective at reducing high-risk behavior.

The idea of threshold analysis is to divide the actual annual cost by the expected monetary benefit per outcome to compute the number of positive outcomes per year needed to break even. Specifically, we assumed that the relevant outcome of the NC CoOp is avoiding a case of HIV infection. The expected monetary benefit of avoiding one case of HIV infection was divided into the annual cost of the program. That threshold is compared to the number of cases that can reasonably be expected to be avoided. Finally, we tested the underlying assumptions of the model to see whether the results are robust.

DATA

Description of the NC CoOp

The NC CoOp is one of twenty-three cooperative sites funded by the National Institute on Drug Abuse. The NC CoOp is directed by researchers at Research Triangle Institute. The goals of the Cooperative sites are to prevent the further spread of HIV infection by conducting community-based outreach and intervention, to target hidden populations of injecting drug users and crack users not in treatment, and to recruit these substances abusers for a more extensive HIV risk reduction intervention. Each program has implemented a standard outreach and intervention protocol and has developed and implemented an enhanced intervention program appropriate for its community.

The NC CoOp began field work in January 1995 in Durham County, North Carolina. Although the program has since expanded to another site, we focus on the Durham site. The Durham site currently employs two outreach workers and two other persons who provide testing and intervention services. The outreach workers screen and recruit drug users at risk of HIV infection to participate in the intervention. The outreach workers follow an outreach protocol in making every effort to locate hidden populations of injecting drug users and crack users who are not in traditional treatment programs. The outreach workers make contact by approaching people on the street, in laundry mats, parks, pool halls, community centers, and informal drug exchange "hot spots." After building rapport with these potential clients, the outreach workers talk about prevention issues and the relationship between substance abuse and HIV. They provide prevention packets containing male condoms, risk reduction kits for injectors, and instructions for both. The outreach workers try to recruit individuals to participate in the research intervention. Several contacts are sometimes necessary before successful recruitment into the study.

Once eligibility is determined, the client spends approximately 45 minutes responding to a standardized data collection instrument used nationally to obtain information on demographics, sexual behavior, drug use, and HIV risk. The information gathered from the survey is used only for research and program evaluation. The key outcomes are changes from risky sexual practices and drug use, which are measured at intake and at follow-up.

After the data are collected, the intervention begins. The intervention is designed to induce positive behavioral changes in the participants. First, the clients are given a short test to determine their working knowledge of HIV and AIDS. The test includes questions which measure the clients' knowledge of HIV transmission routes and basic protection practices. Then they are shown a series of cue cards describing basic HIV information. During this session, they are also given a chance to practice cleaning needles and to place a condom on a dildo. At the end of the session, they are given the option of being tested for HIV. They have the option to refuse the test. The program uses one room for interviewing, one for the intervention, and one for testing blood. In our analysis, we assume that only one of these rooms is necessary. If the phlebotomist were doing both the testing and the intervention, no reason would exist to change rooms. The first follow-up session is used to deliver the HIV test results and to reemphasize the prevention information given in the first session. The third and final session is used to obtain information on how the participants have altered their behavior as a result of the intervention.

Data Collection

We collected the cost information for our analysis from project records, personal interviews, and site visits.[9] Because there is a large research component, the program's financial and client records are complete and are kept in great detail. The records provided us with an accurate assessment of all resources used on the project and the price paid for each item.

We reviewed the monthly financial records for information about costs and resource use. The computerized client tracking system provided information on the number and type of clients served. However, because of the large research component, we distinguished between costs incurred for research purposes and costs incurred for the outreach and intervention. To make this distinction, we conducted personal interviews with the on-site supervisor and the principal investigator for the project. They helped us to determine the aspects of the project which are unrelated to intervention and outreach goals. Subsequently, we conducted site visits to monitor resource use.

Description of the Sample

Through February 1996, the Durham site has recruited and conducted initial interviews with 347 participants (see Table 1). The participants are predominately African-American (91%) and male (65%). Almost 80% of the participants are between the ages of 25 and 44.

NIDA has directed much of its research toward target groups at high risk of HIV infection.[9] Among these groups are injecting drug users who have consistently represented one-third of the AIDS cases in the last decade. Injecting drug users have an incidence of HIV 4.4 times that of men who have sex with men in the New York Metro area.[10] Injecting drug users spread the HIV virus through behavior related to both direct and indirect sharing of injecting equipment and through unprotected sex.[11–13] However, a growing proportion of newly infected persons are women, many of whom report injecting drug use, crack use, or being sexual partners of drug users.[14–18] More alarming is new evidence pointing to the increasing risk that crack-dependent women engage in sex for drug exchange.[19–21]

The NC CoOp study is targeting injecting drug users and crack users as the NIDA target population, with particular emphasis on younger substance abusers, African-American women, and substance abusers in rural areas. More than 90% of participants use some form of crack cocaine. Almost 40% use crack cocaine and inject some form of narcotic. Only 7.5% of the population are injecting drug users who do not use crack cocaine. The population is predominately heterosexual (76%). An additional 20% consider themselves celibate. Less than 5% are either bisexual or homosexual. The population contains a high percentage of people who consider themselves homeless (28.5%). The second most common living arrangement are participants who live with a spouse or partner (27.4%). Nineteen percent live alone and 25% live with some other adult.

Table 1. Population Means[a]

Variable	Percent	Variable	Percent
Demographics		Drug use	
Age		Injection drug user	7.5
18–24	5.7	Crack user	53.0
25–34	39.9	Both	39.2
35–44	39.9	Current pattern of sexual activity	
45+	14.5	Celibate	19.6
Male	65.4	Male-heterosexual	48.1
Race		Male-bisexual/homosexual	3.0
African-American	91.1	Female-heterosexual	27.9
Caucasian	5.4	Female-bisexual/homosexual	1.4
Other race	3.5		
Housing status			
Homeless	28.5		
Living alone	19.3		
Living with spouse/partner	27.4		
Living with other	24.8		

[a]N = 347

METHODS

Costs

We calculated costs for the following categories: labor, rent and utilities, supplies, transportation, and laboratory. We allocated all costs to one of the two major components of the program, outreach and intervention. Research costs were excluded. Because the NC CoOp took a few months to achieve stable personnel and optimal facility use, we used estimates of resource use during the period in which the program was fully staffed and operating as expected. We extrapolated these costs to calculate average monthly and annual costs.

The largest cost category for both outreach and intervention was labor. All personnel are employed through a local temporary employment agency. The employees receive no fringe benefits directly. However, the employment agency charges a fee of 21.44% for its services. The employment agency also pays the FICA tax which is 7.65% for all workers making less than $135,000.[22] We included both the agency fee and the employer tax in the labor cost by multiplying the hourly wage of each worker by 1.2909. We assumed that each employee works 2000 hours per year, or 166.67 hours per month.

The NC CoOp program requires outreach workers to work in teams of two for safety and effectiveness, even though many programs conduct outreach with only one outreach worker. Consequently, we estimated that the outreach labor cost is the cost of two full-time outreach workers. The two outreach workers are paid an average of $10 per hour.

The NC CoOp program currently employs two full-time employees to conduct the intervention. However, we believe that only one person is necessary for the nonresearch component, as long as that person is a phlebotomist. We determined through interviews that a single phlebotomist could conduct the intervention and all blood tests for as much as twice the current case load. The other employee is necessary for the considerable research effort. Therefore, we estimated that intervention labor cost is the cost of one full-time phlebotomist, who is paid $10 per hour.

The next cost category includes rent and utilities. The only outreach utility cost is for the use of a cellular phone. Outreach workers use the cellular phone to improve safety and to allow potential participants to contact them. The phone's basic monthly fee includes one hour of free calls each month. The outreach workers typically use about ninety minutes of phone time per month. We included the average charge for minutes beyond one hour in our calculation of the monthly fee. We amortized the start-up costs over three years, assuming that the cellular phone will be serviceable for three years. The start-up costs include the purchase price, the price of one battery, and the activation fee. The cost of outreach does not include rent because the outreach workers are in the field all day.

The rent and utility costs are larger for the intervention than for the outreach. The NC CoOp rents three rooms from a church in Durham, North Carolina. Currently three rooms are being used for the intervention study, and each room serves a mixture of research and intervention. However, without the research component, only one room would be needed. Therefore, we included only the rent for one room at a cost of $300 per month in our estimate of the intervention cost. Electricity and heat are included in the rent. We calculated that the cost of phone service is the cost of one business line with voice mail. Voice mail is necessary because potential clients often call after normal business hours or when the phone is in use. A post office box is needed for receiving confidential test results because otherwise the mail for the program would go to the church. State confidentiality rules require that the mail come directly to the program.

Outreach supplies consist of prevention packages distributed by the outreach workers to potential participants. These prevention packages include condoms, needle cleaning equipment (bleach and water vials), and instructional and informational pamphlets. Prevention packages were donated by the State of North Carolina, and minimal labor was required by the outreach workers to place appropriate labels on the bleach and water vials. Even though the prevention packages were donated, their cost must be included as an economic cost to society. The State estimated that the prevention packages cost $4 each.

Intervention supplies are needed to furnish one office room, including a desk, chairs, coat rack, filing cabinet, appointment board, and basic desk supplies. The initial purchase of office supplies came to more than $1,600. We estimated the annual supply cost as the depreciation over one year because most supplies were durable goods. All furniture used in the intervention was received used from the Research Triangle Institute warehouse. The warehouse buys and sells goods at prices based on the condition of the furniture. We assumed that all furniture was received in excellent condition and that after one year it would decline by one category to good condition. The monthly cost was calculated as the price in excellent condition minus the price in good condition, divided by twelve. We also included the cost of sample condoms and visual aids used in the educational portion of the intervention.

Outreach workers drive an average of 752 miles each month around Durham County canvass areas for potential participants in primary prevention. This includes some mileage to transport specimens to the State health department. All trips are conducted with personal transportation, and the staff are reimbursed using the federal government's reimbursement rate of thirty cents per mile.

Laboratory equipment is used by the phlebotomist and includes biohazard disposal units, gloves, and a cooler for transporting samples to the local health department. The full price of this equipment is included because, once used, it cannot be resold. We determined the cost of all laboratory equipment from project records. We assumed that the laboratory equipment is replaced annually. The State of North Carolina provides free HIV testing throughout the state. Although these tests are not charged directly to the program, we include them as an economic cost to society. The State estimates that the average cost of HIV testing, including laboratory overhead, is $4.75 per participant.[23] The average cost is an average of the ELISA and Western Blot tests, weighted by the probability of administering the test. Ninety-six percent of all tests result in a single inexpensive ELISA test. If the initial ELISA test is positive, however, then it is repeated twice. The State estimated that the approximately 3% of all persons test positive three times on the ELISA test and go on to receive the more expensive Western Blot test.

We excluded all research costs from our analysis. For example, we do not include the costs of collecting demographic information from participants because that part is not related to the intervention. We also excluded personnel whose sole responsibility is to coordinate research.

We explored the idea of including the client's time of participation, including transportation to and from the intervention, as a cost because, in principle, this should be included, although in practice it is hard to measure. Economists typically assume that people value their time at their wage rate. For example, if a client earns $10 per hour and takes three hours to participate, then the client's time adds $30 to the cost of the program from society's point of view. The project supervisor estimated that only 15 to 20% of the participants are employed and receive an hourly wage of $6 to $7 hour. Assuming that each of the 347 clients participated for three hours and has an average wage of $1.40 (= $7 × 0.2), then the estimated cost of client's time is $486 per year. Including this cost would raise the total program cost by about 0.5%. Therefore, for this program we do not feel these costs are significant enough to include on the basis of this sensitivity test.

Benefits

We used threshold analysis to compare the costs and benefits of AIDs outreach and intervention. Threshold analysis has been used to evaluate programs in which outcomes are too far in the future to estimate benefits accurately.[5–8]

After estimating the costs, the next step in threshold analysis is to identify the benefit measure. Of all possible benefits of AIDS outreach and intervention, the most important is avoiding HIV infection. By encouraging changes in drug use and sexual practice, the NC CoOp aims to avoid further spread of HIV. Avoiding HIV infection and the subsequent full-blown AIDS, has the benefit of avoiding lost utility from life and health expenditures.

Cost-utility analysis has been used to calculate the number of quality-adjusted life years (QALYs) lost due to HIV infection and AIDS. Holtgrave and Qualls[1] use cost-utility analysis to estimate that the value of avoiding one HIV infection is $417,000 in 1993 dollars. They estimate the number of QALYs for a person infected with HIV for each year from the time of infection until age 65. They assume that an uninfected person has a QALY equal to 1.0 and that death has a QALY equal to 0.0. They multiply the difference in QALY by the dollar amount that society would be willing to pay per QALY gained plus a discount factor. Their base-case value of $417,000 is based on societal willingness to pay $45,000 per QALY gained, at a discount rate of 5%, an average age of infection of 26, and an average age of death from AIDS of 38. Therefore, they assume that an HIV infection reduces the number of working years prior to age 65 by 27 years.

In addition to the cost of utility loss, Holtgrave and Qualls estimate that the direct medical costs saved by avoiding an HIV infection is about $56,000 in 1993 dollars.[24] Other studies have estimated much higher treatment costs. For example, Hellinger[26] estimated that the lifetime cost of treating a person with HIV is $119,000 in 1992 dollars. We used the more conservative estimate given by Guinan, Franham, and Holtgrave to avoid overestimating the benefits.[25] Therefore, the total benefit from avoiding an HIV infection is estimated at about $473,000 in 1993 dollars.

We updated Holtgrave and Qualls' figures from 1993 dollars to 1995 dollars to be commensurate with the cost figures. We multiplied $473,000 by the cumulative inflation rate from 1993 to 1995, as measured by the Gross Domestic Product Deflator. The cumulative inflation rate was 6.4% (Federal Reserve Bank of St. Louis). Therefore the combined benefits from productivity and medical care of avoiding HIV infection is about $502,798 in 1995 dollars.

The next step in threshold analysis is to compute the threshold ratio of the cost per year to the benefits of avoiding HIV infection. This ratio gives the threshold number of HIV infections per year needed just to balance the costs and the benefits. If the actual number of HIV infections exceeds this threshold, then the benefits exceed the costs. Alternatively, if the actual number of HIV infections is less than this threshold, then the costs exceed the benefits. We will use the threshold ratios in future research when we estimate the actual benefits of the program.

RESULTS

Costs

We estimated that the total monthly cost of the NC CoOp, excluding research, is $7,899 (see Table 2). On an annual basis the cost is $94,791. Fully 85% of the costs are for labor.

About 60% of the total cost is spent on outreach, about $4,800 per month. The overwhelming fraction of the cost of outreach is spent on labor. The cost of outreach workers is $11.62 and $14.20 per hour, including the fringe rate and employer taxes, a total of about $4,300 per month. Less than 10% of outreach costs are for utilities, supplies, and transportation. The cellular phone costs less than $50 per month, the prevention packages cost $201 per month, and the cost of driving is $226 per month.

The intervention contributes approximately 40% of the total program cost, about $3,100 per month. Again, labor is the greatest cost. The phlebotomist earns $12.90 per hour, including the fringe rate and employer taxes, a total of about $2,200. The largest nonlabor cost is rent, which is $300 per month. Other intervention costs are relatively small in comparison. A phone with voice mail and a post office box costs about $60 per month. Supplies come to less than $90 per month when depreciated over three years. Laboratory equipment costs about $340 per month. The average cost of testing for HIV each month comes to about $81 for 17 tests.

Benefits

We calculated that the benefit of avoiding one HIV infection is about $502,798 in 1995 dollars. The threshold ratio of the cost per year of the NC CoOp program to the benefit per HIV infection avoided yields the number of infections avoided per year to break even (see Table 3). Given the cost per year of about $94,791, the threshold ratio is about 0.19, meaning that, on average, the program needs to avoid only 0.19 cases of HIV per year. Inverting the ratio shows another way to say the same thing—on average, the program must avert one HIV infection about every 5.3 years. Even when compared only to the direct medical costs, the program cost seems relatively small because the threshold ratio is only 1.59 cases of HIV per year.

Can the NC CoOp achieve the threshold of avoiding one HIV infection every 5.3 years? The answer depends on the number of persons who complete the outreach and intervention and how effective the program is in changing behavior. During the first year the NC CoOp program conducted 347 initial interviews. The vast majority who completed the initial interview have already returned for the three-month follow-up interview, providing preliminary data on the program's effectiveness. The answers to four questions about the respondents' change in behavior since the initial interview implies that the NC CoOp has reduced risky behavior (see Table 4). In terms of sexual behavior, 43% decreased the number of encounters with another sexual partner and 31% increased condom use. In terms of drug use, nearly two-thirds of injecting drug users decreased their use of injecting drugs and

Table 2. Monthly and Yearly Costs of NC CoOp Outreach and Intervention

Category	Quantity	Unit Cost	Notes	Monthly Cost	Yearly Cost
Outreach					
Labor	• 2 outreach workers	• 10.00/hour	• Agency fee is an additional 21.44% Taxes are an additional 7.65%	$4,303.00	
Utilities	• 1 cellular phone	• $81.72 • $42.61/month	• Depreciated over 3 years • Monthly fee and extra minutes	$2.27 $42.61	
Supplies	• 30 packages	• $4.00/package	• Prevention packages and pamphlets	$201.54	
Transportation	• 752 miles	• 30¢/mile	• Workers used personal transportation	$225.70	
Total outreach				$4,775.12	$57,301
Intervention					
Labor	• 1 phlebotomist	• $10.00/hour	• Agency fee is an additional 21.44% Taxes are an additional 7.65%	$2,151.50	
Rent and utilities					
Rent	• 1 room	• $300/month	• Includes electricity and heat	$300.00	
P.O. Box	• 1 box	• $58/year		$4.83	
Phone	• 1 business line and voice mail	• $55.95/month		$55.95	
Supplies	• Office furniture • Office supplies	• $1,685.57 • $100/month	• Depreciated 1 condition over 1 year	$87.48 $100.00	
Laboratory					
Equipment	• Phlebotomy equipment			$343.59	
HIV testing	• 17 tests	• 4.75/test	• Weighted average of cost of ELISA and Western Blot tests	$80.75	
Total intervention				$3,124.11	$37,489
Total cost				$7,899.23	$94,791

Table 3. Threshold Ratio for Balancing Costs and Benefits

Costs	
Cost per year (from Table 2)	$94,791
Benefits	
Benefit per HIV infection avoided	$443,214
Direct medical costs	$59,584
Total	$502,798
Threshold ratio	
$\dfrac{\text{Cost per year}}{\text{Benefit per HIV infection avoided}}$	0.19 HIV infections avoided per year to break even
$\dfrac{\text{Benefit per HIV infection avoided}}{\text{Cost per year}}$	5.3 years per HIV infection avoided per year to break even

nearly three-quarters of noninjectors decreased their use of drugs. Although these data are preliminary, they imply that reaching the threshold is a plausible goal for the NC CoOp program. We will answer this question more rigorously in the future research when more definitive data are available.

Sensitivity of Results to Different Assumptions

We tested the sensitivity of our results to the underlying assumptions of the benefits measure because the costs are measured with relatively little uncertainty. In their study, Holtgrave and Qualls[1] estimated the effect of changing each of their assumptions on the expected benefits of avoiding one HIV infection. They concluded that the expected benefits are most sensitive to the number of potential life years and society's willingness to pay per QALY. They also concluded that the expected benefits are modestly sensitive to the QALY value in each health state and the discount rate. We conducted sensitivity analyses on these four assumptions, tailored to the specific differences between their sample and ours. Holtgrave and Qualls based their morbidity and mortality assumptions on the general population with AIDS, and their willingness to pay per QALY on the general population. Our sample differs from theirs primarily in the number of substance abusers, which is higher in our

Table 4. Preliminary Effectiveness Analysis

	Number of Individuals[a]			
	Increased	Stayed Same	Decreased	N
Encounters with another sexual partner	7 (3%)	134 (54%)	105 (43%)	246
Use of condoms	77 (31%)	146 (59%)	24 (10%)	247
Use of injecting drugs (if injecting drug user)	8 (15%)	10 (19%)	34 (65%)	52
Use of drugs (if noninjecting drug user)	14 (7%)	37 (19%)	147 (74%)	198

[a]Percentages are shown in parentheses.

sample. Compared to the benefits, the costs are estimated with relatively little error, and so we focused the sensitivity analysis on the benefits and not the costs.

The expected benefits per HIV infection avoided for our analysis may differ from the expected benefits calculated by Holtgrave and Qualls[1] because of differences between our sample populations (see Table 5). First, our sample has a higher percentage of substance abusers than the general population with AIDS which affects the probability of surviving to age 65 even if the person does not become infected with HIV. Substance abusers are less likely to live as long in the absence of HIV infection. Assuming that our entire population would die ten years earlier at age 55 in the absence of HIV changed the benefits to $353,393. Second, substance abusers are less healthy than the general population while they are alive. Therefore, the value of a QALY for a non-HIV-infected person is likely to be lower for substance abusers than for nonsubstance abusers. If the QALY of a healthy year is changed from 1.0 to 0.9 for our entire sample, then the benefits fall to $386,039. If the QALY is changed to 0.8, then the benefits fall to $328,864. Therefore, although changing these two assumptions reduces the expected benefits, the threshold ratio is still well over three years per HIV infection.

Society's willingness to pay per QALY may be lower for less socially acceptable persons than for the population in general. A lower willingness to pay per QALY would lower the benefits because they are directly proportional. Holtgrave and Qualls[1] assumed $45,000 per QALY, based on the literature for the general population. For obvious ethical reasons, however, economists are reluctant to adjust benefits on the basis of socioeconomic status. We could have conducted sensitivity analysis if we thought that the base-case values were measured with error, but this would merely have repeated what Holtgrave and Qualls had already done. Therefore, we did not conduct any analysis of the sensitivity of the results to willingness to pay per QALY.

Finally, the benefits are modestly sensitive to the discount rate, as shown by Holtgrave and Qualls. An increase in the discount rate from 5 to 6% decreases the benefits to $340,000, whereas a decrease to 4% increases the benefits to $514,000.

There are other possible benefits of avoiding HIV infection not specifically included in the measure of QALYs and direct medical care expenditures. To the extent that the prevention reduces drug abuse, crime may be reduced. Lower crime reduces the costs incurred by the criminal justice system. A prevention program may reduce the need for medical care, other than medical care for treatment of AIDS, by reducing the number of drug related illnesses and injuries. Safer sexual practices avoid sexually transmitted diseases other than

Table 5. Sensitivity Analysis[a]

Assumption	Base-Case Value	Sensitivity Value	Expected Benefits	Threshold Ratio
Benefit per HIV infection avoided	Not applicable	Not applicable	$502,798	0.19
Years of potential life lost	27	17	$353,393	0.27
QALY in healthy year	1.0	0.9	$386,039	0.25
	1.0	0.8	$328,864	0.29
Discount rate	5%	4%	$546,774	0.17
	5%	6%	$362,133	0.27

[a]All financial numbers are based on the Holtgrave and Qualls[1] model updated for inflation from 1993 to 1995 by 6.4%.

HIV, further reducing medical expenditures. Prevention may improve employment opportunities. Substance abuse harms the life of the abuser and also takes a toll on other family members. Prevention may also improve child welfare. Prevention may help to reduce depression and anxiety in drug abusers. The monetary benefits of altered mental health are difficult to measure, but improvement in mental health and self-esteem are clearly positive benefits. Ignoring these other potential benefits biases the estimate of benefits downwards. Therefore, our estimate of the benefits is probably conservative and may overestimate the number of HIV infections needed to balance the costs and the benefits of AIDS outreach and intervention.

For this study we followed the literature and ignored the dynamic aspects of HIV infection and recidivism. The dynamic interaction between persons who may infect each other is extremely complicated to model.[27] Epidemiological models that predict the effect of one person's behavioral change on the probability that another person becomes HIV infected are complex and do not necessarily lead to unique solutions. Solutions are known to simple models of infection within a homogeneous high-risk group, such as injecting drug users or homosexual men, with a known infection rate and rate of transmission. However, epidemiologists are interested in modeling the spread of HIV within groups and also between groups, because in the real world high-risk groups interact. In models with only two groups interacting, the epidemic can die out, stabilize, or infect all persons in both groups depending on the infectiousness of the disease and the rate of contact.[28] Furthermore, with three or more groups, solutions can be found only in special cases because these epidemiological models are governed by a series of differential equations.[29] Any bias caused by assuming static behavioral changes is in an unknown direction. Modeling recidivism is also beyond the scope of this study because it is a form of dynamic behavior.

CONCLUSION

This study shows that the expected benefit of avoiding one HIV infection is quite large relative to the costs of running the NC CoOp program for one year. In particular this study shows how to estimate the costs of an outreach and intervention program. We carefully excluded research costs, amortized fixed costs, considered including client's time cost, and included all other relevant costs in our calculations. We calculated that the cost of such a program is about $95,000 per year. The vast majority of costs are for labor, and about 60% of the costs go for outreach.

For benefits, we focused on avoiding HIV infection. We updated the estimates based on cost-utility analysis made by Holtgrave and Qualls[1] for inflation and added the savings from avoided medical costs. The total benefit from avoiding one HIV infection is about $503,000 in 1995 dollars. We estimated that to break even the program would need to avoid only one HIV infection every 5.3 years. Preliminary data on behavioral change during the three months following the intervention show that this goal is plausible. We plan to build on this research in the future by estimating the actual benefits from the NC CoOp program and comparing those to the costs calculated in this study.

The sensitivity analysis showed that our results are robust to changes in the major assumptions. Adjusting the values of important parameters for differences in our sample population would lower the expected benefits but not by enough to change the conclusions. The threshold ratio would still be several years per HIV infection.

Threshold analysis is an important analytic method for deciding how to spend limited government funds on public health problems. It is fairly simple to apply and can be used to test the financial feasibility of a program under a wide variety of assumptions. For the NC CoOp program, threshold analysis shows that only a few cases of HIV need to be avoided for the benefits to outweigh the costs.

ACKNOWLEDGMENTS.   The authors would like to thank David R. Holtgrave and Gary A. Zarkin for helpful comments. The interpretations and conclusions do not represent the position of NIDA or the Department of Health and Human Services. Portions of this paper were originally presented at the *NIDA AIDS Satellite Conference* in Scottsdale, Arizona, June 1995. This research was supported by NIDA Cooperative Agreement No. 1U01 DA08007.

REFERENCES

1. Holtgrave DR, Qualls NL. Threshold analysis and programs for prevention of HIV infection. *Medical Decision Making* 1995; 15:311–317.
2. Wechsberg WM, Smith FJ, Harris-Adeeyo T. AIDS education and outreach to injecting drug users and the community in public housing. *Psychol Addictive Behaviors* 1992; 6(2):107–113.
3. Zarkin GA, Hubbard RL. *Analytic Issues for Estimating the Benefits and Costs of Substance Abuse Prevention.* Working paper. Research Triangle Institute, Research Triangle Park, NC.
4. Holtgrave DR, Qualls NL, Graham JD. Economic evaluation of HIV prevention programs. *Annu Rev Public Health* 1996; 17:467–488.
5. Holtgrave DR, Valdiserri RO, Gerber AR, et al. Human immunodeficiency virus counseling, testing, referral, and partner notification services. *Arch Intern Med* 1993; 153:1225–1230.
6. Gorsky RD, MacGowan RJ, Swanson NM, et al. Prevention of HIV infection in drug abusers: A cost analysis. *Preventive Med* 1995; 24:3–8.
7. Holtgrave DR, DiFranceisco W, Reiser W, et al. Setting standards for the Wisconsin HIV counseling and testing program: An application of threshold analysis. *J Public Health Manage Prac*, forthcoming.
8. Clark HW, Corbett JM. Needle exchange programs and social policy. *J Mental Health Adm* 1993; 20(1):66–71.
9. Research Triangle Institute. *Drug Abuse Treatment Cost Analysis Program: Cost Interview Guide for Provider Sites.* Unpublished survey instrument; 1994.
10. Brown BS, Beschner GM, eds. *Handbook on Risk of AIDS.* Westport, CT: Greenwood Press; 1993.
11. Holmberg, S. Centers for Disease Control and Prevention. Personal communication with R. Martin, Research Triangle Institute. January 21, 1996.
12. Friedland GH, Harris C, Butkus-Small C, et al. Intravenous drug users and the acquired immunodeficiency syndrome: Demographics, drug users and needle sharing patterns. *Arch Intern Med* 1985; 145:1413–1417.
13. Koester SK, Hoffer L. Indirect sharing: Additional risks associated with drug injection. *AIDS Public Policy J* 1990; 3:100–105.
14. Wechsberg WM, Cavanaugh ER, Dunteman GH, et al. Changing needle practices in community outreach and methadone treatment. *Evaluation and Program Planning* 1994; 17(4):371–379.
15. Booth RE, Watters JK, Chitwood DD. HIV risk-related sex behaviors among injection drug users, crack smokers, and injection drug users who smoke crack. *Am J Public Health* 1993; 83(8):1144–1148.
16. Tortu S, Beardsley M, Deren S, et al. The risk of HIV infection in a national sample of women with injection drug-using partners. *Am J Public Health* 1995; 84(8):1243–1249.
17. Deren S, Davis WR, Beardsley M, et al. Outcomes of a risk-reduction intervention with high risk populations: The Harlem AIDS project. *AIDS Educ Prev* 1995; 7(5):379–390.
18. Hartel D. Context of HIV risk behavior among female injecting drug users and female sexual partners of injecting drug users. In *National Institute on Drug Abuse Research Monograph Series, The Context of HIV Risk Among Drug Users and Their Sexual Partners.* NIH publication no. 94-3750: 1994; pp. 41–47.
19. Wechsberg WM. Strategies for working with women substance abusers. In Brown BS, ed. *Substance Abuse Treatment in the Era of AIDS.* Rockville, MD: Center for Substance Abuse Treatment 1995; 119–152.

20. McCoy HV, Miles C. A gender comparison of health status among users of crack cocaine. *J. Psychoactive Drugs* 1992; 24:389–397.

21. Inciardi JA. HIV/AIDS risks among male, heterosexual noninjecting drug users who exchange crack for sex. In *National Institute on Drug Abuse Research Monograph Series, The Context of HIV Risk Among Drug Users and Their Sexual Partners.* NIH publication no. 94-3750, 1994; pp. 26–40.

22. Ratner MS, ed. *Crack Pipe as Pimp: An Ethnographic Investigation of Sex-for-Crack Exchanges.* New York: Lexington Books; 1993.

23. Bureau of the Census, Statistical Abstract of the United States, 115th ed. Washington, DC, 1995.

24. Rumbough R. North Carolina Department of Environment, Health, and Natural Resources. Personal communication with R. Martin, Research Triangle Institute. February 22, 1995.

25. Guinan ME, Franham PG, Holtgrave DR. Estimating the value of preventing a human immunodeficiency virus infection. *Am J Preventive Med* 1994; 10(1):1–4.

26. Hellinger FJ. The lifetime cost of treating a person with HIV. *JAMA* 1993;270(4):474–478.

27. Rowley JT, Anderson RM. Modeling the impact and cost-effectiveness of HIV prevention efforts. *AIDS* 1994; 8:539–548.

28. Hethcote HW. Qualitative analyses of communicable disease models. *Math Biosci* 1976; 28:335–356.

29. Hethcote HW, Van Ark JW. Epidemiological models for heterogeneous populations: Proportionate mixing, parameter estimation, and immunization programs. *Math Biosci* 1987; 84:85–118.

15

A Few Reflections on the Practicality of Economic Evaluation Methods and Conclusions

DAVID R. HOLTGRAVE

The third section of this book described some key challenges encountered when decision makers attempt to use economic evaluations of HIV prevention programs in their resource allocation decision making. However, solutions to some of the challenges were also offered in this book (e.g., Norton et al.'s coverage of the uses of threshold analyses[1]). Kahn and Washington have previously discussed some ways of making mathematical modeling techniques as relevant as possible to policy making situations.[2] In this final chapter, I provide a few personal reflections on ways of making economic evaluation studies and methods as practical as possible. This chapter includes many statements based on one person's experience and hence should be read with that caveat in mind.

SOME EXPERIENCES FROM THE CENTERS FOR DISEASE CONTROL AND PREVENTION (CDC)

While previously an employee at CDC, I had the opportunity to attempt to answer a number of policy makers' questions regarding CDC's HIV prevention programs. One type of question came from the Office of Management and Budget (OMB) which inquired as to the cost of these HIV prevention programs, their quantitative benefits, the cost-benefit ratio, and possible changes in the ratio if additional funding were made available. A second type of inquiry came from the Office of the Assistant Secretary for Health (OASH) who asked about the cost-benefit ratio for some new programs proposed via budget initiatives by CDC's HIV prevention program. In both cases, the quantitative answers to the questions were required in a matter of just a very few days. Other similar examples could be given.

Answering such important questions by key decision makers is a great opportunity, but answering them in very short order can give pause to an analyst striving for state-of-the-art rigor in the analyses. An academic or person working in another nongovernmental setting might hear such inquiries and feel that the time line for response would be better measured in months rather than hours or days. Still, not responding to policy makers' real questions

DAVID R. HOLTGRAVE • Department of Psychiatry and Behavioral Medicine, Center for AIDS Intervention Research (CAIR), Medical College of Wisconsin, Milwaukee, Wisconsin 53202.

Handbook of Economic Evaluation of HIV Prevention Programs, edited by Holtgrave. Plenum Press, New York, 1998.

wastes opportunities for using economic evaluation methods and findings. A careful balance must be made between relevance, timeliness, and comprehensiveness. Based on these experiences, I have developed a list of ten key "rules" for analysts to consider when they must answer policy questions rapidly. These ten guidelines follow and are meant to be general—not only relevant to the OMB and OASH questions previously mentioned.

1. Review the conditions as to when decision (and other forms of policy) analysis are meaningful (e.g., there are real options among which to choose). If the conditions are not met, no real analysis is possible (or needed).
2. Clearly understand who the key decision makers are. Focus the rapid analysis only on their decision making questions (doing other analyses wastes precious time).
3. When in doubt about parameter values, bias them against the program proposed or examined.
4. Rely heavily on threshold analytic methods.
5. Conduct sensitivity analyses heavily to truly explore the boundaries of the problem.
6. Express the results so that the base-case results are understood with the appropriate level of uncertainty/confidence. Try to couch the results in terms of the sensitivity analyses.
7. Present the results in one to two pages as an Executive Summary, but attach a technical appendix (i.e., "show your work," and keep a copy of it).
8. Even if a decision is made rapidly, work further on the analysis, and subject it to peer review (returning to and overturning the original, rapid decision if necessary).
9. Never oversell the rapid analysis. It is what it is (but that may be better than just using intuition).
10. Prepare in advance! If your job includes this kind of work, keep on hand some central literature on often needed parameters.

These rules focus on giving the policy maker a quick, relevant answer, yet they are also designed to help the decision makers to understand exactly what they are getting and how much uncertainty is in the analyses. These rules also emphasize that rapidly answering a breaking policy question is only the first step in the process. The analyses should continue even after the initial answer is given and should be subjected to full scientific peer review. Of course, this can be a frightening undertaking. The full-scale analysis and subsequent insights of peer reviewers could lead to a revision of the analyses and a different conclusion. If so, the policy maker with the original question must be informed of the new results. Several of the rules listed above were developed with an eye toward making the probability of such an unfortunate event as low as possible.

EXPERIENCE WITH HIV PREVENTION COMMUNITY PLANNING

While working at CDC previously, I was privileged to assist in developing the guidance document for HIV Prevention Community Planning in the U.S. While working at the Medical College of Wisconsin, I was extremely fortunate to be elected to membership in the Wisconsin HIV Prevention Community Planning Group. As noted in the chapters by

Weinstein et al.[4] and Kaplan,[5] in its guidance CDC included instructions that community planning groups should consider the cost-effectiveness of interventions when prioritizing them. However, groups who have attempted to include cost-effectiveness have met with challenges in terms of jargon, literature accessibility, and even literature existence.[4,5] This has prompted attempts to provide alternate ways for community planning groups to consider cost-effectiveness information in their deliberations.[4,5]

Kaplan[5] provides one excellent, alternate method for considering cost-effectiveness information. Based on my community planning experiences, I would like to suggest one even more basic qualitative step that community planning groups might consider as a form of preparation for using Kaplan's methodology. Given their diversity of experiences and expertise, community planning group members may wish to approach the topic of cost-effectiveness by simply asking themselves the following question for each HIV prevention intervention on their list for possible prioritization: Why do we want to do this intervention? Answers might include evidence from the following categories: (a) empirical effectiveness data, (b) client experience, (c) service provider experience, (d) theoretical rationale, (e) affordability, and (f) making the best use of available resources.[6] Other ways to phrase items "e" and "f" are, Can we afford this intervention in terms of available human fiscal resources? and, Is there some better way to spend this pool of resources—that is, could we do a better job of preventing HIV infection by spending the resources in some other way?[6] Qualitative discussion of these questions can help groups to begin balancing the resources consumed by interventions with their consequences. Cost-effectiveness analysis can be as much of a mode of thought as a formal, quantitative technique for policy analysis. Once this focusing begins, the stage is set for using the quantitative technique proposed by Kaplan and for the planning group to consider eventually a literature-based league table of cost-utility ratios for a variety of interventions.

EXPRESSING PREVENTION NEEDS

Recently, federal programs to fund HIV disease treatment have grown much faster than resources available for HIV prevention programs. Clearly, there are many reasons for this differential. One possible reason expressed, for instance, at a July 1997 meeting in Atlanta of the President's Advisory Committee on AIDS is that the needs for further prevention programs are not as easily quantified and expressed as those for treatment programs.

However, the situation is ripe for change. Local HIV Prevention Community Planning Groups have now completed at least one round of empirical needs assessment activities. These assessments are direct expressions of the number and type of HIV prevention services required by persons living in or passing through the locale. Now this information can be merged with the cost analytic findings available in the literature that provide the price tag for a variety of interventions.

For instance, suppose that a community planning group did a series of focus groups and a survey and found that at least 2500 women attending urban primary health care clinics in a particular, large city were at high behavioral risk of HIV infection and might well benefit from a small group, cognitive behavioral, HIV prevention intervention. We know from the literature[7] that such an intervention costs approximately $269 per client (of course, this literature-based estimate could be modified for local circumstances). One reasonable approximation of the quantitative magnitude of this particular prevention need is $672,500 (or 2500 × $269). Given recent estimates of the lifetime costs of treating HIV disease, it could easily be argued via threshold analysis that this program would have to avert only four or five HIV infections to actually be cost saving to society. Such arguments seem much more likely to persuade federal and state legislatures to allocate money for HIV prevention than simply expressing a real but imprecise need.

COMPARING SERVICES IN TERMS OF COST

In July 1997 CDC held a meeting to receive input from a large number and variety of external consultants on the issue of using postexposure prophylaxis (PEP) in nonoccupational settings. I was asked to provide some thoughts comparing behavioral, primary prevention of HIV infection to PEP.[9] I attempted to make a variety of comparisons in terms of effectiveness and cost-effectiveness. Further, I found that now it is possible to compare a number of different types of interventions in terms of their price tags. For instance, it has been estimated that the cost of PEP ranges from approximately $600 to just over $1000.[10,11] From the literature, we know that roughly $600 would buy one person participation in a five-session, cognitive-behavioral intervention ($269),[7] a two-session, small group intervention ($108, or 0.4 × $269), client-centered HIV counseling and testing ($33 to $103 depending on whether the test was HIV seronegative or seropositive),[12] and at least one condom and sterile syringe per day for a year [365 × ($0.25 + $0.17)].[13] When considering the opportunity costs of PEP, having available such cost information on other types of intervention is highly useful.

CONCLUSIONS

In this chapter, I have presented some further thoughts on simple and practical uses of economic evaluation methodologies to address real policy issues. Although it will be helpful eventually to provide decision makers in each locale a custom-tailored league table of various HIV prevention interventions, there are already many practical uses of the economic evaluation studies to date, and there are useful tools for addressing policy questions as they arise. By way of analogy, it is as if we currently have available in the economic evaluation tool chest some hammers, pliers, a good socket wrench set, and a Swiss army knife. We await the addition of the high-speed electronic lathe. Still, one can build a house with basic tools, and the economic evaluation of HIV prevention is already built on a solid foundation.

Although much remains to be done in this area, studies have already shown that HIV prevention can be a cost-saving or cost-effective use of funds, and the studies have provided a great deal of information about the affordability of various HIV prevention interventions. Some limited comparisons of HIV prevention programs to each other on the basis of cost-effectiveness are possible now. We also have a set of practical tools to answer at least some categories of new policy questions as they unfold. This is an excellent beginning for the field.

A new HIV infection occurs every 13 minutes in the United States. The epidemic continues to unfold rapidly. Decisions about how best to slow and ultimately stop HIV infection must be made quickly and have very important consequences. Our analytic work in the economic evaluation of HIV prevention interventions must proceed with dispatch and with these sobering epidemiological facts always foremost in mind.

ACKNOWLEDGMENT.   Preparation of this chapter was supported by grants R01-MH55440, R01-MH56830, and P30-MH52776 from the National Institute of Mental Health.

REFERENCES

1. Norton EC, Martin RF, Wechsberg WM. Threshold analysis of AIDS outreach and intervention. In Holtgrave DR, ed. *Handbook of Economic Evaluation of HIV Prevention Programs*, New York: Plenum; 1998.
2. Kahn JF, Washington AE. Optimizing the policy impact of HIV modeling. In Kaplan EH, Brandeau ML, eds. *Modeling the AIDS Epidemic: Planning, Policy and Prediction*. New York: Raven; 1994; pp. 217–235.
3. Holtgrave DR, Valdiserri RO, Gerber AR, Hinman AR. Human immunodeficiency virus counseling, testing, referral, and partner notification services: A cost-benefit analysis. *Arch Intern Med* 1993; 153:1225–1230.
4. Weinstein B, Melchreit RL. Economic evaluation and HIV prevention decision-making—the state perspective. In Holtgrave DR, ed. *Handbook of Economic Evaluation of HIV Prevention Programs*, New York: Plenum; 1998.
5. Kaplan EH. Economic evaluation and HIV prevention community planning—a policy analyst's perspective. In Holtgrave DR, ed. *Handbook of Economic Evaluation of HIV Prevention Programs*, New York: Plenum; 1998.
6. Holtgrave DR, Pinkerton SD. The economics of HIV primary prevention. *Current Issues in Public Health*, under review.
7. Holtgrave DR, Kelly JA. Preventing HIV/AIDS among high-risk urban women: The cost-effectiveness of a behavioral group intervention. *Am J Public Health* 1996; 86:1442–1445.
8. Holtgrave DR, Pinkerton SD. Updates of cost of illness and quality of life estimates for use in economic evaluations of HIV prevention programs. *J Acquired Immune Defic Syndr Hum Retrovirol*, in press.
9. Holtgrave DR. Behavioral HIV prevention interventions: Effective and cost-effective alternatives to post-exposure prophylaxis. Speech presented at a meeting sponsored by the Centers for Disease Control and Prevention, July 25, 1997, Atlanta GA.
10. Pinkerton SD, Holtgrave DR, Bloom FR. Is post-exposure prophylaxis for sexual or injection-associated exposure to HIV cost-effective? *N Engl J Med* (letter), in press.
11. Pinkerton SD, Holtgrave DR, Bloom FR. The cost-effectiveness of post-exposure prophylaxis in non-occupational settings, under review.
12. Farnham PG, Gorsky RD, Holtgrave DR, Jones WK, Guinan ME. Counseling and testing for HIV prevention: Costs, effects and cost-effectiveness of more rapid screening tests. *Public Health Rep* 1994; 111:44–53.
13. Holtgrave DR, Pinkerton SD, Jones TS, Lurie P, Vlahov D. Cost and cost-effectiveness of increasing access to sterile syringes and needles as an HIV prevention intervention in the U.S. *J Acquired Immune Defic Syndr Hum Retrovirol*, in press.

A Method to Measure the Costs
of Counseling for HIV Prevention

ROBIN D. GORSKY

Cost is one criterion for selecting an HIV prevention program. To have the greatest possible effect on HIV transmission for the limited funds available, it is necessary to know both the costs and effects of programs. Because most HIV prevention programs target risky behavior and many include counseling, it is important to estimate the true resource costs associated with counseling.

HIV prevention programs have only infrequently been subjected to cost analysis. Of almost 300 articles reviewed, only a small proportion included program cost information.[1] Cost is often the limiting factor in selecting HIV prevention interventions for a community. But without cost estimates, it is impossible to plan and justify budgets and expenditures. Therefore, estimating the true costs of HIV prevention programs is critical.

Counseling for HIV prevention is a component of many interventions. The purpose of counseling is varied. It can be (a) to educate clients regarding the results of an HIV antibody test; (b) to enhance the mental health of HIV-positive clients; or (c) to effect reduction of HIV risk behavior, such as unsafe sex or the use of shared drug injection paraphernalia. Regardless of the counseling goal, similar resources are used, and the determination of counseling costs is the same.

Counseling is defined broadly in this chapter as any face-to-face interaction for HIV prevention, regardless of site or situation. Counseling can take place within and outside health care facilities, during clinical care, in group sessions, in drug abuse treatment programs, and in hospitals. Counseling occurs at the worksite, in educational settings, and on the street. It may be at the convenience of the provider or of the client.

The results of HIV counseling cost analyses can be used for resource allocation among prevention programs and to provide cost estimates for cost-benefit, cost-effectiveness, and cost-utility analyses. This chapter provides a simple method to determine the true resource costs of counseling programs for HIV prevention. The results can be used for decision making and planning at program, local, state, and federal levels.

Originally published in *Public Health Reports* 1996, Vol. 111, Supp. 1, pp. 115–122.

ROBIN D. GORSKY • Late of Division of HIV-AIDS Prevention, National Center for HIV, STD, and TB Prevention, Centers for Disease Control and Prevention, Atlanta, Georgia 30333; and Department of Health Management and Policy, University of New Hampshire, Durham, New Hampshire 03824.

Handbook of Economic Evaluation of HIV Prevention Programs, edited by Holtgrave. Plenum Press, New York, 1998.

OVERVIEW OF A COST ANALYSIS

A basic cost analysis includes (a) identifying the resources used in counseling; (b) determining the unit costs of the resources used; and (c) calculating the total costs of counseling. This chapter addresses only the determination of program costs, not program effects or benefits. Economic analysis, such as cost-benefit and cost-effectiveness analysis, which use basic cost analyses, are discussed in *A Practical Guide to Prevention Effectiveness*.[2] A simple economic analysis methodology for disease and injury prevention may be found in the *Morbidity and Mortality Weekly Report (MMWR)*.[3]

The resources and unit costs included in an analysis depend on the perspective taken by the analyst. There are many possible perspectives: societal; service provider (clinic, institution, agency, or individual); business firm; health insurance company and health care reimburser; government; and program participant or client.

The societal perspective is usually taken because all resources associated with the intervention, no matter who pays, are included in the analysis. The actual costs of the resources consumed are used in this perspective, rather than charges to payers or participants, because charges may not reflect the cost to society of the resources used. This perspective is most useful for overall resource allocation decisions.

It is important to recognize that resource costs are not necessarily equal to a program budget. Program resources may include volunteer labor, donated time, and materials funded from other sources. Budgets may underestimate or overestimate the resources required, may include incorrect job categorization of service providers, and may have other factors that obscure true resource costs associated with counseling.

If resources are used in one intervention, the same resources are not available for another societal use. Thus, a particular program, when implemented, should make the best use of the limited health resources available. The focus of this cost analysis is the societal perspective because rational allocation decisions are based on true resource costs to society.

Other perspectives may not use true resource costs. From the service provider's or insurers' perspective, the cost of resources equals the cost to the provider. For example, the charges clinics pay for laboratory tests rather than the actual laboratory costs are often used because providers want to know the cost to *them* for providing a particular prevention service and how much they will be reimbursed. This is the usual managerial or accounting perspective. From the government's perspective, taxes are received and reimbursements are made to service providers. Costs reflect government-defined reimbursement rates for services or budgeted costs to agencies, bureaus, and divisions. From the participant or client's perspective, costs are those actually paid in money, goods, or time for the privilege of participation.

Steps of a Cost Analysis

A cost analysis consists of several steps, each of which will be discussed in detail. These steps include

1. Choosing a time period for the cost analysis
2. Counting the clients served during this time period
3. Inventorying the resources, in specific units, required for all activities comprising the intervention
4. Calculating the cost per unit of each resource used

5. Counting the number of units of each resource used in the time period for the number of clients served
6. Calculating the total costs of the intervention and side effects
7. Calculating the expected cost per client served

A consideration in a cost analysis is whether one is determining the average costs of providing a service or the incremental costs. Average cost is defined as the total cost of a program divided by the total units of services produced and includes a proportion of all resource costs used to produce a service. Some proportion of rent, utilities, and equipment is included in average costs, even if expansion of facilities is not required for the specific intervention. An example is including some proportion of hospital operating expenses, including facilities costs, in the average costs of hospital-based counseling. Incremental cost is defined as the additional cost required to produce an additional unit of service. Incremental costs include only costs directly associated with providing services because it is assumed that, in the short term, an additional unit of service is produced with no increase in facilities or equipment. Thus, preexisting resources, such as facilities, are not included in this type of analysis. An example is adding HIV counseling to an existing clinic without including any clinic space in the incremental costs of clinic-based counseling. This cost analysis uses an incremental cost approach.

DETERMINATION OF COUNSELING COSTS

Choosing the Time Period

The specific time period chosen for the cost analysis is important because costs occur as clients are served. The time period for the cost data collection must be contemporaneous with the time period for which client counts are available. A consideration in choosing a time period for cost data collection is whether seasonality affects either costs or client participation. One year is the ideal time period because all seasons are included. A time period less than one year may bias the result because of seasonal effects on participation and behavior. Time periods greater than one year require a decision about how to incorporate cost increases and changes in technology over time. Studies of interventions lasting longer than one year must also discount to value costs equally in future years.[2]

Counting the Clients Served

Clients of counseling programs can be counted in various ways. The most useful client count in a prevention program is the number of clients *offered* a particular intervention. Using this count allows an administrator or program planner to estimate the cost that a program faces for an estimated number of clients offered the intervention in a particular time period. The fact that some clients do not complete all the parts of a program is an important part of a cost analysis because *any* participation in any part implies some cost to the program.

There are other methods of counting clients, and each provides useful information. Counseling programs may count (a) all persons accepting counseling or (b) only persons offered, accepting, and completing counseling. The appropriate count is that which is consistent with the goal of the cost analysis.

The count becomes the denominator in calculating incremental cost per client. This cost analysis uses the count of clients offered the intervention as the unit of analysis.

Inventorying the Resources Required

Resources are defined as those inputs without which the intervention would not exist. Resources for counseling include counselors' time, materials and supplies, tests, administrative and clerical support, travel, and additional facilities and equipment.

A resource inventory table can be particularly helpful. Each specific resource is a row in the table. The units of each resource, the cost definition of a unit of resource, and the calculated cost per unit represent table columns. Each type of provider should be a separate row of the table. Each specific type of supply, material, test, and so on should also be a separate row. Each resource is used in specific units and has a unit cost. This is the starting point of a cost analysis.

Resources are of three kinds. First, there are program resources consumed on a per client or per service basis, called variable costs. Variable costs vary proportionally with the level of output (clients, services). An example is the time a counselor spends with an individual client. Second, there are program resources consumed on a program basis regardless of the number of clients (in some range, of course), called fixed costs. Fixed costs do not vary with the quantity of output in the short run. An example is a poster board that is used over and over for all clients at a particular stage of counseling or specific facilities used for counseling sessions. Third, there are resources that clients use to participate in the intervention. Examples of these are carfares, lost wages, and child-care costs.

A resource inventory, derived from the list of resources, forms the basis of the cost analysis. From this, the calculation of total and expected costs proceeds.

Calculating the Cost Per Unit of Resource and the Number of Units Used

During a particular time period, specific counts of resource units are used. By multiplying the unit cost from the resource inventory by the number of units used during the time period, the cost of each resource can be determined for the time period.

Each type of resource and the determination of its cost are discussed in the following example. An ongoing clinic-based counseling program for high-risk individuals is used to illustrate the calculations. Resource use and unit costs in the example are hypothetical. The time period chosen for the example is one week. Although this is not the ideal period for data collection, it illustrates how to adapt data from differing time periods to a consistent time period. It is assumed that a resource inventory has been constructed and that 118 clients per week participate in this program. Table 1 illustrates the resource inventory table for this example.

Variable Costs

Provider Time. Provider time can be determined by four methods: (a) direct observation of service duration; (b) random observations of provider activities (snapshots in time); (c) time diaries that providers complete; and (d) patient-flow analysis using time forms that a client carries from provider to provider. The correct sample sizes for estimating provider times can be derived from the statistical and epidemiological references cited subsequently.

Table 1. A Sample Resource Inventory Table for a Hypothetical Counseling Program for High-Risk Clients (Hypothetical Unit Costs)

Resource	Units	Cost Definition	$/Unit
Counselor time	Hours	Salary + fringe	$35,000 + 25%/year
Materials to client	Item	10 items	$2.80
Office supplies	Item	Per client	$0.75
Telephone call	Minute	Phone co. charge	$0.26
Positive test	Each	Laboratory cost	$55
Negative test	Each	Laboratory cost	$15
Facilities	Year	Rent + utilities	$22,500
Computer	Each	Cost to program	$1,900
Travel	Miles	Reimbursement	$0.28
Administration	% time	Salary + fringe	$52,375 + 23%/year
Clerical	% time	Salary + fringe	$12,500 + 15%/year

Direct observation of services is best but requires that each provider be followed by a trained observer who differentiates services from each other and notes the start and stop times of particular services. Direct observation usually requires the consent of the client. At least 25 and perhaps 100 observations may be required to obtain a confident estimate of time durations.[4] Constructing a histogram of times helps determine the number of observations needed. If the histogram has symmetry and small variation, 25 observations may be sufficient. A distribution with the mean equal to the standard deviation suggests 100 observations.

Random observation uses the analogy that the proportion of observations of a particular service equals the proportion of time spent providing a particular service. Providers are given numbers. The analyst chooses provider numbers for an observation list from a random number table. This list is used to find a provider at fixed intervals and to note the service being provided at the exact moment of observation. A beeping computer or a personal digital assistant can prompt the providers to record their activity. At least five observations of each service type must be obtained for the proportionality assumption to hold, based on the multinomial distribution.[5]

A time diaries, which allow self-observation, can be thought of as a piece of paper that represents a day. Rows represent new activities or services. Each row has a check-off list (columns) for the specific type of activity being performed, including personal time, and a large final column for comments or explanations. A pilot observation of a usual day must be completed to construct this check-off list to minimize the provider time required to complete the diary. The provider notes the start time of each activity (one activity = one row) in the first column. Because all activities are included in this continuous stream of activities, only the activity start time is needed. The start time of the next activity is the end time of the previous one. At least 25 observations of each activity are required.[5]

Patient-flow analysis requires a time form that the client carries from provider to provider, beginning with the receptionist when the patient checks in for the program. Ideally this form includes a space to note the time the client arrives at the counseling program, is seen by the first service provider, leaves the provider, sees subsequent providers, and finally leaves the counseling program. Again, at least 25 observations of each activity are required.

Provider cost is determined for each provider type by using the following equation:

Provider cost = [provider salary + fringe] × duration of service
× number of services provided in time period

For example, the hypothetical provider cost per week for group counseling is calculated as follows.

Provider cost per hour = ($35,000 per year + 25% fringe
= $43,750) ÷ (52 weeks × 37.5 hours per week
= 1950 hours per year)
= 22.44

Service time = 25 minutes
= (25 minutes ÷ 60 minutes per hour)
= 0.42 hour

Average group size = 18, and number of clients = 118,

so that there are 6.56 groups per week, on average

Provider cost in the time period of 1 week
= ($22.44 per hour) × (0.42 hours per service) × 6.56 services
= $61.83 per week

Materials, Supplies, and Laboratory Tests. To obtain information about resource use, a discussion with providers or administrators usually suffices. One can review budget and invoices in the time period chosen for the analysis and consult the providers of service(s) to determine the quantities of brochures, office supplies, tests, and other per service resources used.

Materials and supplies cost per unit of service is determined by the following equation:

Materials and supplies cost = specific resource × cost per unit
× number of units used in time period

For example, the hypothetical cost per week for materials to provide ongoing counseling for high-risk clients is calculated as follows:

- Materials handed out to clients cost $0.28 per client
- Office supplies cost $0.75 per client
- Follow-up telephone call costs $0.26 per minute for 3.5 minutes and is necessary for 1 in 5 clients.
- Laboratory test costs $55 for a positive and $15 for a negative result
- The program expects a seroprevalence rate of 10% and expects that 1 in 100 clients agrees to be tested this week.

Total cost during week of data collection
= [($0.28 + $0.75) per client × 118 clients]
+ [$0.26 per minute × 3.5 minutes × (118/5) clients requiring phone call]
+ [$55 × (10%) + $15 × (90%)] × (118/100) clients tested
= $121.54 + $21.48 + $22.42
= $165.44 per week

Fixed Costs

Facilities Costs.   Counseling requires space for the face-to-face interaction and support of that activity. The size of the room in a clinic or the work space in another facility is multiplied by the cost of that space per unit. If the facility is now open for a longer period of time, the cost associated with this additional time as a proportion of total time must be included. If counseling takes place outside of a facility, the cost of any equipment (such as a van) should be included.

The following equation is used to determine the costs of space and utilities:

Facilities costs = additional facility space × (cost of rent and utilities)

for that space or

additional facility time × (cost of rent and utilities) for that proportion
of time spent on the intervention by the program

For example, the facilities costs associated with ongoing counseling are calculated as follows:

Cost per year for rent and utilities = $22,500
Cost per week = ($22,500 ÷ 52) = $432.69

The counseling program is associated with 36% of the time the facility is open.

Program facilities costs = ($432.69 × 0.36)
= $155.77 facilities cost per week for this intervention

Equipment Costs.   Any new equipment purchased for the counseling program, such as a computer or a blood analyzer should be included as a resource. An existing piece of equipment that is used partially for the counseling program should be included on a proportional basis. A van used to transport outreach workers to the counseling sites should be included as equipment. The gasoline and maintenance are a part of the equipment cost.

The following equation is used to determine the cost of equipment associated with the counseling program:
Equipment costs = (total cost of equipment and maintenance ÷ estimated lifetime of equipment) × proportion of that lifetime used for this intervention

For example, the calculation of equipment costs is as follows:

- Cost of computer + software = $1900
- Lifetime of computer = 3 years
- Salvage value of computer = $250
- Computer cost = ($1900 − $250) ÷ 3 years = $550 per year
- Maintenance contract = $45 per month

Computer costs per week = ($550 per year ÷ 52 weeks per year
= $10.58 per week) + ($45 per month ÷ 4.3 weeks per month
= $10.47 per week)
= $21.05

Proportion of time computer used for intervention = 25%

Computer costs to counseling program = ($21.05 × 0.25)

                                    = $5.26 fixed computer costs per week for this intervention

Administrative and Support Costs.   All counseling programs require some administrative and clerical support. Someone acts as a receptionist or makes follow-up telephone
calls or types reports. Someone supervises the counselors or coordinates services. The time
of these persons in support of the counseling program must be included as costs of the
intervention.

The following equation is used to determine the cost of support associated with the
counseling program.

Administration and support costs = proportion of administrators' time spent on intervention
                            × (salary + fringe) + proportion of support staff time
                            spent on intervention × (salary + fringe)

For example, the administrative and clerical support costs associated with this intervention are calculated as follows:

Proportion of time administration and clerical support staff are involved in this intervention
    = 5% and 13%

Administration costs = ($52,375 + 23% fringe) ÷ 52
                    = $1238.87 per week × 0.05
                    = $61.94

Clerical costs = ($12,500 + 15% fringe) ÷ 52
              = $276.44 per week × 0.13
              = $35.94

Cost per week = $97.88 in fixed administrative and clerical costs per week

Other Direct Costs.   Other resources may be required to implement and operate a
counseling program, including travel to street sites, courier service for blood samples, or
charges from outside agencies to perform services that the counselors cannot do themselves.

The following equation is used to determine the cost of other resources associated with
the counseling program:

Other direct costs of providing the intervention (for example, travel, courier,
                    outside agency charges) = actual resource costs

For example, travel costs are calculated as follows:

Cost of travel = 217 miles per week at a cost of $0.28 per mile
              = $60.76 in travel costs per week

Participant Costs

Costs to the participant are important from a societal perspective. Time and money
spent by clients to participate in counseling are time and money unavailable for other
purposes. This cost may be why some clients do not participate in all activities of an HIV
prevention program.

Expense information can be obtained from a survey of the participants. Questions should include

1. How far did you travel (miles)?
2. From where did you travel (home, work, other location)?
3. What time did you leave there, arrive at the clinic, leave the clinic?
4. What expenses did you incur to travel to the clinic?

In addition, one must decide on the salary to use for participant time. One can use either the median salary by occupation or for the region, as listed by the Bureau of Labor Statistics, or the actual salary of participants, if this can be obtained.

The participant costs can be calculated from the following equation:

Participation costs = (Sum of the time that participants spend traveling, waiting, and participating in the service × median salary) + (Sum of the expenses participants accrue for participation)

For example, the clients' costs to participate in this counseling program are calculated as follows:

• Participant time spent in travel, waiting, and service = 115 minutes
• Average participant expenses = $2.59 per client for travel or mileage

Participant costs = (115 mins = 1.92 hours) × $15 per hour median regional wage
= $28.80 time cost + $2.59 for expenses
= $31.39 per participant

Total costs associated with participation
= $31.39 × 118 participants per week
= $3704.02 in participant costs per week

Intervention Side Effects

Almost all prevention interventions can have unintended consequences as a function of participation. Resource costs associated with side effects (consequences) must be considered part of the prevention program costs. These are anticipated costs over time. A hypothetical example follows:

For every 500 persons provided this counseling program for high-risk individuals, one person needs immediate medical attention. The time for the counselor to refer the patient is approximately 35 minutes, and the phone call costs are approximately $1.24. Thus, the total cost of one referral is ($22.44 per hour × 0.58 hours) + $1.24 = $14.26.

In 118 services per week, one would expect fewer than one side effect event. The expected number of side effect events = (118/500) = 0.236 persons with a side effect. Then the expected cost per week for side effects is $3.36.

This cost, $3.36, is a legitimate part of the weekly cost of the intervention because it is paid by the agency, institution, or program.

Calculating the Total and Expected Cost of the Intervention

Once each individual resource and its unit cost are calculated for the time period in question, the total cost of the intervention can be calculated. One presumes that the number of clients served by each part of the intervention has been determined in the resource costing and that the number of clients offered services has been defined as the process measure of clients served.

The calculation of total and expected costs involves the following three steps:

1. Multiply the cost per unit by the number of units used for each resource in the time period, as discussed previously.
2. Add the resource costs for the time period, the participant costs for the time period, and any costs for side effects associated with intervention. This sum equals the total costs associated with the intervention.
3. Divide total costs by the count of clients offered the intervention to determine the expected cost per client offered the intervention.

Continuing the previous example, the calculation of total and expected costs per week for ongoing counseling of high-risk individuals is illustrated in Table 2, based on the calculation table. The total cost per week is $4,254.30, the sum of all resource costs. Dividing this total by the number of clients offered counseling (118), the expected cost per client offered counseling is $36.05 per week.

To estimate the cost to provide this counseling program to 350 participants:

Expected program cost = unit cost of intervention × estimated number of intervention units
= $36.05 × 350 = $12,619

This is correct only *if* there are no changes in fixed costs associated with this number of clients.

DISCUSSION

This paper provides a method for calculating the cost of counseling for HIV prevention. This method can be adapted to estimate the cost of any public health intervention because the basic units of costs and the calculation methods are the same. Public health interventions use similar resources: providers of services (labor); materials; supplies; facilities; utilities; equipment; program support; and other resources.

The strengths of this method for cost analysis are that it (a) provides a systematic approach to estimating the cost of an intervention; (b) standardizes the components of cost; (c) presents tables which simplify calculations; and (d) produces a consistent calculation that is generally accepted. This method of estimating program costs should be particularly useful to nonspecialists in cost analysis for calculating their true program resource costs. Then these costs can be used in conjunction with outcome data to determine the cost of the intervention per unit of behavioral change. This analysis can assist decision makers in allocating resources and funds among prevention programs.

For effective behaviorally based interventions, it is as important to know *how much it costs* as it is to know *what works*. According to Holtgrave[6], one must consider which specific HIV prevention programs have a favorable impact on behavioral outcomes and whether the financial costs of these favorable programs balance the economic benefits. This information allows determining the optimal allocation of HIV prevention funds among specific programs and subpopulations with respect to the greatest number of HIV infections averted.

Table 2. A Sample Calculation Table for a Hypothetical
Counseling Program for High-Risk Clients[a]

Resource (A)	$/Unit (B)	No. Units Used (C)	Resource Cost (D) = (B) × (C)
Provider time	$22.44/hour	0.42 hr × 6.56	$61.81
Materials, supplies	$1.03/client	118 clients	$121.54
Phone calls	$0.91/client	23.6 clients	$21.48
Laboratory tests	$19/test	1.18 tested	$22.42
Facilities	$432.69/week	36% time	$155.77
Computer	$21.05/week	25% time	$5.26
Adminstration	$1,238.87/week	5% time	$61.94
Clerical	$276.44/week	13% time	$35.94
Travel	28¢/mile	217 miles	$60.76
Participation	$13.39/client	118	$3704.02
Side effects	$14.26	0.236	$3.36
Total cost per week			$4,254.30
Expected cost per participant (total cost ÷ 118 participants)			$36.05

[a]Costs per week (hypothetical unit costs from Table 1).

As programs are compared with respect to cost, it is important to compare expected costs per participant rather than total program costs. The size of a program, that is, the number of participants served, is related to total cost. A less expensive program may not necessarily be a better program to fund because it may reach fewer clients.

Cost analyses to determine true resource costs form the basis for realistic decision making and planning in public health. The societal perspective allows determining the true resource costs for an intervention. The method presented here, which minimizes the burden of data collection and calculations, should be useful for program analysts and decision makers at all levels of government.

SUGGESTED READINGS

Borus MEJ, Buntz CG, Tash WR. *Evaluating the Impact of Health Programs: A Primer*. Cambridge, MA: MIT Press; 1982.

Centers for Disease Control: A framework for assessing the effectiveness of disease and injury prevention. *MMWR* 1992; 41 (RR-3):i–iv, 1–12.

Centers for Disease Control and Prevention. A practical guide to prevention effectiveness: decision and economic analysis. Atlanta, GA: U.S. Department of Health and Human Services; 1994.

Cohen DR, Henderson JB. *Health, Prevention and Economics*. Oxford, England: Oxford University Press; 1988.

Drummond, MF, Stoddart GL, Torrance GW. *Methods for the Economic Evaluation of Health Care Programmes*. New York: Oxford University Press; 1987.

Finkler SA: The distinction between cost and charges. *Ann Intern Med* 1982; 96:102–109.

Gorsky RD, Teutsch SM. Assessing the effectiveness of disease and injury prevention programs: Costs and consequences. *MMWR*, in press.

Gramlich EM. *A Guide to Benefit-Cost Analysis*, 2nd ed. Englewood Cliffs, NJ: Prentice-Hall; 1990.

Keeler EB, Cretin S. Discounting of life-saving and other nonmonetary effects. *Manage Sci* 1983; 29(3):300–306.

Luce BR, and Elixhauser A. *Standards for Socioeconomic Evaluation of Health Care Products and Services*. New York: Springer-Verlag; 1990.

Moreau W, Hager CJ. A guide for estimating the cost of services funded by the Ryan White Care Act of 1990.

Washington, DC: U.S. Department of Health and Human Services, Health Resources and Services Administration; 1994.

Petitti DB.: *Meta-Analysis, Decision Analysis, and Cost-Effectiveness Analysis: Methods for Quantitative Synthesis in Medicine*. New York: Oxford University Press; 1994.

Russell LB. *Is Prevention Better Than Cure?* Washington, DC: The Brookings Institution; 1986.

Shepard DS, Thompson MS. First principles of cost-effectiveness analysis. *Public Health Rep* 1979; 94(6): 535–543.

Sugden R, Williams A. *The Principles of Practical Cost-Benefit Analysis*. Oxford, England: Oxford University Press; 1978.

Warner KE. Issues in cost effectiveness in health care. *J Public Health Dentistry* 1989; 49(5):272–278.

Warner KE, Luce BR. *Cost-Benefit and Cost-Effectiveness in Health Care*. Ann Arbor, MI: Health Administration Press, 1982.

Weinstein MC, Stason WB. Foundations of cost-effectiveness analysis for health and medical practices. *N Engl J Med* 1977; 236(13):716–721.

Weinstein MC.: Challenges for cost-effectiveness research. *Medical Decision Making* 1986; 6(4):194–198.

REFERENCES

1. Holtgrave DR, Valdiserri RO, West GA. Quantitative economic evaluations of HIV-related prevention and treatment services: A review. *Risk: Health, Safety, and Environment* 1994; 5:29–47.

2. Centers for Disease Control and Prevention. *A Practical Guide to Prevention Effectiveness*: *Decision and Economic Analysis*. Atlanta, GA: U.S. Department of Health and Human Services, 1994.

3. Gorsky RD, Teutsch SM. Assessing the effectiveness of disease and injury prevention programs: costs and consequences. *MMWR*, in press.

4. Selvin S. *Statistical Analysis of Epidemiologic Data*. New York: Oxford University Press, 1991.

5. Hays WL, Winkler RL. *Statistics*: *Probability, Inference, and Decision*. New York: Holt, Rinehart and Winston; 1971.

6. Holtgrave, DR, et al.: An overview of the effectiveness and efficiency of HIV prevention programs. *Public Health Rep* 1995; 110:134–146.

Updates of Cost of Illness and Quality of Life Estimates for Use in Economic Evaluations of HIV Prevention Programs

DAVID R. HOLTGRAVE and STEVEN D. PINKERTON

The development of new generations of antiretroviral drugs, including protease inhibitors and nonnucleoside reverse transcriptase inhibitors; combination drug therapies; and improved techniques for monitoring disease progression and therapeutic effectiveness have radically altered how HIV disease is perceived. Despite their promise to prolong survival and improve the quality of life of persons with HIV, the new therapeutic regimens are also much more costly than their predecessors. Moreover, as people live longer, they consume greater health care resources, driving the overall health-care costs associated with HIV infection even higher. Resources to fund HIV prevention programs are limited and must be used wisely to maximize their prevention potential.[1] Cost-effectiveness analysis (CEA) and related methods of economic evaluation can be used to help decision makers allocate available HIV prevention funds prudently.[2,3]

The U.S. Public Health Service Panel on Cost-Effectiveness in Health and Medicine issued guidelines for the conduct of economic evaluation studies in which they recommended cost-utility analysis (CUA) as the standard methodology for economic evaluation.[4] The U.S. Centers for Disease Control and Prevention (CDC) defines CUA as: "A type of cost-effectiveness analysis in which benefits are expressed as the number of life years saved adjusted to account for loss of quality from morbidity of the health outcome or side effects from the intervention.[2,p.145]

The most common outcome measure employed in CUA is the number of quality-adjusted life years (QALYs) saved by the health services program under consideration. One QALY equals one year at full health (e.g., two years of survival at a half-diminished quality of life equals QALY). In general, the number of QALYs remaining in a person's life from any given year of life ($i = 1$) until death ($i = I$) is obtained by summing $y_i \, q_i$, where y_i equals

Reprinted with permission from *Journal of Acquired Immune Deficiency Syndromes and Human Retrovirology* 1997, Vol. 16, no. 1, pp. 54–62.

DAVID R. HOLTGRAVE and STEVEN D. PINKERTON • Department of Psychiatry and Behavioral Medicine, Center for AIDS Intervention Research (CAIR), Medical College of Wisconsin, Milwaukee, Wisconsin 53202.

Handbook of Economic Evaluation of HIV Prevention Programs, edited by Holtgrave. Plenum Press, New York, 1998.

unity for each year that the person is alive and q_i is the person's perceived health-related quality of life for that year. One of the principal advantages to the use of QALYs saved by an intervention is that they provide a disease-independent measure of programmatic effectiveness, unlike, for example, the number of HIV infections averted or cases of tuberculosis prevented.

The results of a CUA are typically expressed as a cost-utility ratio that compares the cost per QALY saved of two health service programs.[2,4,5] As a *simplified* example, suppose a decision maker wishes to compare a policy of funding a new HIV testing and counseling program to a "do nothing" option in which the program is left unfunded. The simplified cost-utility ratio would take the form

$$\text{Cost-utility ratio} = \frac{C - AT}{AQ} \tag{1}$$

where C is the cost of the counseling and testing program relative to the do-nothing option, A is the number of HIV infections averted by the program, T is the present value of the medical costs of care and treatment saved by averting an HIV infection, and Q is the number of quality-adjusted life years (QALYs) saved by preventing an infection.

The Panel on Cost-Effectiveness in Health and Medicine recommends that common methods be used across CUA studies to ensure maximum comparability.[4] When applied to a specific illness area, such as HIV prevention, this generic recommendation can be taken a step further. Comparability would clearly be enhanced if all economic evaluations studies of HIV prevention programs used common values of T and Q, at least in referent cases. However, a recent review of the economic evaluation literature on HIV prevention found little evidence of cross-study standardization of analytic methods.[1] This is unfortunate because methodological choices made by the various research teams may limit the comparability of studies across types of HIV prevention programs. If this comparability is limited, so too is the potential for economic evaluation studies to inform public health decision makers responsible for allocating fiscal resources. If methodological choices and certain common parameter values (such as those for T and Q) are employed across studies, the entire literature on HIV-related economic evaluations becomes more useful.

Although carefully estimated T and Q values have been reported in the literature previously,[6,7] they need to be updated to reflect recent, important scientific developments in antiretroviral therapy and the greatly increased costs associated with these breakthrough therapies. A recent panel of clinical investigators convened by the International AIDS Society-U.S.A. (IAS) recommended combination drug therapy with two or more antiretroviral agents for most HIV-infected patients.[8] The recommended treatment regimens (especially those that incorporate one or more protease inhibitors) have dramatically changed the costs of treating HIV disease, and have improved the projected survival of people living with HIV infection.[8–15] As a result, previous characterizations of the course of HIV disease may no longer be valid. As assumptions about disease progression change, so must calculations of the QALYs saved when HIV infections are prevented because these calculations depend on the course of disease progression and its impact on quality of life. Moreover, the empirical literature on measurements of HIV-infected persons' perceptions of their quality of life also has expanded.

In this chapter, first we describe previously published estimates of T and Q then review the literature relevant to the task of updating these estimates. We also compare the available information for calculating Q with the ideal information to meet all recommendations of the Panel on Cost-Effectiveness in Health and Medicine. Several scenarios of HIV disease progression and treatment-related costs are constructed that incorporate explicit assumptions about the impact of protease inhibitors and other promising therapies. Estimates of T and Q for persons undergoing treatment in the United States are calculated for each of these scenarios. This range of estimates provides updated T and Q values appropriate for use in economic evaluations of HIV prevention programs. We also propose a single, paired estimate of T and Q for use as a reference case in all economic evaluation studies of HIV prevention programs. Such standardization in referent case analyses would substantially increase the comparability of important, policy-relevant economic evaluation studies. However, we also emphasize the limitations of the available information to calculate T and Q and the need for further research in these areas.

METHODS

Previous Estimates of Cost of Illness and Quality of Life

Guinan et al. previously estimated the discounted, present value of the cost of medical care and treatment services saved each time an HIV infection is prevented.[6] They assumed that the length of time from HIV infection to death was 12 years. This 12-year survival period was divided into four phases: (a) six years of being unaware of one's HIV-seropositive status; (b) three years of being aware of one's HIV seropositivity with a CD4 cell count of between 200 and 499; (c) one year of AIDS as defined by a CD4 cell count of less than 200; and (d) two years of AIDS as defined by clinical conditions, such as opportunistic infections. In calculating overall costs, Guinan et al. used Hellinger's empirically derived cost of illness estimates[16]—which were based on the AIDS Cost and Service Utilization Survey—for each year that a person is aware of the infection. The total, undiscounted cost of HIV-related illness was $93,696 (in 1992 dollars). Discounting the cost of illness for each year into present value using a 5% discount rate reduces this estimated to $55,640 (also in 1992 dollars).

The number of discounted QALYs saved each time an HIV infection is prevented has also been estimated previously.[7] Holtgrave and Qualls used the survival and disease progression framework employed by Guinan et al. with the additional assumption that the average age at time of HIV infection is 26 years old. Their review of the literature available then on HIV-infected persons' quality of life led to the following estimates for quality of life in each disease stage: (a) full health for persons unaware of their HIV infection; (b) 0.9 of full health for persons aware of their HIV infection with CD4 cells counts of between 200 and 499 (based on one prior, expert judgment study); (c) 0.65 of full health for persons with AIDS, as defined by a CD4 cell count of under 200 (based on three prior, empirical studies with AIDS patients); and (d) 0.40 of full health for persons with AIDS, as defined by clinical conditions (based on four prior, empirical studies with AIDS patients including one international study). Assuming that non-HIV infected individuals enjoy full health, then the average number of undiscounted QALYs saved (before age 65) is 28.85 for each infection averted. When discounted at a 5% rate, this figure is reduced to 9.26 QALYs saved: it is standard practice in economic evaluation to discount health benefits at the same rate as monetary costs.

Holtgrave and Qualls[7] cited three reasons for truncating their analysis at age 65: the number of years of potential life lost before age 65 is a very common measure used in public health research. Given that HIV infection occurs largely among young persons (on average, at age 26 in the United States), *discounted* QALYs saved after age 65 have a very small effect on estimates of QALYs saved by preventing HIV infection. Based on 1991 lifetables, life expectancy at birth would be approximately 69.9 to 71.1 years if adjusted for gender and race/ethnicity matched to demographic characteristics of cumulative AIDS case statistics, and this figure would be lower if it appropriate levels of adjustment were known to account for the detrimental health effects of HIV-related risk behavior, such as injection drug use.

Reasons for Updating *T* and *Q* Parameters

The previously published estimates of *T* and *Q* need to be updated for several reasons. The primary reason is that new drug therapies have dramatically changed assumptions about the course of illness for persons living with HIV infection.[8–15] These promising drugs, however, are also expensive.[14] Combination therapies with two or more antiretroviral agents and especially those that include one or more protease inhibitor can reduce plasma viral load by as much as to several log units.[10,11] Several studies have demonstrated that viral load reductions of one or more log units are associated with significant clinical benefit. Furthermore, it is believed that early treatment with effective antiretroviral regimens can lower the "set point" at which viral levels stabilize after the brief period of primary infection. Additional research has established that this steady state viral load is predicted of long-term clinical outcomes, including time to AIDS.[8,13]

Several different combinations of currently available antiretroviral drugs decrease plasma viral titers below the level of detection. At these low levels of infection, the rate of HIV genetic mutation is slowed, which delays possible development of drug-resistant viral subtypes. Moreover, combination therapy multiplies the number of genetic sites at which HIV must mutate to remain viable, further slowing viral evolution toward resistance.[10,11] Thus, although long-term effects of combination antiretroviral therapy remain uncertain, there is substantial basis for optimism. Besides possible side effects, the most significant downside to these promising therapies is the high cost of the new drugs, which will likely limit their availability to some persons in developed countries, at least for the near future.[11]

Another reason for updating *T* and *Q* estimates is to comply with the recent recommendation of the U.S. Public Health Service's Panel on Cost-Effectiveness in Health and Medicine that all economic evaluation studies employ a 3% discount rate in base-case analysis.[4] (They also recommended performing analyses at 0% and 5% rates as primary comparison cases.) Previous estimates of *T* and *Q* were based on a 5% rate, which results in smaller estimated values. Because HIV disease progresses over more than a decade, the selection of a discount rate value substantially affects derived estimates of *T* and *Q*.

The quality-of-life literature relevant to HIV disease has expanded with the implementation of new therapies. Because the empirical basis for quality-of-life estimates (on which calculations of *Q* rely) has grown, that figure too should be updated now. It should be noted clearly that the Panel on Cost-Effectiveness in Health and Medicine[4] has recommended that quality weights should be empirically measured via a representative sample of the national population. Hence, most respondents would be expressing preferences for health states that (by and large) they have not experienced. As subsequently discussed, no such studies have yet been accomplished. Therefore, our review of the HIV-related quality-of-life literature focused on finding the closest approximations to the Panel's ideal standard for measuring quality weights.

Scenario Analysis

The reasons elucidated above for updating T and Q are interrelated. Hence, we have constructed three different scenarios, each of which is a plausible interpretation of the state of the field regarding HIV treatment and quality of life. The three scenarios are labeled "low-cost," "intermediate-cost," and "high-cost." All costs throughout are expressed in June 1996 dollars.[17]

Table 1 displays the definitions of the disease phases employed in the analyses. Phases 2 through 4 are self-explanatory, but phase 1 is slightly more complicated. For phase 1, there are four different subphases ("A" through "D"), which range from being unaware of one's HIV seropositivity to being aware and receiving viral load monitoring and varying levels of drug treatment. In the three scenarios described later, some of the subphases of phase 1 may be skipped.

Table 2 displays quality-of-life estimates from several empirical studies.[18–23] Because quality-of-life adjustments should be preference-based,[4] we included only empirical studies that purported to measure the perceived value of HIV-related health states (as opposed to studies measuring the health states as such). We focused on studies done in the United States so as not to mix results from patients in different "national" systems of health care. We searched for studies whose results could be matched to one of the disease phases listed in Table 1. In many cases the authors of the original studies labeled disease stages somewhat differently from the scheme outlined in Table 1. However, CD4 cell count levels were used as a matching criterion whenever possible. If a study presented both baseline and follow-up assessments of patients' quality-of-life perceptions, only the follow-up assessment was used. If a study had more than one estimate of the quality of life of a disease phase (using the same assessment methodology), we averaged the two figures.

HIV-infected patients formed the study population of almost all the identified studies. The one exception surveyed physicians as proxies for patients.[23] We included this physician proxy survey because it could be considered the one study that comes closest to the Panel on Cost-Effectiveness in Health and Medicine's recommendation that quality adjustments should be made on the basis of communitywide surveys of persons *not* necessarily living with the particular disease in question.[4] None of the studies met the Panel's recommendation.

Because the studies used varying methodologies to assess quality of life and included different numbers of subjects, we chose the median of the estimates within each disease phase as a summary statistic to minimize the impact of outliers. In this case, an outlier figure

Table 1.   Disease Phases and Definitions

Disease Phase Label	Definition
Phase 1A	HIV infected; unaware of serostatus
Phase 1B	HIV infected; aware of serostatus; receiving viral load monitoring but no treatment
Phase 1C	HIV infected; aware of serostatus; receiving two-drug therapy and viral load monitoring
Phase 1D	HIV infected; aware of serostatus; receiving three-drug therapy and viral load monitoring
Phase 2	HIV infected; aware of serostatus; CD4 cell count between 200 and 499[a]
Phase 3	HIV infected; aware of serostatus; AIDS as defined by CD4 cell count less than 200[a]
Phase 4	HIV infected; aware of serostatus; AIDS as defined by clinical condition (not just by CD4 cell count)[a]

[a]The level of drug treatment and viral load monitoring varies under the three scenarios, as displayed in Tables 3, 4, and 5.

Table 2. Summary of Empirical, Quality-of-Life Studies

Source	Method	Phase 2	Phase 3	Phase 4
Tsevat et al.[18]	Rating scale	0.71	0.71	0.63
	Quality-of-well-being scale	0.72	0.65	0.62
	Time trade-off	0.88	0.74	0.80
	(sample size)	(41)	(34)	(46)
Wu et al.[19]	Quality-of-well-being scale	n/a	n/a	0.60
	(sample size)			(15)
Revicki et al.[20]	Standard gamble	0.81	n/a	0.80
	Rating scale	0.81	n/a	0.74
	(sample size)	(89)		(71)
Wu et al.[21]	Medical Outcomes Study—HIV	0.76	0.67	n/a
	(sample size)	(73)	(44)	
Schag et al.[22]	Medical Outcomes Study—HIV	0.68	0.55	0.57
	Rating scale	0.62	0.49	0.42
	(sample size)	(119)	(65)	(78)
Owens et al.[23]	Physician proxy survey	0.83	0.42	0.17
	(sample size)	(128)	(128)	(128)
Median		0.76	0.65	0.62
Mean		0.76	0.60	0.59

might reflect particular methodological choices of the researchers. The resulting quality-of-life estimates for phases 2, 3, and 4 are 0.76, 0.65, and 0.62, respectively. For an overview of the HIV-related health status and quality of life measurement studies that include but are not limited to those meeting our inclusion criteria, see the work of Holzemer and Wilson.[24] This review and the original articles cited in Table 2, are important sources for psychometric information on the various quality-of-life measures.

Persons living with HIV and AIDS perceive that disease Phases 3 and 4 are approximately equal (0.65 vs 0.62, respectively). This may result from methodological issues of assessments or from patients learning to cope with HIV disease and using these coping strategies to improve or maintain their quality of life even as health problems mount. This finding from the growing literature on the quality of life of persons living with HIV and AIDS is counter to the a priori assumption that quality of life must markedly diminish as disease progresses substantially. If a communitywide survey were done (according to the recommendations of the Panel on Cost-Effectiveness in Health and Medicine), the results might be quite different.

There is very little empiric guidance in the literature on quality-of-life values for phases 1A through 1D. Therefore we assumed that the quality of life in phase 1A is 0.94, in accordance with published estimates of the quality of life of the U.S. population at large, as determined through empirical study.[25] Then we imposed the condition that the difference in the quality of life between phases 1C and 1B should be larger than the difference between phases 1B and 1A (and similarly for phases 2, 1D, 1C and 1B). As disease progresses and additional treatments are imposed (with possibly toxic side effects), quality of life diminishes at an accelerating rate. Although one could argue that monitoring or treatment should prolong survival or enhance quality of life, we have instead assumed that the initiation of treatment marks a decline in overall health and quality of life. The quality-of-life figures of 0.91, 0.87, and 0.82 for phases 1B, 1C, and 1D, respectively, satisfy the assumption previously described. However, we emphasize that these estimates are largely arbitrary.

Low-Cost Scenario

The low-cost scenario is displayed in Table 3. This scenario may be thought of as describing the cost of illness for someone with a very low level of access to current HIV disease treatments. In this scenario, the assumptions on disease progression are exactly those made by Guinan et al. and Holtgrave and Qualls in deriving previous estimates of T and Q values.[6,7] In particular, the scenario assumes that the person is unaware of HIV seropositivity until phase 2 commences. Thereafter, only zidovudine (ZDV) monotherapy is accessed. No viral load monitoring is available.

The costs for HIV disease other than ZDV monotherapy are taken from two sources. The first source is the work of Hellinger (which was based on patients' actual experiences incurring HIV-related costs),[16] and the second source is the work of Gable et al. which was based on expert judgments about the implementation of various protocols for treating HIV disease.[26] The quality-of-life estimates for each disease phase are also displayed in Table 3. This scenario describes a person who receives care and treatment below currently accepted standards and perhaps reflects the experience of someone who has very low access to current state-of-the-art treatment.

Intermediate-Cost Scenario

The intermediate-cost scenario (Table 4), which we consider the base case analysis, reflects current recommendations for the treatment of HIV disease as closely as possible.[8] Still, there is uncertainty in a number of the assumptions made, and we recognize that individual patients' experiences will differ from our illustration of an "average" patient. In this scenario, the time in which patients are unaware of their seropositivity is substantially decreased relative to the low-cost scenario. As more and more persons learn of the

Table 3. Cost-of-Illness Scenario: Low-Cost

Phase	Year	Non-Drug Cost[16]	Non-Drug Cost[26]	Drug Cost	Viral Load Monitoring	Quality of Life
1A	1	n/a	n/a	n/a	n/a	0.94
	2	n/a	n/a	n/a	n/a	0.94
	3	n/a	n/a	n/a	n/a	0.94
	4	n/a	n/a	n/a	n/a	0.94
	5	n/a	n/a	n/a	n/a	0.94
	6	n/a	n/a	n/a	n/a	0.94
2	7	$4,760	$1,981	$3,348	n/a	0.76
	8	$4,760	$1,981	$3,348	n/a	0.76
	9	$4,760	$1,981	$3,348	n/a	0.76
3	10	$12,654	$5,520	$3,348	n/a	0.65
4	11	$35,935	$22,900	$3,348	n/a	0.62
	12	$35,935	$22,900	$3,348	n/a	0.62

Table 4.   Cost-of-Illness Scenario: Intermediate-Cost

Phase	Year	Non-Drug Cost[16]	Non-Drug Cost[26]	Drug Cost	Viral Load Monitoring	Quality of Life
1A	1	n/a	n/a	n/a	n/a	0.94
	2	n/a	n/a	n/a	n/a	0.94
1B	3	$3,092	$1,106	n/a	$175	0.91
1C	4	$3,092	$1,106	$6,036	$175	0.87
	5	$3,092	$1,106	$6,036	$175	0.87
	6	$3,092	$1,106	$6,036	$175	0.87
1D	7	$3,092	$1,106	$12,900	$175	0.82
	8	$3,092	$1,106	$12,900	$175	0.82
	9	$3,092	$1,106	$12,900	$175	0.82
2	10	$4,760	$1,981	$12,900	$175	0.76
	11	$4,760	$1,981	$12,900	$175	0.76
	12	$4,760	$1,981	$12,900	$175	0.76
	13	$4,760	$1,981	$12,900	$175	0.76
3	14	$12,654	$5,520	$12,900	$175	0.65
4	15	$35,935	$22,900	$12,900	$175	0.62
	16	$35,935	$22,900	$12,900	$175	0.62

availability of promising new treatments, we believe that there will be a greater impetus to test individuals earlier in the course of illness.

Consistent with IAS recommendations,[8] we assume that the typical patient progresses through periods of viral load monitoring only; two-drug combination therapy; and three-drug combination therapy. The cost of a viral load test has been estimated at between $71 and $100 U.S.[14,27] Assuming approximately two tests per year, we estimate the annual cost of viral load monitoring at $175 U.S. in this scenario.

For two-drug combination therapy, we assume that the patient receives ZDV and lamivudine (2'-deoxy-3'-thiacytidene [3TC]), in accordance with IAS recommendations. Three-drug therapy adds a protease inhibitor to this regimen. Standard dosing schedules and drug costs (to pharmacists) were obtained from a published source.[12] Saquinavir was selected to represent the class of protease inhibitors because of its intermediate cost (i.e., greater than indinavir and less than retonavir).[12] We assumed that after treatment with a drug was initiated, the drug would not be withdrawn, or, if withdrawn, that another drug of equal cost would be substituted. This yielded a $12,900 U.S. estimate of the annual cost of three-drug therapy. A review of combination therapies[14] estimated that the monthly cost of three-drug therapy ranges from $904 to $1201 U.S. Taking the midpoint of this range and multiplying by twelve months yields an annual estimate of $12,630 U.S. (a figure quite close to our estimate).

The impact of these expanded treatments on survival and disease progression can only be estimated at this point. However, as reviewed previously, there is substantial reason for optimism that combination therapy can extend average survival and prolong the early relatively disease-free phases of HIV infection. The key to this optimism is the pronounced reduction in viral load evident in many patients receiving these therapies.[8] Because increased viral load is associated with immune system deterioration and more rapid progression to AIDS, it is believed that durable suppression of viral levels is crucial for enhanced clinical outcomes. After immune function has significantly deteriorated, however, the benefit of the new therapeutics is likely to be attenuated. We have assumed that phase 1B would last for one year, phase 1C for three years, and phase 1D for three years. The total of all phase 1 subphases is nine years in this scenario, as opposed to the six year duration assumed by Guinan et al.[6] (also compare the low-cost scenario). The length of time spent in phase 2 is increased from three years (as in the low-cost scenario) to four years. Thus, the intermediate-cost scenario expands overall survival from 12 years to 16 years. We are aware of the high level of uncertainty in the survival estimate in this scenario.

High-Cost Scenario

The high-cost scenario describes the possible experiences of an HIV-infected person who has very high levels of access to health-care services (Table 5). This scenario also makes the most optimistic assumptions about the effects of new drug therapies on survival.

This scenario assumes almost instant awareness of HIV seropositivity and continuous access to viral load monitoring services. It also assumes that three-drug therapy is initiated in phase 1D and extends through phase 4, consequently doubling the average duration of phases 1 and 2 (to 12 and 6 years, respectively). The total duration of post-HIV survival in this scenario is 21 years.

RESULTS

The results of the scenario analysis are displayed in Table 6. Results are shown for each of the three scenarios, for each of the two different sources of nondrug costs

Table 5. Cost-of-Illness Scenario: High-Cost

Phase	Year	Non-Drug Cost[16]	Non-Drug Cost[26]	Drug Cost	Viral Load Monitoring	Quality of Life
1D	1	$3,092	$1,106	$12,900	$175	0.82
	2	$3,092	$1,106	$12,900	$175	0.82
	3	$3,092	$1,106	$12,900	$175	0.82
	4	$3,092	$1,106	$12,900	$175	0.82
	5	$3,092	$1,106	$12,900	$175	0.82
	6	$3,092	$1,106	$12,900	$175	0.82
	7	$3,092	$1,106	$12,900	$175	0.82
	8	$3,092	$1,106	$12,900	$175	0.82
	9	$3,092	$1,106	$12,900	$175	0.82
	10	$3,092	$1,106	$12,900	$175	0.82
	11	$3,092	$1,106	$12,900	$175	0.82
	12	$3,092	$1,106	$12,900	$175	0.82
2	13	$4,760	$1,981	$12,900	$175	0.76
	14	$4,760	$1,981	$12,900	$175	0.76
	15	$4,760	$1,981	$12,900	$175	0.76
	16	$4,760	$1,981	$12,900	$175	0.76
	17	$4,760	$1,981	$12,900	$175	0.76
	18	$4,760	$1,981	$12,900	$175	0.76
3	19	$12,654	$5,520	$12,900	$175	0.65
4	20	$35,935	$22,900	$12,900	$175	0.62
	21	$35,935	$22,900	$12,900	$175	0.62

Table 6.   Major Results: Cost of Illness Averted
and Quality-Adjusted Life Years Saved with One HIV Infection Averted

Scenario	Non-Drug Cost Source	Cost of Illness Averted and (Quality-Adjusted Life Years Saved)		
		Discount Rate		
		0%	3%	5%
Low-cost	Hellinger[16]	$118,892 (26.85)	$87,045 (13.18)	$71,143 (8.57)
	Gable et al.[26]	$77,351 (26.85)	$56,595 (13.18)	$46,236 (8.57)
Intermediate-cost	Hellinger[16]	$274,766 (23.87)	$195,188 (11.23)	$157,348 (7.10)
	Gable et al.[26]	$216,544 (23.87)	$154,402 (11.23)	$124,728 (7.10)
High-cost	Hellinger[16]	$424,763 (20.37)	$296,844 (9.34)	$239,945 (5.87)
	Gable et al.[26]	$351,053 (20.37)	$248,224 (9.34)	$202,073 (5.87)

(Hellinger[16] and Gable et al.[26]), and for each of three different discount rates (0%, 3%, and 5%). Cost-of-illness figures (estimates of T) are displayed in pairs with QALYs saved values (estimates of Q). These figures should always be used in pairs, as reflected in the cost-utility ratio (see Eq. 1).

The Hellinger-based (Gable-based) estimates reported in Table 6 range from a low of $T = \$71,143$ ($46,236$) and $Q = 8.57$ to a high of $T = \$424,763$ ($351,053$) and $Q = 20.37$. The intermediate-cost, base-case estimate of T is $195,188 (using Hellinger's nondrug costs), and the base-case value of Q is 11.23. The base-case results reflect a discount rate of 3%. At a 5% rate the corresponding estimates are $T = \$157,348$ and $Q = 7.10$.

DISCUSSION

The base-case results for T (= $195,188$) and Q (= 11.23) are higher than previous estimates for T (estimated at $55,640[6]$) and Q (estimated at 9.26[7]). The increase in T occurs for several reasons. First, even within a particular disease stage, the costs of treatment and disease monitoring are rising. Second, we assume increases in survival due to new therapies (hence, the costs are accumulated for a longer period of time). Third, a lower discount rate is the standard in the field now, and this drives up the discounted cost figure. Fourth, costs now are expressed in June 1996 dollars. As T increases, HIV prevention programs generally appear to be more cost-effective because the numerator of the cost-utility ratio is reduced.

The parameter Q is higher than previous estimates. This occurs primarily because of the lower discount rate now employed. This is true even though two factors tend to decrease the size of Q. First, the new quality-of-life weights employed in our calculations of Q are higher than previous estimates of quality-of-life weights. This decreases Q. Second, our assumption of increased survival from new treatments also decreases the parameter Q. Both of these downward tendencies, however, are more than offset by the change in discount rate.

The resultant higher estimate of Q also makes HIV prevention programs appear to be more cost-effective because as Q increases, the denominator of the cost-utility ratio increases, and the overall cost-utility ratio decreases. In the future, Q may decrease over time if the discount rate and quality weights stabilize in the literature and therapies become more effective at increasing survival.

Increases in the size of T and Q, individually, make HIV prevention programs appear more cost-effective. The *joint* effects of increased values for T and Q are even more pronounced in reducing the size of the cost-utility ratio for any given pairs of values for C and A. To see this, consider the cost-utility ratio introduced previously (see Eq. 1). Although there is no single, universally accepted cost-utility ratio for determining whether or not a program is cost-effective, health service programs with cost-utility ratios less than about $30,00 U.S. per QALY saved are generally considered cost-effective, whereas those with ratios over $140,000 U.S. per QALY saved are difficult to defend as cost-effective.[28-30] Because the cost-utility ratio associated with a particular C and A pair is always smaller when the new estimates of T and Q are used, the ratio using the new T and Q values is more likely to be in the range of cost per QALY saved that is usually considered cost-effective. Now some HIV prevention programs that were not considered cost-effective with the previous estimates of T and Q may be considered to be so.

We propose that the base-case estimates of T and Q derived be used by analysts and others who perform economic evaluations of HIV prevention programs. Such a referent case analysis can render these studies more comparable and more useful to policy makers. Because of the uncertainty in T and Q, economic evaluation studies should include sensitivity analyses in which these parameters are varied over a range of plausible values. Table 6 provides a wide range of values for use in such sensitivity analyses. At a minimum, the range of values reflected in the intermediate case (i.e., the middle rows of Table 6) should be employed in sensitivity analyses of T and Q. For purposes of consistency of assumptions about survival and course of illness, only T and Q *pairs* should be taken from Table 6.

This analysis is subject to limitations. Most important, perhaps, is the present uncertainty about survival and disease progression under the new drug regimens. It will be several years before empirical data are available on actual survival changes over all disease phases induced by the new therapies. However, our assumptions were varied across a wide range of possibilities, and base-case assumptions are cautious rather than overly optimistic. It is important to make these sources of uncertainty explicit so that they can be debated and updated over time. The quality-of-life weights now available in the literature do not correspond with the assessment recommendations of the Panel on Cost-Effectiveness in Health and Medicine. Further empiric research is needed to meet their suggestion for a population-wide survey to assess quality weights. Our estimate of Q should be updated if and when such data become available.

In summary, the results of this analysis suggest that newly developed drug therapies could have a tangible impact on the cost-effectiveness of different HIV prevention programs. Relative to non-HIV health care or health promotion programs, the cost-effectiveness of HIV prevention is enhanced by the increased savings realized each time a case of HIV infection is averted. The estimates reported previously reflect limited foreknowledge of the ultimate effect of novel therapies on the course of HIV disease progression. Moreover, the rapid pace of antiretroviral development assures a limited longevity for even the most accurate estimates of HIV-related treatment costs[31] and quality of life. Nevertheless, HIV policy decisions (especially resource allocation decisions) are being made now, and policy makers deserve the best decision aids possible. Cost-effectiveness analyses can assist their difficult task of making these tough choices, and such analyses should be based on the very best available parameter estimates.

ACKNOWLEDGMENT.   This research was supported by NIMH grants P30-MH52776 and RO1-MH55440. We thanks Drs. Paul Farnham and Mary Guinan for helpful discussions in conceptualizing this project.

REFERENCES

1. Holtgrave DR, Qualls NL, Graham JD. Economic evaluation of HIV primary prevention. *Annu Rev Public Health* 1996; 17:467–488.
2. Haddix AC, Teutsch SM, Shaffer PA, Duñet DO, eds. *Prevention Effectiveness*. New York: Oxford University Press, 1996.
3. Holtgrave DR. Setting priorities and community planning for HIV-prevention programs. *AIDS Public Policy J* 1994; 9:145–151.
4. Gold MR, Siegel JE, Russell LB, Weinstein MC, eds. *Cost-Effectiveness in Health and Medicine*. New York: Oxford University Press, 1996.
5. Holtgrave DR, Kelly JA. Preventing HIV/AIDS among high-risk urban women: The cost-effectiveness of a behavioral group intervention. *Am J Public Health* 1996; 86:1442–1445.
6. Guinan ME, Farnham PG, Holtgrave DR. Estimating the value of preventing a human immunodeficiency virus infection. *Am J Preventive Med* 1994; 10:1–4.
7. Holtgrave DR, Qualls NL. Threshold analysis and HIV prevention programs. *Medical Decision Making* 1995; 15:311–317.
8. Carpenter CCJ, Fischl MA, Hammer SM, et al. Antiretroviral therapy for HIV infection in 1996: Recommendations of an international panel. *JAMA* 1996; 276:146–154.
9. Voelker R. Can researchers use new drugs to push HIV envelope to extinction? *JAMA* 1996; 276:435–437.
10. Ho, DD. Time to hit HIV, early and hard. *N Engl J Med* 1995; 333:450–451.
11. Richman DD. HIV therapeutics. *Science* 1996; 272:1886–1887.
12. Anonymous. New drugs for HIV infection. *Medical Letter on Drugs and Therapeutics*. 1996; 38:35–37.
13. Mellors JW, Kingsley JA, Rinaldo CR Jr, et al. Quantitation of HIV-1 RNA in plasma predicts outcome after seroconversion. *Ann Intern Med* 1995; 122:573–579.
14. Deeks G, Smith M, Holodnly M, Kahn JO. HIV-1 protease inhibitors: A review for clinicians. *JAMA* 1997; 277:145–153.
15. American Health Consultants. Panels to develop standards for antiviral therapy, viral-load testing. *AIDS Alert* 1997; 12:13–15.
16. Hellinger FJ. The lifetime cost of treating a person with HIV. *JAMA* 1993; 270:474–478.
17. U.S. Bureau of Labor Statistics. Consumer price index tables. World Wide Web site, http://stats.bls.gov:80/cgi_bin/surveymost, August 13 1996 (data also available from first author).
18. Tsevat J, Solzan JG, Kuntz KM, et al. Health values of patients with human immunodeficiency virus: Relationship to mental health and physical functioning. *Medical Care* 1996; 34:44–57.
19. Wu AW, Mathews WC, Brysk LT, et al. Quality of life in a placebo-controlled trial of zidovudine in patients with AIDS and AIDS-related complex. *J Acquir Immune Defic Syndr* 1990; 3:683–690.
20. Revicki DA, Wu AW, Murray MI. Change in clinical status, health status, and health utility outcomes in HIV-infected patients. *Medical Care* 1995; 33(suppl):AS173–AS182.
21. Wu AW, Rubin HR, Mathews WC et al. A health status questionnaire using 30 items from the Medical Outcomes Study. *Medical Care* 1991; 29:786–798.
22. Schag, CAC, Ganz PA, Kahn B, Petersen L. Assessing the needs and quality of life of patients with HIV infection: Development of the HIV Overview of Problems Evaluation System (HOPES). *Quality of Life Res* 1992; 1:397–413.
23. Owens DK, Nease RF Jr. Transmission of HIV infection between provider and patient: A quantitative analysis of risk. In Kaplan EH, Brandeau ML, eds. *Modeling the AIDS Epidemic: Planning, Policy, and Prediction*. New York: Raven Press, 1994: 153–177.

24. Holzemer WL, Wilson HS. Quality of life and the spectrum of HIV infection. *Annu Rev Nursing* 1995; 13:3–29.
25. Patrick DL, Erikson P. *Health Status and Health Policy: Allocating Resources to Health Care.* New York: Oxford University Press, 1993.
26. Gable CB, Tierce JC, Simison D, Ward D, Motte K. Costs of HIV+/AIDS at CD4+ counts disease stages based on treatment protocols. *J Acquir Immune Defic Syndr Hum Retrovirol* 1996; 12:413–420.
27. American Health Consultants. Viral-load testing may lower high cost of therapy. *AIDS Alert* 1996; 11:100–101.
28. Laupacis A, Feeny D, Detsky AS, Tugwell PX. Tentative guidelines for using clinical and economic evaluations revisited. *Can Med Assoc J* 1993; 148:927–929.
29. Owens DK, Nease RF, Harris R. Use of cost-effectiveness and value of information analyses to customize guidelines for specific clinical practice settings. *Medical Decision Making* 1993; 13:395 (abstract).
30. Tolley GL, Kenkel D, Fabian R, eds. *Valuing Health for Policy: An Economic Approach.* Chicago: University of Chicago Press, 1994.
31. Pinkerton SD, Holtgrave DR. Lifetime costs of HIV/AIDS medical care (letter). *J Acquir Immune Defic Syndr Hum Retrovirol,* in press.

Cost-Effectiveness of a Community-Level HIV Risk Reduction Intervention

STEVEN D. PINKERTON, DAVID R. HOLTGRAVE, WAYNE J. DiFRANCEISCO, L. YVONNE STEVENSON, and JEFFREY A. KELLY

INTRODUCTION

Successful AIDS risk reduction requires that individuals reduce the sexual and drug use behaviors that place them at risk of becoming infected with HIV or passing the virus to others. A number of carefully conducted experimental and quasi-experimental studies have established the effectiveness of small-group and individual-level interventions that combine risk reduction education with cognitive-behavioral skills-building activities to help participants decrease their sexual risk behavior and foster positive attitudes toward safer sex.[1–9] Unfortunately, the scale and scope of such interventions is necessarily limited by the small-group format. Much larger, *community-level* interventions are needed to prevent the further spread of HIV among at-risk populations.[10] To date, however, comparatively few community-level HIV prevention interventions have been rigorously evaluated.[11–16]

Community-level interventions attempt to alter social norms toward risk behavior and alter the behavior itself, thereby effecting widespread and durable changes throughout the target population. For example, communitywide campaigns to diminish the social acceptability of cigarette smoking have focused on inducing norm changes that encourage smoking cessation.[17] Similarly, community-level HIV prevention efforts have often attempted to induce social norms that encourage risk avoidance and safer sex by members of the target population.

One especially influential community-level HIV prevention model that has received considerable empirical attention is based on "diffusion of innovation" principles.[18] This model hypothesizes that social norms propagate through a population starting with influential "trend setters" who convince others through word and action ("modeling") to adopt the target attitudes and behaviors. In this manner, an intervention of limited scale can have far-reaching, communitywide effects. Because of this, such community-level interventions

STEVEN D. PINKERTON, DAVID R. HOLTGRAVE, WAYNE J. DiFRANCEISCO, L. YVONNE STEVENSON, and JEFFREY A. KELLY • Department of Psychiatry and Behavioral Medicine, Center for AIDS Intervention Research (CAIR), Medical College of Wisconsin, Milwaukee, Wisconsin 53202.

Handbook of Economic Evaluation of HIV Prevention Programs, edited by Holtgrave. Plenum Press, New York, 1998.

have the potential to be highly cost-effective relative to smaller, possibly more intensive, behavioral interventions.

Although recent studies have established the cost-effectiveness of several small-group format HIV behavioral risk reduction interventions,[19–21] the economic efficiency of community-level HIV prevention interventions has not been rigorously evaluated.[22] As a first step toward filling this knowledge gap, in this chapter we assess the cost-effectiveness of an experimental community-level HIV risk reduction intervention conducted at gay bars in a small Southern city.[14]

DESCRIPTION OF INTERVENTION

The intervention was conducted in late 1989 in Biloxi, a small Mississippi city with a population of about 50,000. At the time of the intervention there were two gay bars in the city. These bars were central meeting places and primary social settings within the gay community of Biloxi and the surrounding area.[14,23] The intervention consisted of three main phases. In the first phase, bartenders at the city's two gay bars were trained to observe social interactions among patrons and thereby to identify "popular opinion leaders" (well-respected, influential, socially active men) within the gay community. Thirty-six men received multiple popularity nominations. Twenty-two of these men were recruited into the next phase of the intervention, which consisted of four weekly, 90- to 120-minute sessions led by two to four facilitators. The purpose of these sessions was to instruct the popular opinion leaders in effective communication techniques for endorsing HIV risk reduction and safer sex in conversations with their peers.[14,23] In the final phase of the intervention, the popular opinion leaders were encouraged to engage their peers in conversations about behavioral risk reduction and to visibly endorse safer sex norms over a period of at least two weeks.

At the completion of training, a second wave of popular opinion leaders, consisting of friends of men recruited in the first wave, was enrolled in the four-session training program, and the intervention as described above was replicated with this new group. Thus, the overall intervention consisted of two successive groups of popular opinion leaders who were trained in effective communication skills and then encouraged to engage their peers in conversations about safer sexual practices.

To assess the impact of the intervention, men entering the bars were surveyed about their sexual behavior during the past two months (including frequency and number of partners for insertive and receptive anal intercourse and use of condoms). Surveys were conducted at baseline (before initiating the intervention) and again three months after the second group of popular opinion leaders had completed their training. To control for possible temporal or other confounds, bar patrons in two comparison cities were also given the sexual behavior survey. (Although the comparison cities did not receive the popular opinion leader intervention at this time, safer sex pamphlets were distributed throughout the intervention period at gay bars in all three cities.) Eighty-six percent of the men surveyed were White and 14% were African-American or Hispanic. The mean age of survey respondents in all three cities was 29 years.[14]

Kelly et al. observed statistically significant reductions in the intervention city, from baseline to follow-up, in the proportion of men who engaged in any unprotected anal intercourse or who had multiple sexual partners, and a significant increase in condom use during anal intercourse.[14] These effects were not caused simply by changes in the behavior of the popular opinion leaders, who were excluded from the data analysis. Little or no change was observed in the comparison cities. Thus, Kelly concludes that "it was possible to produce generalized changes in sexual risk behavior within an entire community population—men patronizing gay bars in a city—by enlisting the efforts of popular opinion leaders to visibly and demonstratively recommend, endorse, and support the behavioral change efforts of their friends and acquaintances."[23,p.312]

Cost-Effectiveness

In this study, Kelly et al. documented the effectiveness of a novel community-level intervention for reducing sexual risk behavior associated with the transmission of HIV. Because HIV prevention resources are limited, however, it is not enough that a program be effective. It must also be *cost-effective* (i.e., an efficient expenditure of societal resources). HIV prevention cost-effectiveness studies quantify the economic efficiency of an intervention as the ratio of program costs to the number of infections prevented. Such studies are necessary to enable HIV prevention program planners (including community planning groups) and other public health decision makers to choose between alternative HIV interventions so as to maximize the number of infections averted by funded programs.[24]

The U.S. Public Health Service's Panel on Cost-Effectiveness in Health and Medicine recommends that a variant of cost-effectiveness analysis known as cost-utility analysis also be performed.[25] The outcome variable in a cost-utility analysis is the cost per quality-adjusted life year (QALY) saved by the intervention, rather than cost per infection averted as in a cost-effectiveness analysis. Because QALYs explicitly incorporate possible intervention effects on morbidity and impaired physical, mental, and emotional functioning and reductions in mortality, cost-utility analysis is potentially applicable to a wider class of health promotion interventions than traditional cost-effectiveness analysis. Moreover, because QALYs are not HIV-specific, cost-utility analysis facilitates comparison of HIV prevention interventions with other health-service programs.

The present analysis uses the techniques of cost-effectiveness and cost-utility analysis to evaluate the economic efficiency of Kelly and colleagues' popular opinion leader community-level HIV prevention intervention.[14] This study complements previous economic evaluations of small-group interventions[20,21] and extends the methodology to community-level interventions in which the affected population does not necessarily coincide with the group directly receiving the intervention.

METHODS

Standard methods of cost-effectiveness and cost-utility analysis were employed.[25-28] A societal perspective was adopted. Thus, the analysis incorporates all identifiable costs and consequences, regardless of who pays or who benefits. Monetary costs were adjusted for inflation to 1996 dollars by using the Consumer Price Index (CPI). All costs and the primary outcome measure, quality-adjusted life years (QALYs), were discounted at a 3% annual rate in the base-case analysis and at 0% and 5% in the sensitivity analyses.

The main analytic steps were as follows: (1) retrospective estimation of all intervention-related costs; (2) mathematical modeling to translate observed behavioral effects into an estimate of the number of HIV infections averted by the intervention; (3) estimation of the corresponding number of QALYs saved; and (4) computation of the cost-effectiveness ratio (cost per infection averted) and cost-utility ratio (cost per QALY saved). In addition, multiple sensitivity and threshold analyses were conducted to examine how deviations from base-case assumptions might affect the results and to generalize the results to other contexts (e.g., communities in which the prevalence of HIV is lower than in the intervention city). These five steps are described individually in the following sections (see also Pinkerton and Holtgrave, this volume).

Retrospective Cost Estimation

Intervention cost estimates were obtained retrospectively via interviews with intervention staff and review of original records. Costs were adjusted from 1989 dollars to (June) 1996 dollars using the "all items" index of the CPI (1989 to 1996 scaling factor = 1.26), with the exception of salary and incentive costs, which were adjusted by using the U.S. Bureau of Labor Statistics Employment Cost Index (scaling factor = 1.23).

Principal cost categories included salary for intervention personnel (senior, junior, and administrative staff) and bar staff, incentive payments to popular opinion leaders, travel expenses for intervention personnel, catering, safer sex pamphlets, and the "Stop and Go" posters supplied to the bars, as shown in Table 1. Each of the eight approximately two-hour popular opinion leader training sessions required three hours of senior staff time (including one hour for preparation) and two hours of an administrative assistant's time. Four of these sessions also required three hours of junior staff time. Additional intervention personnel costs were incurred in staff training (96 hours total); contacting and enlisting the support of bar owners and managers (which included paying for lunch) (8 hours); training bar staff to identify popular opinion leader nominees (19 hours); cross-tabulating lists of nominees (2 hours); recruiting the popular opinion leaders into the study (32 hours); and time spent familiarizing bar patrons with intervention staff, and vice-versa (64 hours). Bar staff were each compensated for one hour spent identifying nominees. During the popular opinion leader training sessions, the staff of the intervention bar were also paid to open and close the bar, a total of sixteen hours of bar staff time.

The senior and junior intervention personnel made a total of 36 round trips to the bar (see Table 1). Although extensive travel was not required of the intervention research staff (which stayed at a hotel in the intervention city), a two-hour (about 80 miles) round-trip time was used in the analyses to increase the generalizability of the results to situations in which the agency performing the intervention is located a moderate distance from the intervention city. Travel expenses were calculated at $0.30 a mile, in accordance with practice at the authors' home institution.

The owner of the bar at which the training sessions were held was paid $126 per session (1996 dollars) as rent for use of the bar. The training sessions were also catered at an expense of approximately $63 per session. In addition, the popular opinion leaders (including bar staff) received incentive payments totaling $123 for their participation (in the analysis, these payments were treated as a proxy for client time valuation).

Overhead, including utilities, office rental, maintenance, and general administrative costs, was obtained as a fixed percentage (25% in the base-case) of noncompensation direct costs. Costs associated with the strictly scientific objectives of the intervention study were excluded from the analysis.

Table 1. Intervention Resources Consumed

	Nontravel Time[a]	Travel	Materials and Other Expenses[b]
1. Staff training	Sr: 2 × 28 hrs[c] Jr: 2 × 20 hrs		
2. Contacting/enlisting support of bar owners and managers	Sr: 3 hr/bar × 2 bars Ad: 1 hr/bar × 2 bars	Sr: 1 trip/bar × 2 bars	1 letter/bar × 2 bars × $0.32/letter 2 calls/bar × 2 bars × $0.50/call 1 lunch/bar × 2 bars × $37.80/lunch
3. Training bartenders and overseeing identification of popular opinion leaders (POLs)	Sr: 1 hr/bar × 2 bars Jr: 8 hr/bar × 2 bars Ad: 1 hr total Bar: 1 hr/staff × 8 staff	Sr: 1 trip/bar × 2 bars Jr: 2 trips/bar × 2 bars	2 calls/staff × 8 staff × $0.50/call Recording forms: 8 staff × $0.25/staff
4. Cross-tabulating POL lists	Jr: 1 hr/bar × 2 bars	Jr: 1 trip/bar × 2 bars	Office supplies: $126.00 total (all intervention phases)
5. Recruiting POLs	Jr: 16 hr/bar × 2 bars	Jr: 3 trips/bar × 2 bars	2 letters/nominee × 36 nominees × $0.32/letter 2 calls/nominee × 36 nominees × $0.50/call
6. Training POLs	Sr: 2 × 3 hr/sess × 8 sess Jr: 2 × 3 hr/sess × 4 sess Ad: 2 hr/sess × 8 sess Bar: 1 hr/sess × 8 sess	Sr: 1 trip/sess × 8 sess[d] Jr: 1 trip/sess × 4 sess[d]	Catering: 8 sessions × $63/session Rent: 8 sessions × $126/session Incentives: 43 POLs × $123/POL Handouts: 43 POLs × $6.30/POL Erasable board, markers, etc: $252 total Stop&Go posters: 10 posters/bar × 2 bars × $12.60/poster Stop&Go buttons: $156.50 total Conversation monitoring forms: 43 POLs × $0.51/POL Pamphlets: 750 pamphlets/bar × 2 bars × $0.32/pamphlet + 3 mailings/bar × 2 bars × $5.00/mailing
7. Additional time in bars	Sr: 2 × 8 hr/bar[e] × 2 bars Jr: 2 × 8 hr/bar[e] × 2 bars	Sr: 2 trips/bar × 2 bars[d] Jr: 2 trips/bar × 2 bars[d]	

[a]Senior ("Sr"), junior ("Jr"), and administrative ("Ad") intervention personnel; bar staff ("Bar").
[b]All costs in 1996 dollars.
[c]Senior staff training time includes eight hours to become familiar with intervention and 20 hours to train junior staff.
[d]Assumes senior staff travel together to bars and likewise for junior staff.
[e]Two trips at four hours each.

Mathematical Modeling

A mathematical model was used to translate the observed changes in sexual behavior from baseline to three-month follow-up into an estimate of the number of HIV infections averted by the intervention. Specifically, a Bernoulli-process model of the sexual transmission of HIV was used to estimate the probability that any given respondent would become infected with HIV or pass the virus to another if already infected as a result of the sexual behavior reported on the baseline or follow-up survey.[29–32] By averaging the individual probabilities obtained for the men, populationwide risk estimates at each of the four assessment points can be obtained.

Let B_1, B_2, C_1, and C_2 denote the average probabilities of infection for a survey respondent in the intervention city at baseline (B_1) or follow-up (B_2), or either one of the comparison cities (C_1 and C_2). Then the average reduction in the risk of infection over the two-month period is $\Delta B = B_2 - B_1$ for Biloxi and $\Delta C = C_2 - C_1$ for the pooled comparison cities. The risk reduction difference *between* cities, $\Delta B - \Delta C$, provides an estimate of the average reduction in risk attributable to the intervention.

The overall number of HIV infections averted depends on the effective size (N) of the intervention population, that is, on the number of men who reduced their risk, on average, by $\Delta B - \Delta C$. Once N has been estimated, the number of infections averted is simply $A_p = (\Delta B - \Delta C)N$ (for more on this methodology, see Ref. 33).

Several alternative forms of the basic Bernoulli-process model of HIV transmission risk were considered, and the mean of the values obtained from these models was used in estimating the risk reduction due to the intervention, A_p. In the basic model the probability of transmission is a function of the following factors: (1) the number of acts of unprotected and condom-protected receptive and insertive anal intercourse and the number of partners for each of these four sexual behaviors; (2) the prevalence of HIV among sexual partners (π); (3) the infectivities (per act transmission probabilities) of unprotected receptive and insertive intercourse (α and γ, respectively); and (4) the effectiveness of condoms at reducing the infectivity of anal intercourse (ε). The sexual behavior parameters were derived from the survey results (mean values for these parameters are shown in Table 2). Base-case estimates of the remaining parameters were obtained from the literature, as indicated in Table 3.

In the simplest model, which assumes that all four types of partners are distinct, the probability of transmission is given by

Table 2. Sexual Behavior Data

	Intervention City		Comparison Cities	
	Baseline	Follow-up	Baseline	Follow-up
Frequency of unprotected RAI $(x)^a$	5.35	4.40	3.00	2.67
# of partners for unprotected RAI (X)	0.24	0.17	0.33	0.35
Frequency of condom-protected RAI $(y)^a$	2.44	1.65	1.93	2.58
# of partners for condom-protected RAI (Y)	0.28	0.27	0.37	0.24
Frequency of unprotected IAI $(v)^b$	4.27	3.44	4.32	2.78
# of partners for unprotected IAI (V)	0.30	0.30	0.30	0.40
Frequency of condom-protected IAI $(w)^b$	2.87	2.10	2.16	2.13
# of partners for condom-protected IAI (W)	0.31	0.51	0.44	0.33

[a]Receptive anal intercourse (RAI), per partner.
[b]Insertive anal intercourse (IAI), per partner.

Table 3. Base-Case Parameters Values, Ranges Examined in Sensitivity Analyses, and Sources

	Base-Case Value	Range Examined	Sources
Sexual behavior and epidemiological parameters			
HIV prevalence in community (π)	9%	0%–20%	51,53
Infectivity of receptive anal intercourse (α)	0.009	0.001–0.1	20,43–45
Infectivity of insertive anal intercourse (γ)	0.0009	0.0–0.01	Estimate
Condom effectiveness (e)	95%	69%–99%	49,50
Intervention parameters			
Effective intervention size (N)	449	250–1000	14
Savings estimates			
Discounted medical treatment cost (T)	$87,000	$71,000–$425,000	37,39
QALYs saved per prevented infection (Q)	11.26	4.91–21.21	36,37
Analytic parameters			
Annual discount rate	3%	0%–5%	25

$$P = 1 - \{[(1 - \pi) + \pi(1 - \alpha)^x]^X[(1 - \pi) + \pi(1 - \varepsilon\alpha)^y]^Y \\ \times [(1 - \pi) + \pi(1 - \gamma)^v]^V[(1 - \pi) + \pi(1 - \varepsilon\gamma)^w]^W\}. \tag{1}$$

In this equation, x and X denote the number of acts per partner and the number of partners (respectively) for unprotected receptive anal intercourse and likewise for condom-protected receptive anal intercourse (y and Y), unprotected insertive anal intercourse (v and V), and condom-protected insertive anal intercourse (w and W).

Four other variants of the Bernoulli model were also examined. In two of the variants [1(a) and 1(b)], it was assumed that the partners for protected and unprotected anal intercourse are distinct, but no distinction was drawn between partners for receptive and insertive intercourse. In variant 1(a), the total number of partners for unprotected intercourse was set equal to the maximum of X and V, and likewise for condom-protected intercourse and the maximum of Y and W, whereas variant 1(b) used the minimums. In the other two variants no distinction was made between the four types of partners, and the total number of partners was set to either the maximum [variant 2(a)] or minimum [variant 2(b)] of X, Y, V, and W.

The Bernoulli model previously given provides an estimate of the probability that a previously uninfected person would become infected with HIV. Therefore this model is not applicable to people who are already infected with HIV. The main beneficial effect of sexual behavior risk reduction among already infected persons is limiting the further spread of the virus (there may also be ancillary health benefits, but these are not considered here). A variant of the Bernoulli model can be used to estimate the expected number of "secondary" infections A_s prevented among the partners of an infected intervention participant.[31,34] In the present analysis it was assumed that the prevalence of HIV infection among intervention participants is the same as among the cities' gay community in general. Thus, the total number of infections averted among both intervention participants and their partners is given by

$$A = [(1 - \pi)A_p + \pi(1 - \lambda)A_s]N \tag{2}$$

where N is the effective intervention size and λ is a partnership overlap factor ($\lambda = 25\%$ in the base case) that limits overcounting partners shared by more than one man.[20,21,33]

Although the ostensible target of the intervention is the entire gay community in the intervention city, the behavioral change data collected via baseline and follow-up surveys reflect only the impact of the intervention on a subset of the bar-going population. It is this subgroup, which was randomly surveyed during the data collection and which may or may not have had conversations with the popular opinion leaders, that constitutes the effective target population of the intervention. About 35% of the men in the intervention city who completed the survey did so more than once.[14] Therefore the 606 surveys collected by the research team represent 449 distinct individuals, assuming that each man completed the survey at most twice. This is an *extremely* conservative estimate of the effective intervention size because it assumes that the impact of the intervention is restricted to the sampled subpopulation of bar-going men.

Kelly et al. estimate that they surveyed about 81% of the men entering the bars during the three-night survey period.[14] If it can be reasonably assumed that the surveyed individuals are representative of the overall three-night sample, then the effective intervention size would increase to 554. If instead, the entire bar-going population is included, then the effective intervention size is probably closer to 1,000. However, even this figure is likely to underestimate the true reach of this community-level intervention. Theoretically, the positive effects of the intervention should diffuse beyond the bar-going crowd, as safer sex norms are established and reinforced, reaching others in the gay community who may have few ties to the bars themselves.

The most conservative of these figures, $N = 449$, is used in the base-case analysis. The reader should keep in mind, however, that the true number of affected individuals—hence the true number of infections averted by the intervention—is probably much larger. Similarly, a very brief two-month intervention effect is assumed in the analysis, that is, it is assumed that the positive effects of the intervention persist only during the period monitored by the follow-up assessment. This, also, is a very conservative assumption. Longer term follow-up studies suggest that the intervention effect is quite robust,[15] and significant reductions in risk behavior persisted as long as three years after the conclusion of the original study.[35] Thus, the present analysis is biased *against* the intervention.

Estimation of QALYs Saved

The number of quality-adjusted life years (QALYs) lost to HIV infection can be calculated by dividing the life course of an HIV-infected person into several phases (e.g., unaware of infection; aware, but receiving no treatment; receiving treatment and CD4 count greater than 200; clinically defined AIDS), associating each with a reduction in quality of life as reported in the literature,[36,37] and then summing over years of potential life. The resulting number Q provides an estimate of the number of QALYs saved for each infection prevented. This method yields an estimate of $Q = 11.26$ QALYs, discounted at a 3% annual rate, for someone who is 32 years old (the mean age of survey respondents in the intervention city) at the time of infection and who receives minimal HIV-related medical care, as described further later.[37] Notice that perfect health is assigned a quality valuation of 0.94 rather than the maximum 1.0 because empirical evidence indicates that this value better approximates the average health of an arbitrarily drawn sample at any given time (i.e., perfect health is not necessarily the norm).[38] The total number of QALYs saved by the intervention equals AQ, where A (as before) is the number of infections averted.[19]

Calculation of Cost-Effectiveness and Cost-Utility Ratios

The two main outcome measures of the present study are the cost-effectiveness ratio (cost per HIV infection averted) and the cost-utility ratio (cost per QALY saved by the intervention). The cost-effectiveness ratio is $E = C/A$, where C is the total cost of the intervention and A is the number of infections it prevented. The cost-utility ratio R was calculated from the following formula:

$$R = \frac{C - AT}{AQ} \tag{3}$$

where Q is the discounted number of QALYs saved per prevented infection (see above) and T is the lifetime medical care cost of treating a case of HIV disease and AIDS in the U.S. (Notice that as utilized here, the numerator of the cost-effectiveness ratio is the *gross* program cost, as opposed to the *net* cost, as in numerator of the cost-utility ratio.)

Recently updated estimates of T suggest a range of values from about \$71,000 to \$425,000, depending upon the discount rate and the particular disease progression/access-to-care scenario.[37] The smallest of these estimates is obtained under a presumed HIV care scenario for someone with very poor access to treatment, discounted at a 5% annual rate. Under this scenario, chemotherapy is not initiated until the seventh year of infection, and even then, only zidovudine therapy is available. Therefore the resulting lifetime HIV medical care costs estimate (\$71,000) is quite conservative. (Guinan et al. estimated HIV-related medical costs for a similar scenario at \$56,000 in 1992 dollars, discounted at 5%.[39]) When these cost estimates are discounted at 3% rather than 5%, as recommended by the U.S. Public Health Service's Panel on Cost-Effectiveness in Health and Medicine,[25] lifetime HIV medical care costs grow to about \$87,000, which is the base-case value assumed in the main analysis presented later (as noted in the previous section, under this scenario the number of QALYs lost to HIV infection is 11.26, when discounted at 3%). Alternative scenarios and discount rates are considered in the sensitivity analyses.

If the cost-utility ratio [Eq. (3)] is negative, then the intervention actually saves societal resources and hence is said to be *cost-saving* (ideally, all cost-saving interventions should be funded). Interventions with positive cost-utility ratios may or may not represent sound societal investments. Health-service programs with cost-utility ratios that are less than \$30,000 are generally considered cost-effective, whereas those with ratios over \$140,000 are difficult to justify as cost-effective.[40,41]

Threshold and Sensitivity Analyses

Threshold analyses were performed to determine critical parameter values at which the programs change from being cost-effective (or cost-saving) to being cost-ineffective (or not cost-saving), and vice versa. Multiple sensitivity analyses were also undertaken to examine the effects of variations in key parameters and modeling assumptions. Combined, these analyses provide extensive checks on the reasonableness and robustness of the base-case results and suggest how the results might differ if the intervention were implemented in a different environment (e.g., a community with a lower prevalence of HIV).

RESULTS

The results of the cost analysis and the primary cost-effectiveness and cost-utility analyses are presented in Tables 4 and 5, respectively, and follow in detail. Results of the threshold and sensitivity analyses are also presented.

Costs

Overall, the intervention cost about $17,000, as shown in Table 4. Salary costs accounted for about 39% of total expenses ($6,700, incorporating a 27% fringe benefit rate), and popular opinion leader incentives for about 31% ($5,300; these incentive payments provided a proxy for the opportunity costs associated with the popular opinion leaders' participation in the intervention). Materials and other expenses ($4,100) totaled about 24% of total intervention costs. The largest of these expenses included rental fees paid to the owner of the bar at which the training session were held ($1,000), catering ($500), and staff travel to and from the bars ($860). Overhead accounted for the remaining 6% ($1,000) of the overall cost of the intervention.

Infections Averted and QALYs Saved

As illustrated in Fig. 1, the intervention decreased the expected number of infections, per person, from a baseline level of 0.0017 to 0.0011 at follow-up, a 35% reduction. In con-

Table 4. Intervention Costs

	Unit Costs	Number of Units	Total Cost
Salary			
Senior staff salary	$14.79/hour	200 hours[a]	$2,958
Junior staff salary	$10.35/hour	202 hours[b]	$2,089
Administrative assistant salary	$7.69/hour	19 hours	$146
Bar staff salary	$6.15/hour	16 hours	$98
Total salary cost	–	–	$5,291
Adjusted salary cost[c]	–	–	$6,720
Incentive payments			
Popular opinion leader (POL) incentives	$123 per POL	43 POLs	$5,289
Other expenses			
Rental fees	$126/session	8 sessions	$1,008
Staff travel expenses	$24.00/round trip	36 round trips	$864
Catering	$63/session	8 sessions	$504
Safer sex pamphlets	$0.32/pamphlet	1,500 pamphlets	$480
Stop & Go posters	$12.60/poster	20 posters	$252
Miscellaneous expenses[d]	–	–	$1,005
Total expenses	–	–	$4,113
Overhead (25%)[e]	–	–	$1,028
Ajdusted total	–	–	$5,141
Total cost			$17,150

[a]Includes 56 hours of senior staff travel time.
[b]Includes 56 hours of junior staff travel time.
[c]Includes 27% fringe benefit rate, per standard practice at authors' home institution.
[d]Includes postage, phone calls, printing costs, buttons, office supplies, erasable board, markers, etc.
[e]Includes utilities, office rental, maintenance, and general administrative costs.

Table 5. Results from Primary Analysis

	Discount Rate		
	0%	Base-case (3%)	5%
Intervention cost (C)	$17,150	$17,150	$17,150
QALYs lost per infection (Q)	21.21	11.26	7.62
Lifetime medical care costs (T)[a]	$118,892	$87,045	$71,143
HIV infections averted by intervention (A)	0.262	0.262	0.262
QALYs saved by intervention (AQ)	5.56	2.95	2.00
Medical care costs saved by intervention (AT)	$31,150	$22,806	$18,639
Cost-effectiveness ratio (C/A)	$65,458	$65,458	$65,458
Cost-utility ratio [R; see Eq. (3)]	<0[b]	<0[b]	<0[b]

[a]Low-cost scenario of Holtgrave and Pinkerton, 1997 (Ref. 37).
[b]A cost-utility ratio less than zero signifies that the intervention is cost-saving.

trast, only a modest 7% drop from 0.0015 to 0.0014 was observed in the comparison cities. The overall intervention effect is about 0.0006 infections averted per person. For the base-case intervention size of 449 men, this translates into a total of 0.262 infections averted (about 43% of which were "secondary" infections). Although this effect may appear small, only a very limited two-month period of intervention effectiveness was assumed.

The number of QALYs saved by the intervention depends on the discount rate used in the calculations (see Table 5). Under the base-case assumption of a 3% discount rate, 2.95 QALYs are saved. In contrast, the intervention saves 5.56 undiscounted QALYs, but only 2.0 QALYs when a 5% rate is used.

Cost-Effectiveness and Cost-Utility Ratios

As indicated in Table 5, the base-case cost-effectiveness ratio (cost per HIV infection averted) is about $65,000. Because the lifetime medical care costs associated with HIV disease and AIDS are even greater—ranging from $71,000 to $119,000 (depending on the discount rate) in the low cost scenario of Holtgrave and Pinkerton[37]—it would actually be

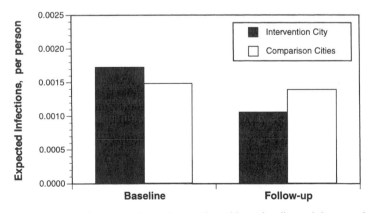

Figure 1. Expected infections for intervention and comparison cities at baseline and three months follow-up.

cost-saving to society to implement this intervention. Moreover, because a cost-saving program is necessarily cost-effective, there is no need to calculate the cost-utility ratio.

Threshold and Sensitivity Analyses

Higher discount rates generally disfavor prevention programs (as opposed to therapeutic interventions) because financial resources are expended in the present whereas benefits are realized only in the discounted future.[42] However, the intervention remains cost-saving at the three discount rates considered here, 0%, 3%, and 5% (see Table 5). The intervention is also cost-saving under each of the nine medical care scenarios (low, intermediate, and high standard of care at 0%, 3%, and 5% discount rates) examined by Holtgrave and Pinkerton,[37] as shown in Table 6.

The results are also not especially sensitive to the particular model selected to estimate the number of infections averted by the intervention. The five models previously described yield estimated numbers of infections averted within a range from 0.241 to 0.283 and a mean of 0.262 (this is the base-case result reported in Table 5). The intervention is cost-saving under any of these estimates.

Indeed, threshold analyses indicate that the intervention remains cost-saving in the base-case (3% discount rate), provided that the total number of infections averted is at least 0.197, as shown in Table 7. Similarly, the intervention would remain cost-saving if the cost of the program were as large as $23,000 or if lifetime medical care treatment costs related to HIV were as low as $65,000. Naturally, the cost-effectiveness thresholds are much less restrictive. For example, the intervention could cost as much as $120,000 or prevent as few as 0.04 infections and still have a cost-utility ratio less than $30,000/QALY (see Table 7). Moreover, it is cost-effective at the $30,000/QALY level, *regardless* of the cost of medical care—that is, it would be cost-effective even if medical care were free.

In the light of these thresholds and because the cost-utility ratio is a linear function of

Table 6.   Cost-of-Illness and Quality-of-Life Sensitivity Analysis

	Discount Rate		
	0%	Base-case (3%)	5%
Low standard of care[a]			
Lifetime medical care costs (*T*)	$118,892	$87,045	$71,143
QALYs lost per infection (*Q*)[b]	21.21	11.26	7.62
Cost-utility ratio (*R*)[c]	<0[d]	<0[d]	<0[d]
Intermediate standard of care[a]			
Lifetime medical care costs (*T*)	$274,766	$195,188	$157,348
QALYs lost per infection (*Q*)[b]	18.23	9.31	6.15
Cost-utility ratio (*R*)[c]	<0[d]	<0[d]	<0[d]
High standard of care[a]			
Lifetime medical care costs (*T*)	$424,763	$296,844	$239,945
QALYs lost per infection (*Q*)[b]	14.73	7.42	4.91
Cost-utility ratio (*R*)[c]	<0[d]	<0[d]	<0[d]

[a]HIV medical care scenario (see Holtgrave and Pinkerton, under review).
[b]Assumes infection occurs at age 32.
[c]Assumes base-case values for infections averted (*A*) and intervention cost (*C*).
[d]A cost-utility ratio less than zero signifies that the intervention is cost-saving.

Table 7. Threshold Analyses[a]

	Base-Case Value	Threshold		
		0	$30,000/QALY	$140,000/QALY
HIV infections averted (A)	0.262	0.197	0.040	0.010
Intervention cost (C)	$17,150	$23,000	$110,000	$440,000
Lifetime medical care costs (T)	$87,045	$65,000	$0	$0

[a]Table values indicate largest (or smallest) parameter value that results in cost-utility ratio less than stated threshold when the other two parameters, together with Q (QALYs saved), retain their base-case values.

both the cost of the intervention and HIV medical care costs, it is unlikely that a moderate error in estimating either or both of these values would alter the general conclusion of the preceding analysis. In contrast, the number of infections A averted by the intervention is derived from a complex multivariate equation [e.g., Eq. (1)] that may magnify small errors arising from estimating constituent parameters. Indeed, past research has shown that the model is sensitive to both the infectivity of HIV (i.e., the per act probability of transmission) and, to a lesser extent, the prevalence of HIV in the intervention population.[19–21,30,31,34]

Published estimates of the infectivity of unprotected receptive anal intercourse (RAI) range from approximately 0.001 to about 0.3.[43–45] HIV is believed to be much more infectious during the brief period that follows initial infection (prior to seroconversion) and again late in the course of infection, when symptoms of AIDS typically appear, but much less infectious during the long asymptomatic period that may last five, ten, or more years.[46,47] The base-case infectivity estimate ($\alpha = 0.009$) represents a temporally weighted average over the course of infection and is consistent with previous analyses.[20,21] Insertive anal intercourse (IAI) is assumed to be less risky and has in infectivity one-tenth that of receptive anal intercourse ($\gamma = 0.0009$ in the base-case).

Table 8 presents the results of a sensitivity analysis crossing three values of the RAI infectivity (α) with three methods for determining the IAI infectivity (γ): either $\gamma = \alpha$, $\gamma = \alpha/10$, or $\gamma = 0$ (this last scenario is included because some investigators have reported little or no association between IAI and HIV transmission[48]). As expected, the number of infections averted is fairly sensitive to the RAI infectivity estimate and less so to the IAI infectivity. However, the cost-utility ratio is less than $43,000—a level generally considered cost-effective[41]—for all scenarios considered in the table. These results are not particularly sensitive to the assumed effectiveness of condoms. For example, reducing the

Table 8. Infections Averted and Cost-Utility Ratio as Function of Infectivity

	Infections Averted			Cost-Utility Ratio		
	Infectivity of IAI (γ)			Infectivity of IAI (γ)		
Infectivity of RAI (α)	$\gamma = 0$	$\gamma = 0.1\alpha$[a]	$\gamma = \alpha$	$\gamma = 0$	$\gamma = 0.1\alpha$[a]	$\gamma = \alpha$
0.001	0.030	0.033	0.034	$43,000	$39,000	$37,000
0.009	0.242	0.262[b]	0.274	<0[c]	<0[b,c]	<0[c]
0.3	2.67	3.13	3.34	<0[c]	<0[c]	<0[c]

[a]α = infectivity of receptive anal intercourse (RAI); γ = infectivity of insertive anal intercourse (IAI).
[b]Base-case value.
[c]A cost-utility ratio less than zero signifies that the intervention is cost-saving.

effectiveness from 95% (the base-case value[49]) to 69%[50] decreases the number of infections averted only slightly from 0.262 to 0.258.

Kelly et al. report that the prevalence of HIV infection among *all* men seeking HIV testing within the intervention city is 2%.[14] However, the prevalence among the gay men in the intervention study is likely to be much higher. Because seroprevalence data were not collected as part of the intervention trial, recent findings for comparably sized cities[5] were used to estimate the HIV prevalence among gay men in the intervention city at 9%. A threshold analysis indicates that the intervention is (1) cost-saving provided that the prevalence of infection is at least 6.7%; (2) cost-effective at the $30,000/QALY level for HIV prevalence in excess of 1.3%; and (3) cost-effective at the $140,000/QALY level if the prevalence is greater than 0.4%. Thus, the intervention is cost-saving in the base-case and would be cost-effective even in very low prevalence populations.

DISCUSSION

The community-level HIV prevention intervention described, in which popular opinion leaders were trained to endorse and model safer sex behavioral norms through conversations with peers, is highly cost-effective—or even cost-saving to society—under most reasonable parameter assumptions. The cost per infection averted ($65,000) compares favorably with other HIV behavioral risk reduction interventions for gay men, such as intensive, small-group cognitive-behavioral skills workshops.[20] Moreover, the overall cost of the intervention ($17,150, or about $40 per affected individual) is likely to fall within the budgetary constraints of many community-based AIDS prevention organizations.

It should be emphasized that these encouraging results were obtained under very conservative assumptions regarding the number of men reached by the intervention and the duration of behavioral change effects. Follow-up studies of the intervention population suggest that the observed change toward safer sexual behaviors endured well beyond the brief two-month period assumed here (see, e.g., the three-year follow-up by St. Lawrence et al.[35]). The analysis also did not attempt to model the diffusion of changes in safer sex norms and behaviors through the gay community, resulting in an underestimation of the number of infections averted by the intervention. Future research is needed to study the diffusion process and to develop better models of community-level effects.[10]

The results presented are generally robust to changes in key parameter values and modeling assumptions. Although the results are somewhat sensitive to the per contact probability of HIV transmission and the prevalence of infection in the intervention population, the intervention remains cost-effective within plausible ranges of values for these parameters. The observed sensitivity to HIV prevalence, however, underscores the importance of targeting interventions to at-risk individuals.

Several limitations of this study should also be noted, including the retrospective collection of cost data, estimation of key epidemiological parameters, modeling to derive outcome data, and reliance on respondents' self-report of their sexual behavior. These concerns are mitigated somewhat by the results of the sensitivity analyses, however, which indicate that the intervention remains cost-effective over a range of reasonable parameter values. It is unlikely that uncertainty in the cost and epidemiological estimates or bias in the self-reporting of sexual behavior data would be sufficient to reverse the overall finding of cost-effectiveness.

Similar comments apply to the results of the modeling exercise. Several variants of the basic model were examined to diminish the impact of modeling-specific assumptions on the results, and multiple sensitivity analyses were performed. Although some investigators prefer a per-partner variant of the Bernoulli model to the per-act version employed here[52], previous analyses suggest that the two models produce similar estimates of the number of infections averted.[19–21] Hence the per-partner model was not pursued here.

External validity is also a critical concern. The intervention was conducted in 1989 among gay men in a small southern city and the results may not generalize to other populations, which differ in preexisting risk levels and motivation to change. The costs to implement the intervention, including possible start-up costs, might also differ by geographical location. Although a large-scale replication study involving 16 medium-sized cities across the U.S. is currently in progress,[51] studies are also needed to assess the "real-world" cost-effectiveness of community-level and other HIV prevention interventions, as implemented by AIDS service organizations in the field.

Despite these limitations, community-level HIV prevention interventions hold great promise as an effective means of curtailing the further spread of HIV in at-risk populations. The response of America's gay communities to the HIV epidemic provides powerful testimony to the potential of such interventions. The history of this response shows that long-term, sustainable change grows from within the community, beginning with influential opinion leaders. Interventions that capitalize on these dynamics by training popular people to be better leaders can affect entire communities and can do so, it appears, in a highly cost-effective manner.

ACKNOWLEDGMENTS. Preparation of this chapter was supported by grants R01-MH55440 and R01-MH42908 from the National Institute of Mental Health (NIMH) and by NIMH center grant P30-MH52776. A condensed version of this research appeared as "Cost-Effectiveness of a Community-Level HIV Risk Reduction Intervention," *American Journal of Public Health*, 1998 (copyright American Public Health Association).

REFERENCES

1. DiClemente RJ, Wingood GM. A randomized controlled trial of an HIV sexual risk-reduction intervention for young African-American women. *JAMA*. 1995; 274:1271–1276.
2. Hobfoll SE, Jackson AP, Lavin J, Britton PJ, Shepherd JB. Reducing inner-city women's AIDS risk activities. *Health Psychol* 1994; 13:397–403.
3. Jemmott JB III, Jemmott LS, Fong GT. Reductions in HIV risk-associated sexual behaviors among black male adolescents: Effects of an AIDS prevention intervention. *Am J Public Health* 1992; 82:372–377.
4. Kelly JA, Murphy DA, Washington CD, Wilson TS, Koob JJ, Davis DR, Ledezma G, Davantes B. The effects of HIV/AIDS intervention groups for high-risk women in urban clinics. *Am J Public Health* 1994; 84:1918–1922.
5. Kelly JA, St. Lawrence JS, Hood HV, Brasfield TL. Behavioral intervention to reduce AIDS risk activities. *J Consulting Clin Psychol* 1989; 57:60–67.
6. Peterson JL, Coates TJ, Catania JA, Hauck WW, Acree M, Daigie D, Hillard B, Middleton L, Hearst N. Evaluation of an HIV risk reduction intervention among African American homosexual and bisexual men. *AIDS* 1996; 10:319–325.
7. Rotheram-Borus MJ, Koopman C, Haignere C, Davies M. Reducing HIV sexual risk behaviors among runaway adolescents. *JAMA* 1991; 266:1237–1241.

8. St. Lawrence JS, Brasfield T, Jefferson KW, Alleyene E, Shirley A. Cognitive-behavioral intervention to reduce African American adolescents' risk for HIV infection. *J Consulting Clin Psychol* 1995; 63:221–237.

9. Valdiserri RO, Lyter DW, Leviton LC, Callahan CM, Kingsley LA, Rinaldo CR. AIDS prevention in homosexual and bisexual men: Results of a randomized trial evaluating two risk-reduction interventions. *AIDS* 1989; 3:21–26.

10. Kelly JA, Murphy DA, Sikkema KJ, Kalichman SC. Psychological interventions to prevent HIV infection are urgently needed. *Am Psychol* 1993; 48:1023–1034.

11. Choi KH, Coates TJ. Prevention of HIV infection. *AIDS* 1994; 8:1371–1389.

12. Centers for Disease Control and Prevention. Community-level prevention of human immunodeficiency virus among high-risk populations: The AIDS Community Demonstration Projects. *MMWR* 1996; 45(RR-6):1–24.

13. Kegeles SM, Hays RB, Coates TJ. The Mpowerment project: A community-level HIV prevention intervention for young gay men. *Am J Public Health* 1996; 86:1129–1136.

14. Kelly JA, St. Lawrence JS, Diaz YE, Stevenson LY, Hauth AC, Brasfield TL, Kalichman SC, Smith JE, Andrew ME. HIV risk behavior reduction following intervention with key opinion leaders of population: An experimental analysis. *Am J Public Health* 1991; 81:168–171.

15. Kelly JA, St. Lawrence JS, Stevenson LY, Hauth AC, Kalichman SC, Diaz YE, Brasfield TL, Koob JJ, Morgan MG. Community AIDS/HIV risk reduction: The effects of endorsements by popular people in three cities. *Am J Public Health* 1992; 82:1483–1489.

16. Rietmeijer CA, Kane MS, Simons PZ, Corby NH, Wolitski RJ, Higgins DL, Judson FN, Cohn DL. Increasing the use of bleach and condoms among injecting drug users in Denver: Outcomes of a targeted, community-level HIV prevention program. *AIDS* 1996; 10:291–298.

17. Hansen WB, Graham J. Preventing alcohol, marijuana, and cigarette abuse among adolescents: Peer pressure resistance training versus establishing conservative norms. *Preventive Med* 1991; 20:414–430.

18. Rogers EM. *Diffusion of Innovations*. New York: Free Press;1983.

19. Holtgrave DR, Kelly JA. Preventing HIV/AIDS among high-risk urban women: The cost-effectiveness of a behavioral group intervention. *Am J Public Health* 1996; 86:1442–1445.

20. Holtgrave DR, Kelly JA. The cost-effectiveness of an HIV prevention intervention for gay men. *AIDS and Behavior* 1997; 1:173–180.

21. Pinkerton SD, Holtgrave DR, Valdiserri RO. Cost-effectiveness of HIV prevention skills training for men who have sex with men. *AIDS* 1997; 11:347–357.

22. Holtgrave DR, Qualls NL, Graham JD. Economic evaluation of HIV prevention programs. *Annu Rev Public Health* 1996; 17:467–488.

23. Kelly JA. HIV prevention among gay and bisexual men in small cities. In DiClemente RJ, Peterson JL, eds. *Preventing AIDS: Theories and Methods of Behavioral Interventions*. New York: Plenum Press; 1994: pp 297–317.

24. Holtgrave DR. Setting priorities and community planning for HIV-prevention programs. *AIDS and Public Policy J* 1994; 9:145–150.

25. Gold MR, Siegel JE, Russell LB, Weinstein MC, eds. *Cost-effectiveness in Health and Medicine*. New York: Oxford University Press; 1996.

26. Dasbach E, Teutsch SM. Cost-utility analysis. In Haddix AC, Teutsch SM, Shaffer PA, Duñet DO, eds. *Prevention Effectiveness: A Guide to Decision Analysis and Economic Evaluation*. New York: Oxford University Press; 1996: pp. 130–142.

27. Drummond MF, Stoddart GL, Torrance GW. *Methods for the Economic Evaluation of Health Care Programmes*. New York: Oxford University Press; 1987: pp. 112–148.

28. Haddix AC, Shaffer PA. Cost-effectiveness analysis. In Haddix AC, Teutsch SM, Shaffer PA, Duñet DO, eds. *Prevention Effectiveness: A Guide to Decision Analysis and Economic Evaluation*. New York: Oxford University Press; 1996: pp. 130–142.

29. Hearst N, Hulley SB. Preventing the heterosexual spread of AIDS. *JAMA* 1988; 259:2428–2432.

30. Pinkerton SD, Abramson PR. Evaluating the risks: A Bernoulli process model of HIV infection and risk reduction. *Evaluation Rev* 1993;17:504–528.

31. Pinkerton SD, Abramson PR. The Bernoulli-process model of HIV transmission: Applications and implications. In Holtgrave DR, ed. *Handbook of Economic Evaluation of HIV Prevention Programs*. New York: Plenum Press; in press.

32. Weinstein MC, Graham JD, Siegel JE, Fineberg HV. Cost-effectiveness analysis of AIDS prevention programs: Concepts, complications, and illustrations. In Turner CF, Miller HG, Moses LE, eds. *AIDS: Sexual Behavior and Intravenous Drug Use*. Washington, DC: National Academy Press; 1989: pp. 471–499.

33. Pinkerton SD, Holtgrave DR, Leviton LC, Wagstaff D, Cecil H, Abramson PR. Toward a standardized minimum sexual behavior data set for the evaluation of HIV prevention interventions. *Am J Health Behavior*, in press.

34. Pinkerton SD, Abramson PR. An alternative model of the reproductive rate of HIV infection: Formulation, evaluation, and implications for risk reduction interventions. *Evaluation Rev* 1994; 18:371–388.

35. St. Lawrence JS, Brasfield TL, Diaz YE, Jefferson KW, Reynolds MT, Leonard MO. Three-year follow-up of an HIV risk-reduction intervention that used popular peers. *Am J Public Health* 1994; 84:2027–2028.

36. Holtgrave DR, Qualls NL. Threshold analysis and HIV prevention programs. *Medical Decision Making* 1995; 15:311–317.

37. Holtgrave DR, Pinkerton SD. Updates of cost of illness and quality of life estimates for use in economic evaluations of HIV prevention programs. *J Acquired Immune Defic Syndr* 1997; 16:54–62.

38. Patrick DL, Erikson P. *Health Status and Health Policy: Allocating Resources to Health Care*. New York: Oxford University Press; 1993: p 263.

39. Guinan ME, Farnham PG, Holtgrave DR. Estimating the value of preventing a human immunodeficiency virus infection. *Am J Preventive Med* 1994; 10:1–4.

40. Laupacis A, Feeny D, Detsky AS, Tugwell PX. Tentative guidelines for using clinical and economic evaluations revisited. *Can Med Assoc J* 1993; 148:927–929.

41. Fabian R. The Qualy approach. In Tolley GL, Kenkel D, Fabian R, eds. *Valuing Health for Policy: An Economic Approach*. Chicago: University of Chicago Press; 1994: pp. 188–136.

42. Phillips KA, Holtgrave DR. Using cost-effectiveness/cost-benefit analysis to allocate health resources: A level playing field for prevention? *Am J Preventive Med* 1997; 13:18–25.

43. Brookmeyer R, Gail MH. *AIDS Epidemiology: A Quantitative Approach*. New York: Oxford University Press; 1994: p 50.

44. DeGruttola V, Seage GR III, Mayer KH, Horsburgh CR Jr. Infectiousness of HIV between male homosexual partners. *J Clin Epidemiol* 1989; 42:849–856.

45. Grant RM, Wiley JA, Winkelstein W. Infectivity of human immunodeficiency virus: Estimates from a prospective study of homosexual men. *J Infect Dis* 1987; 156:189–193.

46. Jacquez JA, Koopman JS, Simon CP, Longini IM Jr. Role of primary infection in epidemics of HIV infection in gay cohorts. *J Acquired Immune Defic Syndr* 1994; 7: 1169–1184.

47. Pinkerton SD, Abramson PR. Implications of increased infectivity in early-stage HIV infection: Application of a Bernoulli-process model of HIV transmission. *Evaluation Rev* 1996; 20:516–540.

48. Ostrow DG, DiFranceisco WJ, Chmiel JS, Wagstaff DA, Wesch J. A case-control study of human immunodeficiency virus type 1 seroconversion and risk-related behaviors in the Chicago MACS/CCS cohort, 1984–1992. *Am J Epidemiol* 1995; 142:875–883.

49. Pinkerton SD, Abramson PR. Effectiveness of condoms in preventing HIV transmission. *Soc Sci Med* 1997; 44:1303–1312.

50. Weller SC. A meta-analysis of condom effectiveness in reducing sexually transmitted HIV. *Soc Sci Med* 1993; 36:1635–1644.

51. Kelly JA, Murphy DA, Sikkema KJ, McAuliffe TL, Roffman RA, Soloman LJ, Winett RA, Kalichman SC, and the Community HIV Prevention Research Collaborative. Randomised, controlled, community-level HIV prevention intervention for sexual-risk behaviour among homosexual men in US cities. *Lancet* 1997; 350: 1500–1505.

52. Kaplan EH. Modeling HIV infectivity: Must sex acts be counted? *J Acquired Immune Defic Syndr* 1990; 3: 55–61.

53. Holmberg SD. The estimated prevalence and incidence of HIV in 96 large US metropolitan areas. *Am J Public Health* 1996; 86:642–654.

HIV Prevention and Cost-Effectiveness Resources on the World Wide Web

MARY E. TURK, STEVEN D. PINKERTON, DAVID R. HOLTGRAVE, and HEATHER CECIL

INTRODUCTION

HIV prevention science, like the HIV epidemic itself, progresses at a rapid pace. The Internet, and especially the World Wide Web, permits expeditious dissemination of scientific results, HIV-related news, and current events, as well as a forum for HIV-infected persons, at-risk or affected individuals, and HIV prevention researchers to share information, thoughts, and fears. Sites are run by governmental agencies (e.g., the Centers for Disease Control and Prevention); academic institutions (e.g., the University of California, San Francisco); AIDS activists (e.g., ACT UP); and other private organizations (e.g., Society for Medical Decision Making); among others. Many of these sites include resources, discussions, and information pertinent to evaluating HIV prevention interventions.

A number of useful tools are available on the Web to assist researchers and others in assessing the economic efficiency of HIV prevention programs. For example, the Consumer Price Index (available at the U.S. Bureau of Labor Statistics' web site) is used to adjust medical care and other costs for inflation, and the Employment Cost Index is used to determine the average wage rate in a particular region of the country. Other sites can be consulted for the latest epidemiological data or to access behavioral or hospital utilization and cost surveys.

Several print journals (including the *Journal of the American Medical Association*, *AIDS*, the *American Journal of Public Health*, *Medical Decision Making*, and *Pharmacoeconomics*) maintain sites that make available tables of contents, abstracts, and in some cases, the text of recent articles that have appeared in the journal. A number of on-line reference databases (including MEDLINE and AIDSLINE) also can be accessed via the Internet, as can a variety of other reference materials. In addition, many governmental agencies have web sites at which the user can obtain information about currently funded research projects and new funding initiatives. In short, the Web offers a wealth of information of interest to researchers concerned about HIV/AIDS and the economic efficiency of HIV prevention programs, in particular.

MARY E. TURK, STEVEN D. PINKERTON, DAVID R. HOLTGRAVE, and HEATHER CECIL • Department of Psychiatry and Behavioral Medicine, Center for AIDS Intervention Research (CAIR), Medical College of Wisconsin, Milwaukee, Wisconsin 53202.

Handbook of Economic Evaluation of HIV Prevention Programs, edited by Holtgrave. Plenum Press, New York, 1998.

This appendix provides a partial listing of free resources that are available through the Internet. There is a great deal of information relevant to the topic of HIV/AIDS prevention and cost-effectiveness analysis that is accessible with a few key strokes and mouse clicks. Because the Internet is a constantly changing entity, Uniform Resource Locators (URLs), or web addresses, often change. The URLs provided in the following lists may change but are accurate as of the publication of this book.

In the General Interest HIV/AIDS Sites we have chosen some of the top sites that offer a broad range of information pertaining to HIV/AIDS prevention and related topics. The sites listed under Sites with Prevention Resources and Information are exceptionally strong on the topic of prevention, although they may offer more than prevention information. Listed under the heading Sites for Economic, Population, and Health Care Information and Data are sites that offer the kind of data necessary for cost-effectiveness analyses. A wealth of detailed information and data relevant to the topic of HIV/AIDS prevention and cost-effectiveness analysis are also available at the sites listed under United States Government Sites for Information and Data. The Other Sites of Interest section contains information on a variety of sites relevant to HIV/AIDS prevention and economic analysis. Finally, a list of scholarly journals related to HIV/AIDS and/or cost-effectiveness/economic analyses can be found under Sites for Relevant Journals.

GENERAL INTEREST HIV/AIDS SITES

AIDS Education Global Information System (AEGIS)
http://www.aegis.com/
AEGIS began as a grassroots bulletin board system and now purports that it is the largest HIV/AIDS database in the world. AEGIS's mission is to "seek to relieve some of the suffering and isolation caused by HIV/AIDS and foster the understanding and knowledge that will lead to better care, prevention, and a cure." The site is searchable, provides many links to other relevant sites, and is an excellent source for current news stories about HIV/AIDS. AEGIS LIVE! is available for those using Internet Explorer V4 or Windows 98. AEGIS LIVE! is a free service that will automatically email the latest HIV/AIDS news to a subscriber's desktop computer. Another news service at the AEGIS site is a continuously updating 24-hour News Bot, an Internet robot that scans major news sources for news stories and feature articles. Also available is *The AIDS Daily Summary*, produced daily by the Centers for Disease Control and Prevention (CDC). The *Daily Summary* contains brief summaries of recent scientific advances, news, and current events related to HIV/AIDS. AEGIS makes available the most recent summary and past issues (the *Daily Summary* is also available in text format at the CDC's own website described below).

Centers for Disease Control and Prevention National AIDS Clearinghouse (CDC NAC)
http://www.cdcnac.org/
The Centers for Disease Control (CDC) National AIDS Clearinghouse is the CDC's main site for information on HIV/AIDS. The site is designed "to facilitate the sharing of HIV/AIDS and STD resources and information about education and prevention, published materials, research findings, and news about related trends." This site offers a broad range of information on HIV/AIDS, including publications, databases, and clinical information. Databases available online include Resources and Services Database, a database of community-based organizations providing services for HIV/AIDS patients and their fami-

lies; CDC NCHSTP Daily News Update Database, a service that provides abstracts of HIV/AIDS-related articles from major news services updated daily; Funding Database, a database of funding opportunities for organizations working in the areas of HIV/AIDS; and Educational Materials Database, a database of over 15,000 descriptions of HIV/AIDS educational materials. The CDC NAC has prepared their own guide to the Internet and its resources. This *Guide to Selected HIV/AIDS-Related Internet Resources* provides an excellent tutorial on the Internet and useful suggestions for searching the web. It also includes lists of HIV/AIDS-related web sites, news groups, and list servers.

HIV InSite
http://www.hivinsite.ucsf.edu/
   This University of California San Francisco AIDS Research Institute site is a very well developed and maintained web site. This searchable site organizes information into the following areas: Medical Information, Prevention and Education, Social Issues and Resources. The Medical Information section offers a comprehensive on-line textbook on HIV, a database of all HIV clinical trials in the United States, a database of antiretroviral drugs, a glossary of medical terms, treatment guidelines, case studies, clinical fact sheets in English and Spanish, and information on programs that help people with HIV to pay for medications. A variety of medically oriented publications unique to HIV InSite and links to other publications are also available. The goal of the Prevention and Education section is "to help service providers, researchers, educators, and others build stronger programs and studies in the effort to prevent HIV infections." This section is especially rich in information on program development and evaluation. Also included is basic information on HIV and safer sex, what works and what does not in prevention, examples of cutting edge prevention programs, and information about the course of the epidemic and those at risk. The Social Issues section contains materials related to HIV/AIDS policy, legislation, legal services, governmental agencies, advocacy resources, and links to other related sites. The Resources section provides a variety of useful links to databases and other data sources. Finally, the site offers CDC case counts by state and metropolitan area.

John Hopkins AIDS Service
http://www.hopkins-aids.edu/
   This site offers scholarly articles on topics such as outcomes and cost-effectiveness and provides on-line access to *The Hopkins HIV Report* newsletter. Treatment information includes guidelines for managing HIV infection and an on-line version of the book *Medical Management of HIV* that is updated monthly. A large number of national and international links related to HIV/AIDS also can be found at this site.

Medscape
http://www.medscape.com/
   This commercial site is searchable and provides full text from a variety of peer reviewed journals. Free registration is required for complete access. The journal, *The AIDS Reader*, is available in full text format from March/April 1995 to present. Access is provided for searching MEDLINE, AIDSLINE, and TOXLINE.

The WWW Virtual Library Index
http://vlib.stanford.edu/overview.html
   The WWW Virtual Library is a distributed subject catalog of Internet sites maintained by volunteers. Although the library contains numerous subjects, the following subjects are relevant to HIV/AIDS and cost-effectiveness analysis:

AIDS: http://planet.com/aidsvl/index.html
Biostatistics: http://www.bistat.washington.edu/Xvlib/
Demography: http://coombs.anu.edu.au/ResFacilities/DemographyPage.html
Economics: http://www.hkkk.fi/EconVLib.html/
Epidemiology: http://chanane.ucsf.edu/epidem/epidem.html
Medicine: http://www.ohsu.edu/cliniweb/wwwvl/
Public Health: http://www.uni-ulm.de/public_health/vl/
Statistics: http://www.stat.ufl.edu/vlib/statistics.html

SITES WITH PREVENTION RESOURCES AND INFORMATION

Center for AIDS Prevention Studies (CAPS)
http://www.epibiostat.ucsf.edu/capsweb/
This site from the University of California, San Francisco Center for AIDS Prevention Studies focuses on prevention from an applied, community-based perspective. This searchable site offers a comprehensive listing with detailed descriptions of select Center projects in the following areas: Studies of AIDS Risk Behaviors; AIDS Prevention Among Youth; Primary Prevention and Early Intervention; Stress, Coping, and HIV; Substance Abuse and HIV; International Research; Improving Health Care and AIDS Risk Assessment; Policy and Ethical Issues; Epidemiological Research; and Directions in HIV Research. Information on the Center's researchers is available, as is a bibliography by author or topic of the Center's articles and reports including some abstracts. Prevention fact sheets are also available (in English and Spanish), as are press releases and CAPS newsletters. Like its sister site HIV InSite (CAPS manages both sites), the CAPS web site is a good source of information for program development and evaluation. Both sites also maintain excellent collections of links to other relevant web sites.

Critical Path AIDS Project
http://www.critpath.org/
This site was founded by people with AIDS to provide treatment, resource, and prevention information. The site offers information on a broad range of topics and many links. The prevention section provides general information in the areas of prevention resources, harm reduction strategies, and community-based interventions.

Managing Desire: HIV Prevention Strategies for the Twenty-First Century
http://www.managingdesire.org/index.html
As a grassroots prevention site, "this site aims to break down the barriers to AIDS prevention knowledge by offering everyone access to prevention resources and discussions in a non-clinical, non-didactic manner." The major sections reflect the diversity of audience that the site wishes to attract. A Relationships and Safer Sex section answers frequently asked questions at the personal level. The Counselor Resources section provides methods and materials for HIV test counselors, health educators, and outreach workers. The Theorizing Desire section consists of original research in desire in the context of AIDS prevention and includes forums for discussions about HIV prevention. An extensive listing of links is also provided.

National Center for HIV, STD & TB Prevention (NCHSTP)
http://www.cdc.gov/nchstp/od/nchstp.html

This web site provides general information on HIV/AIDS, sexually transmitted diseases, and tuberculosis. The Division of HIV/AIDS Prevention has its own site which is accessible directly (http://www.cdc.gov/nchstp/hiv_aids/dhap.htm) or through the NCHSTP main menu. Features of the prevention site include basic statistics, general information on HIV/AIDS, and slides and graphics of surveillance data. A public use database with analysis software containing AIDS cases reported through 1996 is available for downloading.

Rural Center for AIDS/STD Prevention
http://www.indiana.edu/~aids/

The Rural Center for AIDS/STD Prevention is a joint project of Indiana University and Purdue University. With a focus on HIV/STD prevention in rural America, the center develops and evaluates educational materials and approaches, examines barriers to prevention, and provides prevention resources to professionals and the public. The site offers a newsletter and a variety of fact sheets.

SITES FOR ECONOMIC, POPULATION, AND HEALTH-CARE INFORMATION AND DATA

AIDS in Canada
http://www.hwc.ca/hpb/lcdc/publicat/aids/index.html

This site from Health Canada's Health Protection Branch of the Laboratory Centre for Disease Control provides data on AIDS in Canada. This information includes annual reports for 1994 and 1995 and a surveillance report for the period 1985 to 1995. The most current data are available through a quarterly surveillance update.

Cost of Living Calculator
http://www.newsengin.com/neFreeTools.nsf/CPIcalc

This handy calculator, provided by News Engin Inc., allows users to compute the real buying power of historical dollar amounts adjusted for inflation by using data from the Bureau of Labor Statistics. Separate categories available for calculation include Medical Care and Medical Care Services.

The Health Services Research Discovery Zone
http://ascorpnt.mda.uth.tmc.edu/disczone.htm

The Health Services Research Discovery Zone consists of a sample data set from The Ambulatory and Supportive Care Oncology Research Program (ASCORP) at the University of Texas M. D. Anderson Cancer Center. This data set is provided so that students and other researchers can conduct simulated outcomes and cost-effectiveness studies. The data are presented in several illustrative reports.

HIV/AIDS and the World Bank
http://www.worldbank.org/html/extdr/hivaids/default.htm

The World Bank, a funder of HIV/AIDS-related projects in low-income countries, provides valuable information at their web site about HIV/AIDS in underdeveloped and developing countries—countries severely effected by HIV/AIDS. The site has a page on AIDS economics that includes World Bank reports, a bibliographic database, an electronic newsletter, and a list of links to other related web sites.

Organization for Economic Cooperation and Development (OECD)
http://www.oecd.org/
        This OECD site provides a global perspective on health and economics. The Organization for Economic Cooperation and Development consists of 29 member countries from North America, Europe, and the Asia-Pacific area. The OECD collects and analyses data that allows comparisons of statistics across countries. These statistics include health expenditures, life expectancy, in-patient care, and infant mortality. Various papers and data tables are available in PDF (Adobe Acrobat) format.

Society for Medical Decision Making
http://www.nemc.org/SMDM/Welcome2.html
        The Society for Medical Decision Making is "an international, interdisciplinary society dedicated to the study and improvement of all aspects of medical decision making." Their quarterly on-line newsletter is available at the web site and issues go back to March 1996. The table of contents and abstracts from the quarterly journal *Medical Decision Making* are available back to October/December 1996.

World Health Organization
http://www.who.ch/
        Worldwide HIV/AIDS surveillance data and other HIV/AIDS and health information are available through the WHO web site. The areas of particular interest include annual World Health Reports for 1995, 1996, and 1997 and the WHO *Weekly Epidemiological Record* (WER) that provides information on cases and outbreaks of diseases and health problems. Also available is the *HIV/AIDS and Sexually Transmitted Diseases Newsletter* from the WHO Office of HIV/AIDS and Sexually Transmitted Diseases in issues from June 1996. The newsletter of the World Health Organization Global Programme on AIDS and information from their Task Force on Health Economics are available through the WHO gopher.

U.S. GOVERNMENT SITES FOR INFORMATION AND DATA (NOT LISTED PREVIOUSLY)

Agency for Health Care Policy and Research (AHCPR)
http://www.ahcpr.gov/text.htm
        The AHCPR is "the lead agency charged with supporting research designed to improve the quality of health care, reduce its cost, and broaden access to essential services." Information available at this site includes the results of the Medical Expenditure Panel Survey and the AIDS Cost and Services Utilization Survey (ACSUS).

Bureau of Labor Statistics (BLS)
http://www.bls.gov/
        BLS is the principal agency in the field of labor economics and statistics. This site is organized into the following sections: Data; Economy at a Glance; Keyword Search;

Surveys and Programs; Publications and Research Papers; Regional Information; About BLS; Other Statistical Sites; and What's New. Under the Data section are form-based applications that allow the user to define BLS time series data. Available data include statistics on employment and unemployment, compensation and working conditions, productivity and technology, and price and living conditions. A form-based "Most Requested Series" application allows users to obtain easily consumer price index (CPI) data for specific time periods, regions of the country, or cost categories (including Medical Care and Medical Care Services). Select data are available at the international, national, and local levels. Another useful BLS area is the Employment Cost Trends page (http://stats.bls.gov/ ecthome.htm) which provides access to the Employment Cost Index.

Centers for Disease Control and Prevention (CDC)
http://www.cdc.gov

The homepage of the CDC offers sections on Publications, Software and Products, and Data and Statistics. Under the section on Data and Statistics is a link to CDC and ATSDR (Agency for Toxic Substances and Disease Registry) Electronic Information Resources for Health Offices. This link provides information on the important resource offerings of the CDC via computer and electronic media. There is also a link to CDC WONDER. The CDC has developed CDC WONDER to provide access to its data on mortality, natality, population, AIDS and other sexually transmitted diseases, and a variety of other topics and data sets. Software is provided for tabulation and graphing, or data can be exported in one of 10 common formats. CDC WONDER allows for searches and queries and provides guidelines and reports.

Surveillance data available from the CDC include:

Behavioral Risk Factor Surveillance System
    http://www.cdc.gov/nccdphp/brfss/
    State and sex specific prevalence of select characteristics are available for 1994 and 1995.
HIV/AIDS Surveillance Report
    http://www.cdc.gov/nchstp/hiv_aids/stats/hasrlink.htm
    Surveillance reports are available in PDF format from second quarter 1993 and in ASCII text format from mid-year 1994.
Sexually Transmitted Disease Surveillance Report
    http://wonder.cdc.gov/rchtml/Convert/data/Reports.html
    Surveillance reports are available from 1993.
Youth Risk Behavior National Survey
    http://www.cdc.gov/nccdphp/dash/yrbs/ov.htm
    Selected summaries of 1995 data are available.

Publications available include:

Morbidity and Mortality Weekly Report
    http://www.cdc.gov/epo/mmwr/mmwr.html
    The publication *Morbidity and Mortality Weekly Report* is available in PDF (Adobe Acrobat) format on-line with a searchable index of publications from 1993. Tables from these issues can be queried by year, week, and location. The publication is also available for on-line subscription.

Department of Health and Human Services (DHHS)
http://www.hhs.gov/
Many governmental agencies with information relevant to cost-effectiveness and HIV/ AIDS fall under the auspices of the DHHS. The DHHS offers several means of searching its site and those of its subagencies. The search utility Healthfinder (http://www.healthfinder. gov/) is a health and human services information utility aimed at consumers. The Government Information Locator Service (http://www.usgs.gov/gils/index.htm) is a search utility that maintains descriptions of publicly available information and identifies how to assess the information. A direct electronic line is provided in some cases.

Economic Statistics Briefing Room
http://www.whitehouse.gov/fsbr/esbr.html
Social Statistics Briefing Room
http://www.whitehouse.gov/fsbr/ssbr.html
These sites are ideal for a quick look at federal economic and social statistics. Selected data are displayed in chart form, with previous data and the most current data provided for comparison. Links are provided to the site that is the source of the data for further information.

Fedstats
http://www.fedstats
The Federal Interagency Council on Statistical Policy maintains this searchable site to provide easy access to the full range of statistics and information produced by more than 70 agencies of the United States Federal Government. In addition to keyword searching capabilities, topics can be selected from an alphabetical listing or from a program listing. Topics include demographics, economics, and health.

Food and Drug Administration (FDA)
http://www.fda.gov/fdahomepage.html
This searchable site offers information on HIV/AIDS testing, articles, brochures, barrier products, and therapies. Also available is a listing of other HIV/AIDS web sites.

Health Care Financing Administration (HCFA)
http://www.hcfa.gov
The HCFA administers the Medicare, Medicaid, and Child Health programs. Expenditure and utilization data are available for these programs.

Health Resources and Services Administration (HRSA)
http://www.hrsa.dhhs.gov/
Abstracts of reports and publications related to HIV/AIDS are available from HRSA's HIV/AIDS Bureau at this site. It is possible to obtain profiles by state that include demographic and health-care statistics through the Bureau of Primary Health Care.

National Center for Health Statistics (NCHS)
http://www.cdc.gov/nchswww/nchshome.htm
NCHS is the federal government's principal health and vital statistics agency. NCHS data systems include data on vital events, health status, lifestyle and exposure to unhealthy influences, onset and diagnosis of illness and disability, and health-care utilization. Available HIV/AIDS related data include the following:

National Health Interview Survey
    http://www.cdc.gov/nchswww/about/major/nhis/nhis.htm
National Health and Nutrition Examination Survey
    http://www.cdc.gov/nchswww/about/major/nhanes/nhanes.htm
National Health Care Survey—National Hospital Discharge Survey
    http://www.cdc.gov/nchswww/about/major/nhcs/nhcs.htm
National Vital Statistics System
    http://www.cdc.gov/nchswww/about/major/nvss/nvss.htm

National Institute of Allergy and Infectious Diseases (NIAID)
http://www.niaid.nih.gov/
    One of the four divisions that comprise NIAID is the Division of AIDS. Included in the section for the Division of AIDS are conference and meeting summaries, research resources, supported programs, and publications. A listing of AIDS-related data sets available for a fee are included under research resources.

National Institute of Mental Health (NIMH)
http://www.nimh.nih.gov/home.htm
    The NIMH Office on AIDS Research (OAR) supports "research activities related to the primary and secondary prevention of AIDS and the neurobehavioral sequelae that develop as a result of HIV infection." Information pertaining to the office's activities are available at this site and at the NIMH OAR (http://www.nimh.nih.gov/oa/index.htm).

National Institutes of Health (NIH)
http://www.nih.gov/
    This searchable site includes information in a wide variety of health areas. Sections include News and Events, Health Information, Scientific Resources, Institutes and Offices, and Grants and Contracts. The section on Institutes and Offices includes the Office of AIDS Research (OAR) in its listing. Abstracts of AIDS related research projects "officially funded as AIDS research" are available from the OAR homepage (http://www.nimh.nih.gov/oa/index.htm). Access to these abstracts is through NIH's AIDS Research Information System (ARIS) gopher server in text-only format. The section on Grants and Contracts includes a link to the CRISP system. This Computer Retrieval of Information on Scientific Projects (CRISP) includes information on both extra- and intramural projects supported by the NIH and select other agencies. The CRISP database is updated weekly.

National Library of Medicine (NLM)
http://sis.nlm.nih.gov/index.htm
    This searchable site offers the resources of the world's largest medical library. HIV/AIDS resources are available under the Special Information Programs. These resources include conference abstracts, publications, and databases. A Guide to NIH HIV/AIDS Information Services is also available. This guide draws together details in a single resource about the many HIV/AIDS information-related activities of the National Institutes of Health. Free access to MEDLINE is also available at this site.

U.S. Census Bureau
http://www.census.gov/
    The Census Bureau offers data and reports based on the census and other surveys. In addition to census information, the following information is available:

1996 Statistical Abstract of the United States
    http://www.census.gov/ftp/pub/prod/www/abs/msgenlld.html
Annual Demographic Survey
    http://www.bls.census.gov/cps/ads/adsdes.htm
Current Population Survey
    http://www.bls.census.gov/cps/cpsmain.htm
Survey of Income and Program Participation
    http://www.census.gov/pub/dusd/MAB/sipp~l.html

OTHER SITES OF INTEREST

ACT UP Golden Gate
http://www.actupgg.org/
    The AIDS Coalition to Unleash Power (ACT UP) is one of the premier HIV/AIDS activist organizations. This site from one of the San Francisco chapters of ACT UP offers a variety of news releases, abstracts, reports and articles on HIV and AIDS.

ACT UP New York
http://www.actupny.org/
    This site from the New York chapter of ACT UP is quite extensive. Offerings range from an on-line civil disobedience training video to an index of AIDS treatments called Real Treatments for Real People. The site also offers numerous links to other web sites.

AIDS Economics
http://www.worldbank.org/aids-econ/
    This site "focuses on the economics of HIV/AIDS prevention and treatment." Its aim is "to help researchers and policy makers to define and implement effective AIDS policy." Although the site is in the early stages of development, plans are to include the following content areas: the economic impact of HIV/AIDS; the role of government in prevention and mitigation; the nature of government partnerships; and the cost-effectiveness of specific interventions. The site also will be home to the AIDS & Economics Network, "an informal association of researchers and policy makers working to improve policy options for combating HIV/AIDS."

The Body
http://www.thebody.com/cgi-bin/body.cgi
    The Body: A Multimedia AIDS and HIV Information Resource is a site that provides on-line forums, expert answers to questions about HIV/AIDS, information about organizations and hotlines, and basic information on HIV/AIDS and its treatment. The site's mission includes: "use of the web to lower barriers between patients and clinicians; demystify HIV/AIDS and its treatment; improve patients' quality of life; and foster community through human connection." The site is a good source of information for HIV-infected individuals and others affected by HIV.

Gay Men's Health Crisis (GHMC)
http://www.gmhc.org/
    GMHC purports that it is the "oldest and largest not-for-profit AIDS organization in the United States" and offers support services for persons with AIDS and their families in

New York City as well as education and advocacy nationwide. This web site is a good source of basic prevention and treatment information.

International Association of Physicians in AIDS Care
http://www.iapac.org/

The IAPAC site is geared primarily toward physicians and other health professionals caring for people living with HIV/AIDS. The site is searchable and offers tables of contents and select full text for their *Journal of the International Association of Physicians in AIDS Care* dating from February 1995. This site includes several rather unique sections. The Consumer Information section offers booklets and articles in multiple languages and provides answers to inquiries from the Internet. IAPAC's section on Minority Issues offers *A Legislative Report on African Americans and AIDS* in the inaugural issue of a new on-line publication called *Themis*. Finally, there is a section on Women's Health Issues that includes abstracts from the 1997 National Conference on Women & Aids, conference reports, and a variety of articles from their publications. One of these publications is *DemiMondaine*, a magazine exclusively for immunocompromised women.

International Health Economics Association (iHEA)
http://cbix.unh.edu/ihea/ihea.htm

iHEA was formed "to increase communication among health economists, foster a higher standard of debate in the applications of economics to health and health care systems", and to "assist young researchers." A worldwide directory of member health economists, an electronic newsletter, and a print newsletter are available at this site. The electronic newsletter *eHEAL* is published every two months. Current and past issues of *eHEAL* (from December 1996 to present) are available as ASCII text files. Past issues (dating back to 1995) of the print newsletter *HEAL* are available as PDF (Adobe Acrobat) files.

JAMA HIV/AIDS Information Center
http://www.ama-assn.org/special/hiv/hivhome.htm

This searchable site is produced by the *Journal of the American Medical Association*. The site contains information useful to those affected by HIV/AIDS and to health professionals. Daily updates, special reports, background reports, and analyses are provided by an HIV/AIDS correspondent in Newsline. A JAMA & Archives Libraries offers full text articles from *JAMA* and other publications on the topics of HIV/AIDS. Updated weekly, Journal Scan provides a review of HIV/AIDS articles from the scientific literature presented in full text as available. Through an agreement with HealthGate Data Corporation, this site offers unlimited access to the following databases: AIDSDRUGS, AIDSLINE, AIDS-TRIALS, and BIOETHICSLINE.

Population Index
http://popindex.princeton.edu/

The Population Index provides an annotated bibliography of published books, working papers, journal articles, and other materials related to demography. The entire published database for 1986 to 1997 is available on-line and can be searched and/or browsed.

WebEc
http://www.helsinki.fi/WebEc/webeci.html

"WebEc is an effort to categorize free information in economics" on the World Wide

Web. This international site contains numerous links to other web sites, including sites relating to Health, Education and Welfare. WebEc is a good "jumping off point" to search for health economics information.

SITES FOR RELEVANT JOURNALS

AIDS
http://www.chapmanhall.com/ai/default.html
Searchable abstracts from May 1997 to present.
http://adref.com/adref/aids/0192/issues.htm
Searchable tables of contents from August 1992 to present.

AIDS Care: Psychological and Socio-Medical Aspects of AIDS/HIV
http://www.carfax.co.uk/aic-ad.htm
Tables of contents from December 1996 to present.
http://adref.com/adref/aids/0292/issues.htm
Searchable tables of contents from June 1992 to present.

AIDS Education and Prevention
http://adref.com/adref/aids/0392/issues.htm
Searchable tables of contents from spring 1993 to present.

AIDS Patient Care
http://adref.com/adref/aids/0492/issues.htm
Searchable tables of contents from August 1992 to present.

AIDS Research and Human Retroviruses
http://adref.com/adref/aids/0592/issues.htm
Searchable tables of contents from November 1992 to present.

American Journal of Public Health
http://www.apha.org/news/publications/Journal/AJPH2.html
Tables of contents and abstracts from January 1997 to present.

British Medical Journal
http://www.bmj.com/bmj/
Tables of contents and select full texts from March 1995 to present.

The European Journal of Public Health
http://www.oup.co.uk/eurpub/
Searchable tables of contents and select abstracts from March 1996 to present.

Health Education & Behavior
http://www.sph.umich.edu/group/heb/
Abstracts from October 1997 to present.

Health Policy
http://www.elsevier.com:80/inca/publications/store/5/0/5/9/6/2/
Searchable tables of contents from January 1995 to present.

Health Policy and Planning
http://www.oup.co.uk/jnls/list/heapol/
Searchable abstracts from March 1996 to present.

Health Psychology
http://www.apa.org/journals/hea.html
Searchable tables of contents and select abstracts from November 1996 to present.

Health Services Research
http://www.xnet.com/~hret/hsr.htm
Tables of contents and abstracts from April 1995 to present. Searchable subject and author 10-year indexes.

HIV Policy & Law Newsletter
http://www.odyssee.net/~jujube/elements/bulletinE.html
Abstracts from fall 1994 to October 1995.

International Journal of STD and AIDS
http://adref.com/adref/aids/1392/issues.htm
Searchable tables of contents from July/August 1992 to present.

Journal of Acquired Immune Deficiency Syndromes and Human Retrovirology
http://adref.com/adref/aids/1692/issues.htm
Searchable tables of contents from August 1992 to present.

Journal of Epidemiology & Community Health
http://www.bmjpg.com/data/echb/htm
Tables of contents from February 1996 to present.

Journal of Health and Social Policy
http://bubl.ac.uk/journals/soc/jhasp/
Searchable abstracts from 1994 to present.

Journal of Health Economics
http://www.elsevier.nl/estoc/publications/store/6/01676296/
Searchable tables of contents from May 1995 to present.

Journal of HIV/AIDS Prevention and Education for Adolescents and Children
http://bubl.ac.uk/journals/soc/jhapaefaac/
Searchable abstracts from 1997 to present.

Journal of Research in Pharmaceutical Economics
http://bubl.ac.uk/journals/bus/jripe/
Searchable abstracts from 1995 to present.

The Journal of the American Medical Association
http://www.ama-assn.org/public/journals/jama/jamahome.htm
Searchable abstracts from July 1995 to present.

The Lancet
http://www.thelancet.com/
Searchable tables of contents and select abstracts from June 1996 to present. Requires free registration.

Medical Decision Making
http://www.uic.edu/orgs/mdm
Tables of contents and abstracts from January/March 1996 to January/March 1997.
http://www2.hanleyandbelfus.com/hanleyandbelfus/journals/mdm.html
Tables of contents and abstracts from January/March 1997 to present.

Morbidity and Mortality Weekly Report
http://www.cdc.gov/epo/mmwr/mmwr.html
Searchable tables of contents and full texts from 1993 to present.

The New England Journal of Medicine
http://www.nejm.org/
Searchable tables of contents, abstracts, and select full texts from January 1995 to present.

PharmacoEconomics
http://biomednet.com/library/pjo
Searchable abstracts from September 1996 to present. Requires free registration.

Preventive Medicine
http://www.apnet.com/www/journal/pm.htm
Searchable tables of contents from January/February 1996 to present.

Public Health
http://www.stockton-press.co.uk/ph/index.html
Tables of contents from most recent issue.

Social Science & Medicine
http://www.elsevier.com:80/inca/publications/store/3/1/5/
Searchable tables of contents from January 1995 to present.

Index

ISBN 0-306-45749-0

90000